Diet, Drugs,
and Dopamine

ALSO BY DAVID A. KESSLER, MD

A Question of Intent
The End of Overeating
Capture
Your Food Is Fooling You
Fast Carbs, Slow Carbs

Diet, Drugs, *and* Dopamine

The New Science of Achieving
a Healthy Weight

· · · · · · · · · · · ·

David A. Kessler, MD

FLATIRON
BOOKS
NEW YORK

The information in this book is not intended to replace the advice of the reader's own physician or other medical professional. You should consult a medical professional in matters relating to health, especially if you have existing medical conditions, and before starting, stopping, or changing the dose of any medication you are taking. Individual readers are solely responsible for their own healthcare decisions. The author and the publisher do not accept responsibility for any adverse effects individuals may claim to experience, whether directly or indirectly, from the information contained in this book.

The fact that an organization or website is mentioned in the book as a potential source of information does not mean that the author or the publisher endorses any of the information they may provide or recommendations they may make.

To Paulette

For Rosie

Contents

. . . .

Introduction

I am average. I am like everyone else. For most of my life, I have been in a battle with my body. I have been fat, and I have been thin, and I have been every size in between.

I am like the nearly three-quarters of the population who are either overweight or obese and have had their health jeopardized because of it. Since I was a kid, I've gained and lost weight repeatedly, putting on twenty pounds, taking it off, putting on thirty pounds, returning to the drudgery of restraint until I'd lost it again, only to gain the weight back once more. It has been a cycle of despair, repair, and back to despair.

No longer.

We can reclaim our health. Dramatic and lasting weight loss is possible. Anyone struggling with weight can lose the toxic fat that threatens our health—and keep it off. Let me be clear: It is this toxic fat—also known as visceral fat—that we carry in and around our organs that is the problem, not how big or small our bodies are.

We now have highly effective anti-obesity medications, otherwise known as GLP-1 (glucagon-like peptide-1) agonists. These drugs have revolutionized our understanding of weight loss, and of obesity itself. For too long, body weight has been shrouded in mystery. Why have so many of us gained weight? Why is it so hard to lose weight? And, if we do manage to lose it, why does it feel so impossible to keep it off?

The fact that the new anti-obesity drugs are highly effective underscores the fact that being overweight or obese is not a product of lack of discipline or willpower—a bias that has long prevailed, even within the medical profession. It is instead a product of biology. We know from clinical studies that these medications work largely by increasing satiety—or feelings of satisfaction or fullness after eating—and quieting "food noise," that clamorous, food-focused chorus in our heads that plays on repeat throughout the day. Food noise comes from a preoccupation with and craving for food. When people stop taking anti-obesity drugs, these unpleasant experiences reemerge.

Preoccupation with and craving for food are also hallmarks of the addictive process. That chorus that plays in our heads is a result of the ultra-formulated food that has increasingly become the mainstay of our diets. Over the last fifty years, the food industry has glutted our grocery stores, delis, and corner markets with the irresistible, highly processed, highly palatable, energy-dense, high-glycemic foods—ultraformulated foods—that have quietly commandeered the reward centers of our brains. Put simply, these foods are addictive.

The widespread availability of these foods has created an ongoing insult to our brains, triggering our addictive circuits—causing cravings that can arise outside of awareness, as well as compulsive eating—and altering the neurohormones that control weight. As a result, our average weight settling point—that is, the weight range that the body naturally tends to gravitate toward—has increased. We are now caught between what the food industry has done to the American diet and what our metabolisms can accommodate. Being overweight or obese has essentially become our default setting, and, consequently, we have experienced a rise in the diseases and conditions that toxic fat causes, including arthritis, certain forms of cancer, blood clots, type 2 diabetes, hypertension, increased blood lipids, atherosclerotic heart disease, dementia, and stroke. It is a health catastrophe that has reached its apex on every level. Current projections do not indicate a significant change in longevity over the next three decades, but there *will* be a substantial rise in morbidity due to obesity. The culprit is not weight or body mass index (BMI) but visceral fat. By decreasing chronic diseases caused by visceral fat, we can improve lifespan and quality of life. In other words, a major key to our longevity is linked to losing this toxic fat.

And we have underestimated the very important role that food addiction plays in controlling our weight. Ultraformulated food is our new cigarette, and it is critical that we understand the changes that need to occur—in our lives, in our bodies—through this lens. "There is no free ride in the brain when you take drugs. No matter what drug you take," as Dr. George Koob, director of the National Institute on Alcohol Abuse and Alcoholism, puts it. "If you keep eating highly palatable foods, you are changing the physiology of the body."

Now, for the first time in medical history, using these anti-obesity medications, we can specifically modify the addictive neural pathways, allowing us to change our body weight in a decisive way. It is not uncomplicated, and it is not without risks. It is also not for everyone. And yet, for many people who have struggled long and hard with their weight—myself included—these drugs offer significant health and emotional benefits.

But make no mistake: There are no magic pills here. Prescribing these medications alone does not meet the standard of good medical care, and we have not yet figured out how to safely and practically use these drugs over the long term. Anti-obesity medications only work for the duration they are administered; appetite and weight return when they are stopped. Because of this, the pharmaceutical industry has positioned them as "forever drugs"—taken until death do you part—as, indeed, that strategy offers them billions in profits. For some people, this may be the right course of action. But I consider these drugs as only one powerful tool we can now use to manage our weight and our health. The other tools have been there all along: nutrition, behavioral therapies, and physical activity. When used together as a system, it is possible to reset weight in a healthy way in the modern world, and the change can be dramatic.

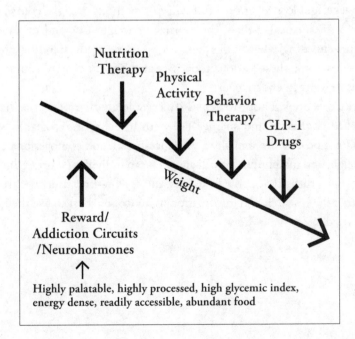

All these options, either on their own or in conjunction with one an-other, grant us the space we need—slowing us down enough to make more mindful choices—to bypass our addictive circuits and rebuild our eating patterns. "I think it's really difficult for people to conceive of how hard it is to exist when you're that obese," said a patient advocate who studies nutrition and who himself lost more than 200 pounds by changing his eating pattern, but never took an anti-obesity drug. "The way I eat now is so much easier." To a greater or lesser extent, this idea holds true for all of us. We have an array of tools to choose from to push back against the food addiction that characterizes our modern era. We can use these tools to disrupt that addiction and create the opportunity for sustainable weight loss.

Now that we have effective anti-obesity medications, the ways in which we engage with all these methods have changed. For example, because these drugs alter our food preferences, as well as drastically reduce the amount of food that we eat, it is critical that doctors who prescribe them also provide nutrition guidance. Unfortunately, most doctors are not trained in nutrition; there is a great deal about weight management that they are not equipped to handle.

Perhaps most crucially, effective treatment *does* require a lifelong com-mitment, but not in the way the pharmaceutical companies portray. Sus-tainable weight loss relies on a full range of methods over the course of our lifetimes. Realistically, then, the journey of weight loss and management requires choosing what works best for you, and understanding not only how to combine these various tools, but also how to change course if one begins to wane in effectiveness.

With this book, I hope to demystify a physiological process that has long provoked confusion and shame. The path to achieving a healthy weight should not be obscure, but clear, evidence-based, and compassionate. Los-ing weight and maintaining it will always be an individual journey, but there are certain truths that apply to us all. And for the first time, we are accu-mulating the research and information to know how best to use them. Let's get started.

Part I

· · · · ·

ADDICTION

1

. . . .

Environment Is Destiny

It was hailed as a nutritional nirvana. The word was that people tended to live longer in Sardinia, an island west of mainland Italy in the Mediterranean Sea offering a landscape that presents both vast mountains and captivating coastlines, donkeys grazing in fields of yellow wildflowers, and a population comprised of shepherds, dairy farmers, and cheese makers that have lived there for generations.

Some believe the seclusion of the island was the secret to its inhabitants' health. In addition to being geographically remote, Sardinia did not receive electricity until 1936. As a result, during this period, the mountainous areas—which have shown the highest clusters of longevity—were the most isolated. "The diet was extremely simple," nutritionist Dr. Ivo Pirisi told me as we drove up a craggy road to visit the mountain village of Seulo. Dr. Pirisi, who has lived on the island his entire life, met with me during my visit to Sardinia in May 2024. "By simple, I mean extremely poor," he continued. "Legumes, goat's milk, bread, lard, cheese, and vegetable soup. We'd been living the same way for hundreds of years. There were periods of calorie restriction and sometimes famine, especially in those mountain areas that could not cultivate cereal grains. Also, in the mountains, where they'd settled to avoid potential attacks from enemies, they did not have access to fish. We are in the center of the Mediterranean; the diet of the Sardinian centenarians is a Mediterranean diet."

The Mediterranean diet, in fact, is not as uniform as many presume; there are, as Dr. Pirisi points out, different types of diets practiced in different

Mediterranean regions. The Sardinian "Mediterranean" diet traditionally consisted of vegetables, pulses, bread, cheese, cereals, potatoes, lard, pasta, and dairy. There was another secret to this diet, however, that would be lost to future decades. Despite the limited calories and periods of famine, these vegetables, legumes, and lard made the Sardinians feel full. The high fiber, protein, and fat were not rapidly absorbed; these foods provided satiety. There were no processed foods.

But, as industrialization and economic progress increased on the island throughout the 1950s and 1960s—in large part, due to the post–World War II *piani di rinascita*, or "rebirth plans," which initiated major infrastructure projects and the creation of large industrial complexes, such as oil refineries—there was a shift in their eating. People who for generations had lived in scarcity were no longer living that way, both economically and nutritionally. During these years, there was a progressive change in dietary habits. People's diets began to include more simple sugars and refined carbohydrates. The consumption of meat and fruit increased. Researchers sometimes refer to this period on the island as the "nutrition transition." In the decades that followed, the increase in fast and processed food that had occurred in the United States slowly made its way overseas. McDonald's, for instance, opened in Rome in 1986 and expanded from there, reaching across the Mediterranean and onto the shores of Sardinia. Now there are more than a dozen McDonald's scattered across the island.

"Those who grew up in the hard lifestyle of the 1920s and 1930s retained a sense of moderation," Dr. Pirisi explained. It was not just the change in the composition of the diet that mattered. According to Dr. Pirisi, when the economic boom finally arrived in Sardinia, it meant there were new possibilities. New jobs, cars, more eating opportunities. In contrast to the meager conditions of previous generations, the younger population embraced and enjoyed abundance and, as a result, gained weight. Now, according to him, many among them have begun to develop type 2 diabetes and other health complications brought on by visceral adiposity, or toxic body fat. Over the course of three decades, as one study found, the prevalence of men struggling with obesity and being overweight more than doubled, from 4.33% and 0.55% in 1969 to 9.8% and 3% in 1998. In 2022, the number of people in the overall population contending with these issues rose to 32.7% among those who were overweight and 10.1% for those who were obese. Additionally, on my visit there, I noted that the lifestyle that had once been touted as naturally supporting the general health of this population had also drastically shifted: The Sardinian shepherds who once walked upwards of five miles a day, for instance, can now be seen herding sheep from their trucks.

Ultimately, within one generation, the environment had changed dramatically and, along with it, the Sardinians, heralded for their health and longevity, had also altered their bodies' natural weight range.

The New Cigarette

Our brains are not always under our control. That is, the brain can be influenced by its interactions with our environment as well as our bodies, often outside of our own awareness. Dr. Kevin Hall, a senior investigator at the National Institute of Diabetes and Digestive and Kidney Diseases, explores how people's environment relates to their eating habits and health by creating highly controlled nutrition trials. In 2019, Dr. Hall and his colleagues published one such trial in which twenty adults lived at the National Institutes of Health (NIH) full time and spent two weeks following a diet comprised of ultraprocessed foods—defined by one researcher as "formulations mostly of cheap industrial sources of dietary energy and nutrients plus additives, using a series of processes"—and two weeks in which they ate unprocessed foods. Both diets had similar nutrient levels, and with each one, the participants were told that they could eat as much as they wanted.

The people being studied were unaware of why they were being observed; there were no instructions to try to gain or lose weight. And yet, in the end, participants gained an average of two pounds over the two weeks they were eating the ultraprocessed diet, whereas they lost an average of two pounds on the minimally processed diet; during both periods, they reported the same level of appetite. Something about the food environment, when it was filled with ultraprocessed food, caused people to consume more calories—on average 500 extra calories per day—than when it was otherwise. "People can achieve very different energy intake levels, leading to either weight gain or weight loss, over relatively short periods," Dr. Hall explains. But the critical point for him about this study was that the "environment interacts with the system that regulates appetite and body weight in such a way to change where we equilibrate in terms of body weight." That is, like the Sardinians, the environment the participants lived in changed their bodies.

We have seen before how the environment drastically and detrimentally affects our habits and our health. In 1991, when I was the commissioner of the FDA, we took on the tobacco industry to halt what I considered to be a man-made epidemic: Big Tobacco had quietly and insidiously coaxed Americans into taking up a habit that, still to this day, is one of the leading causes of preventable disease and death. We set out to examine the addictive qualities of nicotine and, as we did, it became clear that the meteoric rise in accessibility of cigarettes and a forceful marketing campaign—that is, a change in our *environment*—had caused a significant portion of the population to shift their perceptions, and habits, to accommodate a behavior that was deeply corrosive to their health.

In the beginning, cigarette smoking was mainly viewed as a "dirty habit." For much of the 1800s, primarily men smoked—it was seen as inappropriate for women—and they rolled their cigarettes by hand. Even so, cigarettes made up a relatively insignificant portion of the American tobacco market as compared to cigars, chewing tobacco, and pipes. Starting in the 1880s, however, cigarettes shifted from being hand-rolled to being mass-made by machines, which created a production capacity that quickly outstripped demand. Consequently, the tobacco industry realized that they would need to mount an aggressive marketing campaign to attract new smokers. There was nothing in cigarettes that the nonsmoker would naturally desire, as one tobacco executive would later explain, so, instead, they had to convince people to smoke by wholly irrational reasons.

And convince them they did. The tobacco companies created massive marketing and promotion campaigns meant to associate smoking with fun, adventure, independence, sexiness, and glamour. Manufacturers began putting pictures of women in lingerie on cards that they inserted in cigarette packs; celebrities such as Lucille Ball and Desi Arnaz, Frank Sinatra, and Joan Crawford sang the praises of Philip Morris and Chesterfield; and of course there was the cultural icon the Marlboro Man. This became the promotional playbook of the tobacco industry for much of the twentieth century. To attract female smokers, the industry consulted with psychoanalyst A. A. Brill, who helped to conceive campaigns linking smoking with women's emancipation, creating slogans that rebranded cigarettes as "torches of freedom." In 1929, the American Tobacco Company organized a march down Fifth Avenue in New York City—women smoking their torches of freedom the whole way. But then, alarming studies began to emerge linking smoking to cancer and heart disease and the Public Health Cigarette Smoking Act of 1970 was passed and went into effect in the following year. At which point, the tobacco industry set its sights on children and young adults—using cartoon characters, for example, Joe Camel—to replenish the ranks of adult smokers who were now dying.

Still, the industry strenuously denied that nicotine was addictive, asserting that this poisonous chemical compound was in cigarettes simply for the taste and flavor. They created just the right amount of doubt about tobacco causing cancer. Between this uncertainty and the mistaken belief by the public that if cigarettes were indeed dangerous, the government would outright ban them, smokers felt justified in continuing the habit. Addiction continued to take hold of a considerable percentage of smokers, who only discovered that this was the case when they tried to quit smoking.

Finally, in the 1990s, our FDA investigation showed how the industry manipulated the level of nicotine in cigarettes to addict smokers and target young people and helped change how the product was viewed by society at large. Even tobacco industry executives finally admitted this dangerous truth, and lawsuits resulted in a settlement of billions of dollars. In the end, it took a century to shift the public perception of using tobacco back to what it really was—a deadly, addictive, disgusting habit. And yet, by commercializing a psychoactive substance and promoting it in a way that convinced people they needed it, they still managed to make addicts of millions of people. When the FDA first took on the tobacco industry, the Centers for Disease Control and Prevention estimated that 89.8 million adults in the United States—nearly half the adult population—were, or had been, smokers. Essentially, tobacco companies achieved this by creating an environment that encouraged people to smoke, and addiction compelled them to keep coming back for more.

Similarly, over the last three decades, the food industry has increasingly created an environment that is brimming with irresistible, highly processed, highly palatable, energy-dense, high-glycemic foods. (Note that in this book I do not call them "ultraprocessed" foods, the more common term, because I prefer to be more direct about what these foods are and why they exist. From here on out, I will refer to them simply as "ultraformulated," which focuses attention on the fact that much of what we are eating has been deliberately engineered to manipulate our brain's reward systems.) In many ways, ultraformulated foods have become the new cigarette. These foods deliver just the right combinations of fat and salt or fat and sugar—or that potent trifecta: fat, sugar, and salt—to trigger the reward centers of our brains, filling a void that keeps us in their thrall. But there is another component to these foods that has created a change in our brains and bodies; this component is, in fact, the key energy supply for our brains and bodies. This is glucose, one of two simple sugars that create sucrose, a naturally occurring sugar in food. Over millions of years, our bodies have developed and engaged mechanisms and hormones to handle glucose. But over the last one hundred years, all of that has changed. Our bodies are not designed to handle the excessive loads of glucose (as well as fat) that we're ingesting from ultraformulated foods. Consequently, we are flooding the receptors in the gut and increasing central nervous system reinforcement, which are parts of the addictive circuits in our brains.

There is a more beneficent view of our recent shift in the environment with ultraformulated foods, largely offered by the food industry. This argument is that, throughout the 1950s and 1960s, manufacturers simply took dishes that families had been cooking in their kitchens and made them shelf-stable, not just so that they would last longer but also to sell them more readily in supermarkets; essentially, these foods were created for modern convenience. And yet, while this might have been the initial impulse, the food industry has continually upped the ante, over the last fifty years in particular, until the hedonic aspect of these foods—driving us not only to eat more but also more quickly and more often—has become the norm. And, at the same time, these products have become available *everywhere*. What began as an effort to make certain types of home-cooked foods, primarily desserts, readily available at the grocery store transformed into 24/7 access to a wide array of ultraformulated foods, effortlessly found at the local deli, gas station, or corner market. "The immediate access at one's fingertips to various sources of gratification brings the addictive phase to its most dangerous . . . outcome," Frank Schalow, the late professor of philosophy at the University of New Orleans, wrote, in explaining how such constant accessibility makes it difficult for a person to avoid the "allure of his/her addiction."

Alongside this change, not coincidentally, the obesity rate in the United States has steeply and continuously climbed. Today, 41.9% of the adult population struggles with obesity; by 2030, about half of us will. Though research shows that older age groups have a higher incidence of obesity, young and middle-aged adults (ages twenty to thirty-nine and forty to fifty-nine, respectively) experience the greatest weight gain. This means that many of us who are not yet overweight or obese may find ourselves there at some point during our lifetimes. The average adult gains approximately seventeen pounds from their twenties through their late thirties, making them more likely to be overweight. Another fourteen or so pounds are gained from age forty to fifty, which pushes many into the obese category. The additional ten pounds gained from age fifty to sixty further escalates health risks.

And yet it should be noted that changing one's environment from one that facilitates addiction to an environment that does *not* can have a hugely positive impact on health. In 1971, on an official visit to Vietnam, Congressmen Robert Steele from Connecticut and Morgan Murphy from Illinois discovered that a significant number—15%—of US servicemen were addicted to heroin. The drug was widely accessible, cheap, and potent. Then-president Nixon created the Special Action Office for Drug Abuse Prevention and laid out a program for rehabilitation of these servicemen. Those who were addicted remained in Vietnam for detoxification; only then were they allowed to return home. Remarkably, a very well-conducted study by Dr. Lee Robins, a psychiatric researcher and professor at Washington University in St. Louis, showed that upon returning home to the United States, only a small percentage remained addicted. An estimated 5% of these men relapsed in the first year, as opposed to the two-thirds relapse rate generally seen in the United States.

But treatment of these soldiers was not the reason for their marked recovery, since treatment—other than the detoxification they'd gone through in Vietnam to come home—wasn't readily available. "This surprising rate of recovery . . . ran counter to the conventional wisdom that heroin is a drug which causes addicts to suffer intolerable craving that rapidly leads to re-addiction if re-exposed to the drug," Dr. Robins wrote, reflecting on her findings. The main conclusion of the study was that "narcotic use and narcotic addiction were extremely common in Vietnam (although not as common as the use of alcohol and marijuana); availability was the main explanation." In other words, when the soldiers changed their environment—to a place where the heroin was less accessible than it had been in Vietnam—there were also fewer unconscious prompts directing these men's actions. (Similarly, it has been found that smokers' cravings for cigarettes decrease when they know it is impossible to smoke in certain environments—such as on an airplane—and then return when the possibility of smoking is reinstated.) So, change can happen spontaneously if the environment changes.

Ultimately, nicotine, opioids, and ultraformulated foods provoke consumption when they are widely available in the environment and trigger the addictive circuits of the brain. Some experts say nicotine and opioids are psychoactive and therefore different from ultraformulated foods. But I believe all three are psychoactive. A substance is psychoactive when "it affects how the brain works and causes changes in mood, awareness, thoughts, feelings, or behavior." Most crucially, these three substances—nicotine, opioids, and ultraformulated foods—change how we *feel*.

Our addiction to ultraformulated foods results in widespread overeating, which has physiologically changed our brains and bodies, leading to both weight gain and an unceasing desire to eat *more* of this type of food. There is no doubt that our environment—with its widespread accessibility to these foods, along with the influence of billion-dollar advertising campaigns aimed at making us aware of them—has tipped us in the direction of declining health.

The challenge now is that, even if we do manage to lose weight, we struggle mightily to keep it off. Research has shown, for instance, that people who lose 10% of their weight must consume 300 to 400 fewer calories per day, depending on their weight, or exercise so that they are burning off that same number of calories to maintain their reduced weight, as compared to people who weigh a similar amount but didn't have to lose weight to arrive at that number. In other words: When you reach your ideal weight, you can't just go back to doing what you did before.

Why is it so difficult to reset body weight? The inability to reset our weight occurs due to both metabolic adaptation (i.e., your metabolism slows down) and what I consider to be the "relapse" of food addiction. Food addiction affects many of us on a continuum, changing our bodies and minds. These foods take hold of us on a variety of different levels—by commandeering our cognitive processes and the reward center of our brains, as well as disrupting key hormones and neurotransmitters—so that we now find ourselves locked in a fierce and continuous battle with our own physiologies. The mysteries of weight loss have plagued us for so long because we didn't understand that food addiction plays a role in detrimentally altering multiple biological systems that were once meant to stabilize our weight. This is the heart of addiction.

2

· · · ·

The Addictive Power of Food

For me, the cravings were always worse in the evening. It was as if there were an alarm clock in my mind primed to go off a few hours after dinner, around 10 p.m. I would be working at my computer and I'd have this sudden feeling of unease and restlessness. The discomfort would grow. A conflict would ensue in my head. *Should I go downstairs and eat? Why can't I control myself?* I needed food—to make me feel better, to make the unease go away. As I tried to resist this impulse, a pain would develop in my head, not knife-like, but intensely discomforting. I couldn't shake the feeling. No matter how much I would try to distract myself, only eating could quiet the noise. Once I finally relented, going down to the kitchen for a snack, it was as if there were an electrode in my brain—urging me forward, insisting that I pursue pleasure—bite after bite.

A Small Desire Made Large

Addictions can encompass both substances and compulsive behaviors. "Both substances and behaviors can be considered to be forms of addictions, understood as an abnormal, long-lasting pattern of use or practice that is reinforcing and may be repeated to excess, to the point that it endangers the individual," write Dr. Marc Auriacombe and a group of professors and psychiatrists who specialize in addiction. Or, put more succinctly, as

Professor Schalow writes, "The simplest desire can be exaggerated . . . and thus cross over to form the 'hook' of addiction."

The *DSM*-5 (*Diagnostic and Statistical Manual of Mental Disorders*), long considered the "bible" for assessment of mental health disorders, doesn't yet include a classification for food addiction. Instead, it offers four groupings of diagnostic criteria to diagnose substance use disorder: impaired control; social impairment; risky use; and pharmacological adaptation. But these categories do not capture the essence of addiction.

Seeking criteria for addiction's signs and symptoms to better identify those suffering, Dr. Auriacombe and his colleagues propose a model for addiction diagnosis that challenges that of the *DSM*-5. These authors argue that we should put "impaired control" and craving at the center of addiction.

Craving as I have experienced it—a pressing unease—is also how it is often described by participants in more general addiction research. Addiction psychiatrist Dr. Omar Manejwala pointedly defines cravings as distinct from urges and desires: An urge might be strong but is usually fleeting, while a desire doesn't necessarily register as a *physical* need (for example, you wouldn't say you "crave" a promotion). By contrast, cravings, Dr. Manejwala says, can "produce unpleasant mental and physical symptoms if not satisfied." In the model put forth by Dr. Auriacombe, *craving* is suggested to be the critical link among behavior, brain, and environment.

The authors also propose a broader, simplified model for addiction comprised of three components: cues, craving, and relapse. Cues—signals in the environment that influence behavior and decision-making—prompt craving which, in turn, is a "precipitating factor" for relapse. I would add that the inability to stop—occurring after craving has taken hold—is another universal symptom of addiction.

More specifically, with food addiction, the allure and power of ultraformulated food comes from anticipating it as a reward, making it difficult for us to deny ourselves. Because these ultraformulated foods are now nearly ubiquitous, this presents us with an even steeper challenge. Sights, smells, locations, times of day—anything we might associate with the pleasure of eating these foods—can become cues. This might be something as obvious as glimpsing a chocolate chip cookie in the kitchen or as subtle as passing a street corner where we once ate a delicious hamburger. These cues grab our attention and stimulate arousal; they provoke emotions. And they incite cravings. Perhaps unsurprisingly, those who identify as "food addicted" report more intense and frequent cravings than those who do not. Crucially, this entire process can happen outside of our awareness. So, even if we *do* become conscious of having been triggered, reversing the consequent behavior is very difficult. In other words, cues provoke a craving, motivating us to get our hands on that chocolate chip cookie and devour it before we've even become aware enough to change our minds. The next time you find you have a craving for something to eat, try to identify the cue that stimulated you. There is always a cue.

Many years ago, I traveled to meet Dr. Nico Frijda, a Dutch psychologist who spent his entire career studying emotion. He identified "action tendencies," or the urge to engage in certain behaviors linked to specific emotions. It is generally accepted in psychology that there are seven basic emotions—anger, surprise, disgust, fear, happiness, contempt, and sadness—each with its own expression, or action tendency. The action tendency of fear, for instance, is an urge to escape. I would argue that, with food addiction, and addiction more generally, "wanting" is an emotion unto itself, and *its* action tendency is craving. "There is an awareness of urge. There is an awareness of what one wants to do before doing it and of being set for a given action," according to Dr. Frijda.

Which brings me back to my own late-night conundrum. I wanted to know more about what was going on in my brain when I had this 10 p.m. craving rendering me powerless night after night. I called Dr. Eric Zorrilla, an associate neuroscience professor at the Scripps Research Institute, and his mentor and colleague, Dr. George Koob, also a neuroscience professor at Scripps as well as the director of NIH's National Institute on Alcohol Abuse and Alcoholism. Both of these men are very familiar with the power of craving in addiction and have written extensively about it.

When someone—in this case, me—eats ultraformulated food and later experiences an episode of distress, or craving, this is what the two doctors refer to as an "opponent process." This theory posits that drug use of any kind can activate, after the initial pleasurable response, an anti-reward reaction. These "a" and "b" processes, as Drs. Koob and Zorrilla conceptualize them—"a" being the pleasurable phase and "b" being the feeling of withdrawal—are fully contained, in the case of drugs, within the reward circuitry and within the extended amygdala, the almond-shaped part of the brain that processes emotions and links them to memories, among other duties. "It's the downregulation in the reward circuitry," Dr. Zorrilla explains, "and the upregulation of the amygdala stress circuits."

With food, homeostatic signals—biochemical processes that allow cells to sense and respond to changes in their environment—also interact with the brain's reward system. "You're getting an 'a' process from all the homeostatic signals," Dr. Zorrilla explains, "and then because of the nature of the reward circuitry and because of the nature of those meal-related signals going down, you get a letdown." Essentially, in every addiction, for each high, there is a corresponding low. Eating ultraformulated food, for me, is the "a" process and my 10 p.m. unease is the "b" process, or what Dr. Koob describes as "hyperkatifeia," derived from the Greek *katifeia*, meaning dejection or a negative emotional state.

According to Drs. Koob and Zorrilla, the opponent process can result from both acute and chronic experiences, such as a single meal or a long-term habit of eating ultraformulated foods, respectively. And either state can build on itself. "If a person . . . got some sort of food reward associated with eating under conflict," Dr. Zorrilla expounds, "then they would tend to be biased toward eating again under conflict, from having experienced that food reward." So, what I decide to do during my 10 p.m. craving will be determined by what I did in the past (which, I confess, was to eat). And what I do in the future will be influenced by what I do now.

The negative withdrawal state can also grow in intensity and duration with repeated exposure. "One of the things that's been shown is the more you've done this—the more you've engaged in palatable eating or the more you've engaged in substance use," Dr. Zorrilla explains, "the opponent process happens earlier, and it lasts longer and it's more severe." Put more succinctly, the more you eat ultraformulated food, the more quickly cravings will reoccur, and with increased intensity. In this phase, the brain's circuitry doesn't return to the earlier steady state as easily; it sustains the negative state for longer. Dr. Koob calls this "the dark side." He explained that this part of the addiction cycle is "the negative urgency that drives one into impulsive behavior, especially regarding food." Higher levels of impulsivity, experts believe, is one of the main drivers of overeating and is a characteristic of addictive behavior. I never plan to overeat. I'm driven to do so by the impulse that comes over me, and the illusory feeling that I'm going to satisfy myself once and for all.

Resisting Temptation

As it happened, at this time, I had also been experimenting with a continuous glucose monitor, or a CGM, a patch that I wore on the back of my upper arm. As the name implies, this device continuously measured my blood glucose levels—the amount of sugar in my blood, which mainly comes from carbohydrates. Glucose sensitivity is the counterpart to insulin resistance. It refers to the body's ability to efficiently regulate blood sugar levels in response to eating. If glucose sensitivity is high, the body can manage blood sugar spikes and dips effectively after meals. Impaired glucose sensitivity, which is often seen in people with insulin resistance, means the body does not effectively control these fluctuations, leading to higher blood sugar levels. Glucose sensitivity reflects how well the body handles frequent changes in blood glucose levels. Disruption of blood glucose regulation complicates weight management. Understanding insulin resistance and impaired glucose sensitivity is vital, because these disruptions raise the risk of type 2 diabetes and cardiovascular problems, along with other conditions. I was experimenting with the monitor in hopes of better understanding my cravings. At first, there didn't seem to be any rhyme or reason to my results. I couldn't tell what, if anything, in my diet correlated with my hunger or cravings. Although I'm not diabetic, there was great variability in the measurements throughout—all kinds of spikes and troughs, showing my blood sugar level steeply rising and falling.

I was about to toss the CGM when I decided to try a different diet. I ended up experimenting with the protein-sparing modified-fast diet used by Bruce Bistrian and George Blackburn in the 1980s, which was very effective for weight loss then and is still used in obesity medicine today. And I found that this low-calorie, relatively high-protein, low-fat, low-carb diet *did* flatten my glucose curve. And it seemed that when I flattened the curve, I was less under the sway of food. My 10 p.m. cravings didn't entirely go away, but they *did* decrease.

I decided to test this new tolerance with what is, for me, the ultimate temptation. One night, I walked into The Baked Bear in San Francisco's North Beach neighborhood, where customers create customized ice cream sandwiches by mixing and matching from a variety of cookies, ice cream flavors, and toppings. I'd made any number of my own creations here in the past, piling ice cream and candy between chocolate chip and M&M cookies, and then voraciously eating these concoctions on the spot. But this time, I wasn't tempted. I walked in and then back out again without ordering.

While looking at the flat blood glucose results that I'd achieved on the protein-sparing diet, I recalled a PowerPoint slide I'd once seen when I was one of the lead experts for the cities, states, and counties that had sued the opioid manufacturers. One of the big drug companies had a slide to illustrate how methadone had tamed the roller coaster of oxycodone addictions and cravings, flattening *its* curve. In addition, I remembered that when I'd been at the FDA, we'd treated nicotine addiction with nicotine replacement patches to level out the blood nicotine level; these had reduced the cues and dopamine surges that accompanied cigarette cravings. It occurred to me that by flattening my blood glucose level, I was experiencing something similar to what had been achieved with opioids and nicotine.

Glucose is certainly not the only metabolic signal to set off the brain's reward circuits or its addictive circuitry with ultraformulated food. And my experience was certainly not evidence of a simple causal mechanism—but leveling out those peaks and troughs and experiencing fewer cravings gave credence to the biological and physiological underpinnings of my feelings of loss of control around ultraformulated food.

It became clear to me that homeostasis—a state of balance among the body systems—is the key to loosening the grip of food addiction. In any addiction, there is a hunger for ecstasy, for something to lift you out of the mundane. But this is always an illusory goal because that same hunger, or desire, eventually becomes your downfall. You think you want more and more, but, as Drs. Zorrilla and Koob point out with their opponent process theory, what really happens is that the pleasure decreases and negative mood increases. Your craving comes to demand something that you will never be able to deliver. But if you can achieve homeostasis—flattening the curve, so to speak—you will be able to eliminate the cravings. It is in this absence of wanting that achieving a sense of balance becomes possible.

Food Addiction Is Part of Being Human

Food addiction is real, and it impacts many of us. Only by confronting this fact can we successfully help people to lose weight and maintain weight loss. Although there are references to food addiction dating back to the late nineteenth century—when, for instance, the case of a "chocolate inebriate" appeared in *The Journal of Inebriety*, the first journal of addiction medicine, describing a man whose "only thought night and day is how to get chocolate"—a concentrated focus on the subject began in earnest in the early 2000s. And the interest in it is urgent enough that the FDA commissioner under President Biden, Robert Califf, recently addressed it in an Alliance for a Stronger FDA meeting, saying, "I am personally convinced that there's a significant part of ultraprocessing which creates addictive behavior . . . It seems to me it would make a lot more sense to make food which doesn't create that problem in the first place. And so we're really anxious to have more research done on this, so that we can be more specific about how to label food . . . We're last in high income countries in life expectancy . . . How can that be? . . . We've got really smart people, but something's wrong with the way that we're taking care of our health." And the notion has become embedded in our culture, enough so that Adam Platt, former restaurant critic for *New York* magazine, gave a relatively accurate explanation of the phenomenon to the *New York Times* in describing the consequences of being a professional eater: "You have this giant distended belly which wants to be filled. All those weird sensors in your brain that cry out for deliciousness are at DEFCON 1 all day. You become an addict." (Platt also suffered many of obesity's attendant ailments: gout, hypertension, high cholesterol, and type 2 diabetes.)

Over the past two decades, food addiction has gained academic recognition through extensive research, including brain imaging, animal models of addiction-like sugar intake, and applying substance dependence criteria to eating, including the development of the Yale Food Addiction Scale. Twenty years ago, I began investigating how the food industry had done an astonishing job designing potent ultraformulated food that delivers just the right combinations of sugar, salt, and fat, or "the three points of the compass," as one leading food consultant referred to these ingredients. This became the subject of my 2009 book *The End of Overeating*. In the intervening decades, despite continual debate about what diets work or the quickest ways to lose weight, a consensus was reached that these artificial products, contrived to be more desirable than anything we could experience naturally, have driven us not just to eat unhealthy food but to eat more of it than we need. This has created "a continuum of addiction," as Dr. Andrew Tatarsky, founder of integrative harm reduction psychotherapy, describes it. In other words, "reward-based eating"—the compulsive drive to eat to light up the reward circuitry of the brain—affects, in varying degrees, many who eat the ultraformulated food that is now a mainstay of the American diet. We think we can stop at any time, that it's just a bad habit we'll break one day, that once we diet, we'll get back on track. Meanwhile, the ability to lose weight and maintain it continues to elude us.

There is a newly emerging concept in the addiction world—introduced by Drs. George Koob, A. T. McLellan, founder and chairman of the board of directors at the Treatment Research Institute, and Dr. Nora Volkow, the director of the National Institute on Drug Abuse—that we should create a classification of pre-addiction. They have proposed that if a person checks off two to five symptoms in the *DSM*-5 under substance abuse disorder—as opposed to the six or more that qualifies a person for addiction—that could serve as the operational definition for pre-addiction. The aim of this would be to achieve a similar effect as the term "prediabetes," which the American Diabetes Association created to initiate an early intervention strategy for type 2 diabetes. I believe this classification would be enormously helpful in relation to food addiction specifically; it would capture the full scale of those of us who are drawn to the ultraformulated foods that surround us—perhaps not to the degree of full-blown addiction, but enough to cause potential harm.

And yet, for decades, scientists have largely refrained from applying the concept of addiction to ultraformulated foods for fear that it would sound inflammatory; some worried that labeling people living with obesity as "addicts" would further the stigma attached to excess weight. But given the manipulation of our food and the biological susceptibility that makes us all vulnerable, food addiction is clearly *not* a reflection of personal failure, or a loss of willpower, but rather a human process. Indeed, the psychological and biological pathways that allow food addiction to take hold reside within all of us; it is only *how* they manifest in each of us that is unique. Still, a vast majority of people—85% in fact—believe that obesity is entirely their responsibility.

Some scientists have questioned how food, required for survival, can be considered an addictive substance. But the very fact that food is necessary to live makes it a thornier addiction than, say, tobacco or opioids. With other substances, it is possible—not easy, but *possible*—to stop using them altogether, whereas with food, as the saying goes, you've still got to take the beast out of its cage three times a day. And though it's true food is required for survival—as it was thousands of years ago in hunter-gatherer culture, when our ancestors hunted animals and foraged plants for their meals— none of the ultraformulated foods we eat today are found in nature.

Although the public and medical community—and, most of all, the food companies—have known for decades that these ultraformulations hook us with sugar, fat, and salt so that we are guaranteed to keep eating them in unhealthy quantities, food addiction is still treated as an outlier in medicine. But, after going out into the field and interviewing a wide variety of doctors and health professionals, I found that I am not the only one who has made a connection among my own physiology, cravings, and weight-gaining behavior. There is, in fact, an emerging group of pioneering physicians and health professionals who have made food addiction a central focus of their practices based on their own lived experiences and struggles—and who offer real-world examples of how the medical system could better address the needs of those who similarly struggle.

I spoke extensively with many of these obesity medicine experts, all of whom discovered food addiction, and its destructive consequences, in themselves before incorporating its treatment into their professional lives. Dr. Claire Wilcox, for instance, a psychiatrist in Placitas, New Mexico, found that, because the addiction and eating disorder worlds had not yet fully embraced food as a habit-forming substance, she was long able to rationalize her compulsive eating as simply a reward for her grueling workdays. Dr. Robert Cywes, a specialist in weight management and bariatric surgery for adults and adolescents in West Palm Beach, Florida, reached 300 pounds before he realized addiction had been passed on intergenerationally in his family, although *his* drug of choice was carbohydrates whereas his father's had been nicotine. After Dr. Erin McArthur, a pediatrician practicing in Anchorage, Alaska, was diagnosed with type 2 diabetes—and ended up in the ICU in a diabetic crisis—it still took her another year before she stopped secretly eating "all the cookies and chips and diet sodas and Snickers I could." Dr. Tro Kalayjian, founder and medical director of Toward Health in Tappan, New York, only realized that he was suffering from addiction when he administered a questionnaire to one of his patients to assess whether he might have an alcohol use disorder. "While I was asking these questions of my patient, I thought, *Wait a minute, I'm four out of four on this survey*," Dr. Kalayjian told me. That's when he realized he had a substance abuse issue too—with food.

Many of these doctors discussed the difficulty of determining their own food addiction, given the high degree of shame and stigma attached to it. This is another reason that it took Dr. Wilcox—despite having completed both her internal medicine and addictive psychiatry residencies—longer to recognize that her compulsive eating was an addiction. Wilcox's excessive behaviors began all at once—smoking, drinking, and eating—when she was fifteen years old. But because there isn't yet the same fundamental understanding of, or structure for, food addiction as exists for smoking and drinking, it was difficult for her to discern when her eating habits had veered into a more precarious realm. Even after she successfully quit smoking and drinking, it took her many more years to face her issues with food. "I really did blame myself for that behavior in a way that I didn't blame myself for drinking and smoking," she says.

Dr. McArthur too considered her food addiction to be a failing, even as she treated children with obesity, exploring the addictive pathways that ultraformulated foods had forged in their brains. "I had this idea that I must be a bad person; I didn't have willpower. Forget the fact that I'd made it through med school, and I'd been successful at every other thing I've tried in my life for the most part," she explains. "But I wasn't having any success [overcoming my food addiction] because I was attacking the wrong problem. It didn't have anything to do with my moral uprightness. It's a disease."

Many of these doctors I spoke with came to deeply understand the science of food addiction not with a group of researchers doing rigorous randomized trials but by closely studying their own habits and behaviors, as well as those of their patients, over time. Dr. Nathaël Leduc is a family doctor in Quebec, Canada, who runs a food addiction and obesity treatment program. She discovered, as I did, that extreme variability in glucose seemed to exacerbate her cravings. And, in describing "delay discounting"—an addiction term that signifies a person's "tendency to choose small immediate rewards over larger delayed ones"—Dr. Wilcox also further illuminated Dr. Koob's "b" stage of the opponent process theory. "If you take a person who's never smoked a cigarette and give them cigarettes for a week or two, they develop a tolerance and withdrawal symptoms related to the nicotine," she explains. "At that point, they have a problem and want to keep going back to use it. This causes conditioning to take place in the brain, which causes more negative emotions and discomfort. But it is also this same psychological pain syndrome that leads to its continued overuse. I think food is the same way." In other words, the ultraformulated food meant to relieve suffering ends up causing it instead.

Several of the doctors I interviewed have either trained with or taken a workshop from Bitten Jonsson, a Swedish internal medicine nurse and American-trained addiction specialist. Jonsson—who also has her own personal story of overcoming compulsive eating—offers courses for professionals. She was an early proponent of abstinence, or becoming "drug free," which is the term she prefers with food addiction, meaning getting rid of the parts of the diet—sugar, carbs, flour—that can provoke compulsive eating. Accordingly, Drs. McArthur and Wilcox both found that cutting sugar out of their diets meant that they were able to lose weight and reduce their cravings. Once she stopped eating sugary foods, Dr. Wilcox says, it was like "night and day," and she is at a healthy weight now. "Not everybody is like that though," Dr. McArthur points out. "There are people who can eat [sugary foods] in moderation. There are others who will deprive themselves and it will make them binge. But for me, when I practice abstinence, that's when I feel true freedom."

As these doctors came to understand how best to treat themselves, they made food addiction treatment a focus among their patients. Dr. Leduc created the first program of its kind in French, incorporating her neuro-scientific understanding of the brain's reward center, her clinical observations of patients with food addiction, and her strong sense that consistent psychological support is necessary to maintain positive changes. Dr. Leduc also believes that group therapy works best for this type of treatment. "The group setting really moves people to open up. The connection with others makes you feel like you can go on and you're able to do it."

Dr. Kim Dennis, another doctor whom I spoke with among this group, is a psychiatrist specializing in treating eating disorders, addiction, and trauma. Dr. Dennis binged and purged throughout her college years—"It felt like what I imagine an 8-ball of cocaine would be like," she says, "the high came during the eating, then the purging was like nodding off"—and struggled with what felt like a one-size-fits-all approach to her treatment. "Research shows that 80% of people with bulimia also meet the criteria for food addiction based on the Yale Food Addiction Scale," and yet, Dr. Dennis points out, "when you talk to any clinician in the eating disorder world, if you even mention 'food addiction,' people lose their minds." It raises questions of diet culture and restriction, she explains, and conjures up a strict twelve-step abstinence model. The philosophy of her practice, with integrated outpatient and residential treatment centers, distinguishes between standard eating disorders and eating disorders with food addiction, as well as offers a holistic approach with a staff that includes psychiatrists, dietitians, nurses, therapists, and counselors.

Similarly, Dr. Kalayjian offers a variety of support at his center, including a wellness coach, to help patients recognize eating patterns and vulnerabilities. There is also an education component, not only about hunger and appetite, but also about food addiction. The patients' health is continually and remotely supervised. "We have continuous glucose monitors, scales, blood pressure cuffs that all link up to our office, so we're always reviewing that data."

These conversations have made even clearer to me that we need to create a new paradigm for addiction altogether. The stereotypical perception that addiction takes hold of the weak or those who have fallen on hard times misses the biological nature of addiction and only further marginalizes those captured by it. Addiction is what happens in a normally functioning brain; that is, it occurs when our brains, which are wired to meet our needs, become maladaptive. Indeed, "research in the area of neurobiology is beginning to demonstrate that drug taking behavior is controlled by brain mechanisms developed through evolution to ensure the reinforcing effects of biologically essential activities of eating, drinking, and copulation," as a scientific report for the National Institute on Drug Abuse recognized as early as 1996. "The implication of these research findings is that, were it not for countervailing influences"—meaning societal forces—"drug use would be the norm, not the aberration."

In other words, the maladaptive shift in the brain that occurs because of addiction doesn't take place because the brain is not working properly, but rather because it is working too well. It has the appearance of a pathological state but it begins because the brain is doing what it does best: adapting to its environment. And yet what started as a canny adaptation has now created a variety of new problems. By eating more ultraformulated food, we are triggering the addictive circuit, which not only makes us want to eat more but also robs us of the ability to feel full. And these behaviors lead, of course, to weight gain and obesity, which puts us at heightened risk of a number of diseases that threaten lifespan and life quality.

3

· · · ·

Betrayed by Our Own Biology

The human brain evolved to deal with scarcity, not abundance. For much of human history there was no guarantee as to when our next meal would arrive, and so our biological systems are designed to seek out the sweetest and most energy-dense foods. These systems are also designed to hold on to body fat for survival. Put simply, we are programmed to eat energy-dense foods, which are never—in our modern food environment—scarce. This mismatch of biology and environment explains why, over the last fifty years, obesity rates have skyrocketed. In fact, the real question is not why do we gain weight but how can we *not*?

"It's taken us a long time to realize the clinical implications of biology that drive weight regain. Traditionally, we've always blamed our patients," says Dr. Arya Sharma, professor emeritus and past chair in obesity research and management at the University of Alberta, Edmonton, Canada. "I think we have not fully acknowledged that there are very powerful biological drivers that actually almost guarantee that our patients will not be able to keep weight off."

The problem, as Dr. Sharma points out, is that our biological systems are no longer working *for* us. Scientists who study such biological systems have traditionally divided them into two categories—the homeostatic and hedonic systems—with the brain in control of both.

The function of the homeostatic system is to keep the body in balance and to meet the body's energy needs. In addition to regulating our food intake, this system achieves internal balance by constantly adjusting other factors in its external environment—such as blood pressure, blood sugar, and body temperature—to keep them within relatively narrow ranges. The brain receives and integrates hormonal signals that control both energy intake as well as expenditure. These signals originate in several organs. Some gastrointestinal hormones give rise to hunger, others to satiety, or the feeling of fullness that occurs between meals, and satiation, the feeling of fullness during ingestion of a meal. Fat cells relay how much energy is stored. Muscle relays energy needs. Once low on energy, the brain increases hunger; when there is too much stored energy, appetite should decrease. The gastrointestinal tract relays the type of nutrients in the environment that are ingested. The vagus nerve, a main nerve in the body, is a key transmitter of information from other organs to the brain. It's a sophisticated system that works because many parts of the body communicate with each other in tandem.

Ideally, the homeostatic system keeps body weight and fat mass within a given range. By keeping food intake and energy expenditure closely aligned, we had been able to consume hundreds of thousands of calories every year without significant fluctuation in weight. That is, until relatively recently. Astonishingly, until the modern era's changes to our food environment, body weight was stable through most of our adult years—until we entered our sixties, when weight typically began to fall slightly. Starting in the 1980s, however, body weight increased in most people throughout their lifespan. In other words, our most fundamental biological system—the homeostatic system—broke.

This is because the homeostatic system, as Dr. Sharma explains, serves "one purpose, and one purpose alone. That purpose is to defend us *against* weight loss." Or, as other obesity experts put it, the brain defends its highest fat mass, meaning that once you've introduced a higher weight, this becomes the number your body yearns for, and it will fight you tooth and nail to stay there. Which puts the homeostatic system at odds not only with our environment but also the other biological system involved in our eating behavior: the reward system.

The body's reward system—also known as the hedonic system— evolved to ensure our survival by focusing our attention on the most important objects in our environment. Evolutionary psychologists suggest that, biochemically, pleasure served to induce behavior that increased the chances of survival by making food and sex salient so that we would prioritize those objects. But in this era of abundance, the reward system can promote maladaptive pursuits instead. With its powerful circuits operating automatically—directing our attention, thoughts, and behavior toward important cues in our environment—the reward system prompts us to eat beyond our hunger and energy needs. And this thwarts the homeostatic system's goal of keeping weight within a functional range. Although the field has been reluctant to use this term, these are also our *addictive* circuits.

"Your hedonic system can override the homeostatic system. It doesn't care about body weight or energy balance or whether you've had enough to eat or not," Dr. Sharma says. "It cares about pleasure, physical reward, emotion. It's a whole different part of the brain."

Dr. Cywes, whom I interviewed about food addiction, also pointed out that "starting at a very early age, we now learn to override the homeostatic feedback system to the brain that is meant to let us know, *Hey, you've had enough.*"

And yet these two systems—homeostatic and reward—also communicate in other ways. "One of the tricky things that the homeostatic system can do is activate the hedonic system," Dr. Sharma explains. "If you've not eaten all day, you'll come home in the evening and enjoy cold pizza. It'll be the most delicious food you've ever eaten. Why? Because your hedonic system is now ready to eat whatever there is because your homeostatic system has woken up and kicked the hedonic system and said, *Do your job. Let's go find food. That's why you're craving.* The two systems talk to each other." In fact, many neurohormones work not only on the homeostatic system, but also the hedonic system.

There is another way that the homeostatic system can be disrupted by food addiction. Interoception, which is the sensory processing that gives us information about our bodily condition, is also involved with the homeostatic operations of the body. Hunger, for instance, is an interoceptive cue that can motivate us to eat, just as feeling too cold will urge us to seek warmth. One model of food addiction builds on the established research on conditioning, showing that interoceptive sensations *other* than hunger—such as fatigue and boredom—can become cues to eat. As such, ultraformulated foods become incorporated into the homeostatic operations of the body in that we habitually use this substance to decrease negative affect and increase arousal.

Beyond the homeostatic and reward circuits, there are executive control areas of the brain. The executive control circuits allow us to choose how to act, but the problem is that the homeostatic and hedonic systems operate beneath our conscious awareness. So, the addictive machinery constantly undermines the executive control functions of the brain. "It's really not a surprise we would not have a lot of success," says Dr. Sharma. "All of our so-called lifestyle and behavioral interventions rely on the executive function to do their job. And we know that the executive system is very poor at doing the job. We've been addressing the weakest part of the system."

If we want to reset weight, it is critical that we recognize that obesity is not simply the result of the cognitive elements of addiction: cue reactivity, craving, and relapse. We need to confront the biology of both the homeostatic and addictive circuits of the brain. What gets set is our appetite. Start feeding a laboratory animal a highly palatable diet for three weeks or longer and a long-term memory for that preference stays with them. Emotional memory is a big part of addiction. Prolonged eating of ultraformulated food robs us of the ability to feel full from traditional foods; essentially, it steals our satiety. This lack of satiety, as well as the reward system driving us to eat ultraformulated foods, makes obesity an incredibly complex disease to treat.

The Wanting Molecule

The hedonic system involves both the pleasurable sensation of reward and the neurotransmitter dopamine, which is focused on "wanting," or the desire for this reward. One of the neural pathways that dopamine travels, which is called the mesolimbic dopaminergic circuitry, also plays a critical role in food addiction by creating a hypersensitivity to the cues that become associated with and predict reward. Although several neurotransmitters are involved, dopamine is the most critical. Dopamine—which, beyond its starring role as the "desire" chemical, is also involved in memory, movement, motivation, and attention, among other functions—helps strengthen the connections of neurocircuits that lead to the pursuit of salient stimuli. (We are evolutionarily wired to focus our attention on the most salient stimuli in our environment.) Dr. Kent Berridge, professor of psychology and neuroscience at the University of Michigan, proposed a model of incentive salience—the psychological process by which we are drawn toward rewards such as food and sex—in which dopamine circuits are sensitive to salient stimuli. Dopamine firing is also associated with positive *reinforcement*, which means that when a behavior leads to a rewarding outcome, the brain releases this neurotransmitter, encouraging the repetition of that behavior to seek similar reward in the future; essentially dopamine acts as a "reward signal" in the brain and begins a feedforward process that strengthens habitual behavior. Once experience teaches us that a cue is linked to a certain food—say, a donut—the cue, rather than the donut itself, initiates the dopamine response, whetting the appetite.

"For me, the problem is I keep wanting more and more and more, or one extra bite," says Dr. Roy Wise, a scientist who spent his career at the NIH's National Institute on Drug Abuse, and whose work showed that dopamine, in part, strengthens the neurocircuits that are responsible for the compulsive pursuit in people sensitized to drugs of abuse. "The brain is looking for a target to pin dopamine activation on and, once it learns that target, it becomes narrowly focused on it," Dr. Berridge says. The allure and power of food, in large part, come from anticipating it as a reward. Foods that are high in fat, sugar, or salt, or any combinations of these ingredients, powerfully capture these circuits.

But dopamine does not act alone. It interfaces with the neurotransmitter GABA (gamma aminobutyric acid) and glutamate neural circuits. These circuits continue to exist even in the absence of dopamine. Months later, if you eat a certain food that you have enjoyed in the past—like that donut—those connections will be strengthened, and eventually the impulse to eat it will become habitual. Dr. Wise considers this "stamping in" of a habit to be a critical part of our food addiction.

There is another view of dopamine's role in creating a kind of memory; this one involves a variation in levels of the neurotransmitter that is more emotionally driven. "You might think our brains would learn a lot every time we get a big reward, but in fact, we are wired to learn only when the outcomes don't match up with our expectations," writes Dr. Charan Ranganath, a professor of psychology and neuroscience at the University of California, Davis. "Dopamine activity ramps up when we are expecting a reward, and that expectation determines how the brain will respond to that reward. If we get a reward that is exactly what we expect, like a paycheck, there might be no change in dopamine levels. If we get a reward, but it is less than what we expected, like if our pay was docked, we might see a drop in dopamine levels, and if we receive more than expected, like a surprise bonus, we might see an increase in dopamine levels." Ranganath goes on to point out that "a cup of coffee or an oven-baked cookie could get you excited, leave you with nothing, or be bitterly disappointing based largely on your expectations from past experiences. This variation in dopamine levels can keep us on a hedonic treadmill, sometimes working hard and joylessly to escape that feeling of deprivation."

There are many nuanced debates about how the reward circuits capture our attention and trigger our desires. And yet, despite the varying theories within the field of just *how* dopamine behaves, there is no doubt that ultra-formulated food can affect the dopaminergic circuitry.

Scientists such as Dr. Koob and Dr. Anna Lembke, who is professor of psychiatry at Stanford University School of Medicine, argue that the first step—that rise in dopamine that creates desire—is inevitably followed by a second step, bringing us into the darker side of addiction. This is essentially the opponent process theory applied to dopamine: For every rise, there is a drop. And the drop in dopamine causes dysphoria, a state of unease or general dissatisfaction. "It could be mild dysphoria, but that generates, through rumination, greater dysphoria," Dr. Koob explained. "You start thinking about all the negative things happening. Conditioning kicks in. You go get immediate relief from a candy bar or a cookie, or Häagen-Dazs ice cream, or whatever is your favorite substance."

I talked to Drs. Koob and Zorrilla about my 10 p.m. craving. "I have this visceral sensation and I have this rumination about whether I should eat something," I said. "Is that because my dopamine is waning? Am I in a dopamine trough?"

"If we think of the dopamine trough as certain neurons, the more repetitive ones, under-signaling," Dr. Zorrilla replied, "then I would say yes."

Dr. Lembke describes it this way: "What happens right after I do something that is really pleasurable and releases a lot of dopamine? My brain is going to immediately compensate by downregulating my own dopamine receptors, my dopamine transmission. That's the comedown, or the hangover . . . There is the single use, which easily passes, but it's the chronic use that can really reset our dopamine threshold. And then nothing is enjoyable—then everything sort of pales in comparison to this one drug that I want to keep doing."

Dr. Koob, among other experts, believes addiction gets locked in when substances that trigger dopamine firings—in this case ultraformulated foods—are used to cope with unpleasant feelings, caused either by decreases in dopamine firing itself or other negative emotions.

And yet, Dr. Mitch Roitman, a professor in the psychology department and director of the Laboratory for Integrative Neuroscience at the University of Illinois, believes that rather than drops in dopamine, there are *pauses* in dopamine firing. "I don't know how much empirical evidence there is for a trough relative to 'baseline' that occurs before the next 'hit' of food," Dr. Roitman told me. "It's very difficult to assess the actual dopamine concentrations and how they might change over days, weeks, months."

Dr. Roitman believes that on a moment-to-moment basis, the concentration of dopamine in specific regions of the brain is highly variable. He views dopamine, within a pool of dopamine neurons, as firing at various, or asynchronous, times. But rewarding stimuli, such as ultraformulated foods, he explained, cause synchronous bursting, which creates a widely broadcast dopamine signal.

Some experts place more emphasis on other parts of the brain at work in the addictive machinery. According to Dr. Antoine Bechara, a professor of psychology at the University of Southern California, there are ac   ⸯ three systems involved in addictive behavior: the dopamine signaling system; the insula, a part of the brain that helps determine how effective dopamine is in steering us toward a salient stimulus; and the reflective system, those executive control circuits that allow us to assess the consequences of engaging in such behavior.

Dr. Bechara explains that the insula—which not only responds to internal body signals but translates those signals into feelings of urge and craving—hijacks executive control, usually responsible for inhibiting the reward system. That inhibition is markedly diminished in addiction. It subverts attention, reasoning, planning, and decision-making.

Indeed, damage to the insula can dramatically disrupt addictive behavior. In 2023, for instance, doctors at the University of Iowa hospitals and clinics reported on the case of a fifty-three-year-old female who had suffered damage to her insula region due to a large benign brain tumor. Throughout her life, the woman had always struggled with her weight. After the damage to her insula, however, she no longer felt the urge to eat large meals and experienced gradual, sustained, effortless weight loss.

In this sense, how we act and feel results from how different parts of the brain interact—and whether one can dominate the other. Dr. Sami Schiff at the University of Padova explains that "in many situations of daily stress, individuals may have uncomfortable feelings of internal imbalance which they wish to suppress as soon as possible." In these cases, he suggests, food can quickly mitigate discomfort. More specifically, he sees this as an imbalance in the brain. The mesolimbic dopaminergic circuits drive increased attention toward food and the executive control functions, when confronted with ultraformulated foods, fail to prevent impulsive behavior. "All these factors contribute to an obese cognitive profile that favors the development and maintenance of loss of control over eating," Dr. Schiff says.

The Addiction Cycle

"How does addiction take hold?" I asked Dr. Koob. I returned to him to discuss the overall cycle—the cognitive and biological drivers—behind addiction. We worked together to apply to food the trajectory that has generally been accepted for drugs. We agreed that the addiction cycle begins with exposure to ultraformulated foods. This leads to an increase in energy intake—or consuming more calories (energy) than your body is using—leading to chronic use and dopamine release, as well as amygdala activation and increased sensitivity to cues, motivating us to seek out pleasurable foods. This process can be conceived of as "incentive salience," "food reward," or "reward sensitivity." It results in weight gain, which, in turn, means the body's energy balance is maintained at a higher level and its "settling point" increases.

Here, Dr. Koob asked me about the subtle difference between the terms "set point," which suggests that the body regulates weight within a certain range, and "settling point," which suggests that the body settles at an equilibrium point. I prefer the term "settling point," as I see weight as a balance of forces with no predetermined point. There is no thermostat. Additional forces that can affect the body's weight settling point include environment, sleep deprivation, chronic stress, and medications that cause weight gain.

Dr. Koob and I agreed that following the establishment of incentive salience, when craving is expressed as a symptom of withdrawal, there is a rise in negative mood. Ultraformulated foods are used as a relief; they become a coping mechanism. Essentially, we start using food as a drug. Early dependence sets in, resulting in compulsive use, which incites more negative moods. And with that, the addiction cycle is well underway.

What Makes Modern Food Addictive

The multilayered addictive process that plays out in our brains and bodies begs the question: *How* did ultraformulated food hook us so deeply in the first place? Again, my experience at the FDA battling the tobacco industry helped me to better understand this phenomenon. To find out what the tobacco companies knew about nicotine, our investigators found a behavioral psychologist who'd been employed by Philip Morris from 1980 to 1984. To protect his identity, they gave him a code name: Cigarette. Cigarette told our investigators that while at Philip Morris, he'd done research into what made nicotine "reinforcing"—meaning what made people keep coming back for more—by working with laboratory animals.

He gave the animals two levers to press: one for nicotine, the other for saline. The animals conditioned themselves to self-administer nicotine. This was a critical piece of information for us: Self-administration is the test that all federal agencies use to decide whether a drug should be a controlled substance. Cigarette also told us that he'd written a paper with these results and submitted it to the *Journal of Psychopharmacology*, but Philip Morris had forced him to withdraw it before it was ever published. Moreover, the company had instructed Cigarette to kill all his lab animals and suspend further research. As luck would have it, though, the editor of the *Journal of Psychopharmacology* had saved a copy of Cigarette's paper—and we were able to track it down. Given that self-administration is the sine qua non of addiction, this became one of the central pieces of evidence that allowed us to assert jurisdiction over nicotine in cigarettes as an addictive drug delivery device.

Bearing this history in mind, in 2007, Dr. Jeffrey Grimm, director of Western Washington University's Behavioral Neuroscience Program, and I undertook experiments to determine what, if anything, in food is self-administered in laboratory animals. We specifically looked at whether fat, sugar, or flavoring were self-administered by laboratory rats. We found sucrose—table sugar, which is made up of a molecule of glucose linked with a molecule of fructose—to be the dominant reinforcing component of novel foods containing mixtures of sucrose, fat, and flavor. Although we found fat to be synergistic—meaning it had a greater physiological effect in combination with other food components—sucrose was more motivating. The data have also been replicated in a dose-dependent manner, showing that higher doses of sucrose are *more* reinforcing. In addition, using a more homogenous fat than we did, Dr. Anthony Sclafani, emeritus distinguished professor of psychology at Brooklyn College, found that fat was another substantial reinforcer.

There are also "secondary reinforcers"—stimuli or cues that gain reinforcing value through their association with a primary reinforcer—that help deepen sucrose's draw. As such, sucrose can condition an animal to want to be in certain places, referred to as "conditioned place preference"— essentially, when a location becomes a cue for an animal—and obtain certain flavors, known as "conditioned flavor preference." Studies also demonstrate that humans will work for sweet-tasting rewards. Children generally prefer simple exposures of sugar, fat, and flavor, but as they get older, they tend to prefer more complex mixtures and combinations. One of the key hallmarks of reinforcers is that they are psychoactive, meaning they can change how people feel. Studies show that sweetness, for instance, is one of the most effective ways to alleviate infant distress.

The most potent reinforcers—urging people to keep returning for more—however, are the *combinations* of fat, sugar, and salt. These supernormal stimuli are rarely found together in foods in nature, but when artificially combined, they become the ingredients that give ultraprocessed foods their appeal. They stimulate the brain's food reward circuits and result in consumption of more calories. Indeed, as one very senior food industry designer told me, "The shock and surprise of addictiveness and crave-ability is an open secret in the food industry. I've been to many of those meetings. It's on the table."

Additionally, the processing changes the structure of ultraformulated foods by removing fiber and water, so the foods are ingested more rapidly.

"The poison, so to speak, is in the food," as Dr. Tera Fazzino, associate director at the Cofrin Logan Center for Addiction Research and Treatment, puts it. Dr. Fazzino and her team sought a data-driven approach to developing a quantitative definition of palatable foods based on combinations of nutrients; the effort was meant to bring specificity to the term. So, Dr. Fazzino and her team conducted a systematic review of all the foods in the literature that were identified as being highly palatable. They then entered these items into nutrition software, pulled all the nutrient data, and were able to graph them to identify some of the commonalities. This also allowed them to develop criteria for defining hyperpalatable foods. They categorized three combinations of nutrients that tend to be most reinforcing: fat and sodium (greater than 25% calories from fat plus more than 0.30% sodium by weight), fat and simple sugars (more than 20% calories from fat and more than 20% calories from sugar), and carbohydrates and sodium (greater than 40% calories from carbohydrates and more than 0.20% sodium by weight).

Dr. Fazzino highlights that while much literature focuses on sweets and high-fat, high-sugar foods, their criteria found most hyperpalatable foods had elevated sodium levels.

The combinations of these nutrients are essential. On their own, the addictive nature of each of these ingredients is limited. Sucrose, for instance, is reinforcing but if I just gave you a packet of sugar and said, "Have a good time," it's probably not going to do much for you. But there is another key component: the *experience*. Which is to say, the sensory properties of hyperpalatable foods are also a draw: the succulent crunch of a piece of fried chicken or the silken pleasure of a milkshake. The color, temperature, texture, and smell of these foods are also integral to their irresistibility. "The ultimate food is bacon," explains Gail Vance Civille, founder and president of Sensory Spectrum, a management consulting firm that studies the sensory-consumer experience. "It's not about the fat, sugar, and salt as much as about pure pork that's browned . . . delivering the fat, sugar, and salt." Civille asserts that the food industry assembles expert panels to test the sensory experience with certain foods to create products with the greatest hedonic response.

And yet, despite the addictive strength of these supernormal stimuli, this knowledge can also be used to counter their effect. That is, if you eliminate fat, you also eliminate the combination of fat and sugar, or the combination of fat and salt. Eliminate sugar and you eliminate the combination of fat and sugar. Fat plus sugar, fat plus salt, fat plus sugar and salt—these all provide reward and stimulate eating. Therefore, eliminating one of the components—sugar, fat, sodium, or any of these combinations—goes a long way toward quieting the addictive circuits.

The Lure of Sugar

Why is sugar so addictive? When I published *The End of Overeating*, I hypothesized that sugar was reinforcing—I wasn't ready to use the word *addictive* then—because when we eat ultraformulated food that is rich in sugar, fat, and salt, we are stimulating taste neurons directly connected to the reward centers of the brain. The evidence then showed that those neurons "encoded" palatability.

This means, as Dr. Howard Fields, a professor of neurology and physiology at the University of California, San Francisco, explained to me then, that "if a neuron encodes the color red, it will fire more when a red light is showing than when any other color is showing... The neuron shows a preference by firing more." Therefore, neurons encoded for sucrose respond to sweet foods. The more sucrose is consumed, the more these neurons fire. Animals in studies consume sucrose for "orosensory self-stimulation," where eating tasty foods signals the brain to want more. This process involves opioid circuits—chemicals like endorphins that create rewarding effects similar to opioid drugs, making such foods highly pleasing. The stimulation or calming effect of these circuits contributes to sugar's addictive nature.

But, while I still think palatability is important in food addiction, it is not the whole story. Yes, sucrose exerts its rewarding properties by activating hardwired taste receptors in the mouth linked to the brain's reward circuitry. But glucose on its own—which is released after carbohydrate-containing foods are digested and is the body's preferred carb-based energy source—has also been the focus of a variety of critical studies, showing that it not only can originate from the taste receptors, but also other parts of the body. And—as I, too, found in my experience wearing a continuous glucose monitor—reducing its highs and lows may help regulate the brain's addictive circuits.

Work done by Dr. Anthony Sclafani, as well as others, shows that when triggered by glucose, cells that are part of the digestive tract—specifically, the duodenum, the first part of the small intestine, and jejunum, the middle part of the small intestine—can activate the body's vagus nerve which, in turn, activates the brain's reward circuits. In experiments in which glucose is put directly in the intestine, bypassing the mouth, Dr. Sclafani has shown that mice and rats can be conditioned to prefer specific flavors. This supports the understanding that there are receptors in the digestive tract, located beyond the mouth, that can activate the brain's reward pathway. When carbohydrates are digested, glucose molecules encounter certain receptors in our intestines, ultimately triggering the reward circuits.

One of the most important advances of the last decade is understanding the intricate nature of the cells that line the intestine that sense and prepare the body for the nutrients being ingested and absorbed. These enteroendocrine cells (endocrine cells in the intestine) help signal to the brain which nutrients are rewarding or aversive; they can also help the brain spot nutrients that are useful for survival in times of nutrient uncertainty, as well as those that are potentially toxic. Dr. Zach Knight, a professor of physiology at the University of California, San Francisco, has written that these cells are critical for guiding animals toward safe and nutritious food sources in the wild.

Additionally, Dr. Diego Bohórquez at Duke University discovered neuropods in the intestine that can sense glucose and signal the brain's reward circuits via the vagus nerve. Drs. Molly McDougle and Guillaume de Lartigue at the University of Pennsylvania identified gut-brain circuits for fat and sugar, showing that their combination triggers dopamine release and overeating.

These post-ingestive signals in the intestine are part of the feedforward signal that encourages us to seek out food. "Most people are eating because they want that hit," Dr. Mitchell Roitman says. "That hit in the gut also signals the reward circuitry to keep eating." There are also glucose-sensing neurons in the liver and brain. Dr. Roitman's lab has shown how drops in glucose affect the dopamine reward circuit.

About a decade ago, my colleague Dr. Dana Small, with my assistance, showed that in patients who experienced challenges including loss of control, lack of satiety, and preoccupation with hyperpalatable food, those with higher body weight struggled more with eating behavior. Upon consumption of a chocolate milkshake, this group had greater continued activation of the amygdala region of the brain, which regulates appetite. For the higher weight participants, drinking the milkshake actually stimulated appetite instead of decreasing their craving.

When I talked to Dr. Small more recently, she suggested that the critical finding of the research was that the primary reinforcer related to food, such as glucose, is generated during digestion and is crucial for cellular survival and function. Dopamine levels increase when animals seek glucose, making it highly reinforcing. These reinforcing signals are subliminal and not consciously perceived. Dr. Small highlighted that glucose and fat pathways are separate but more reinforcing when consumed together, noting that many foods have high energetic signals.

Dr. Ivan de Araujo, director at the Max Planck Institute for Biological Cybernetics, has spent the last fifteen years using animal experiments to study how the glucose that enters our body every time we eat sugar stimulates brain dopamine. "When dopamine levels are the lowest, that's when the animals have the motivation to press the lever. Whenever the glucose level or stimulation of the brain by glucose goes down, the reflexive behavior is to seek more glucose," Dr. de Araujo explains, based on his experiments. "The animals are seeking a dopamine hit." And glucose delivery in the early part of the intestine is driving much of the reinforcing behavior.

"So, once I start eating sugar or carbohydrates, it is hard to stop?" I ask.

"Yes, you should be careful when you start. And particularly careful how many times you stimulate yourself. In that sense, it's very similar to drugs, tobacco, or alcohol. If you start a relatively regular schedule of stimulation, you will change your brain to trigger the same behavior." Meaning you will be driven to keep eating that sugary or starchy treat—be it ice cream or soda or pasta—to keep getting the dopamine hit, just like the animals continually pressing the lever.

This is true of glucose above and beyond other types of sugar. "Glucose produces more dopamine release than all other sweet things even though it's not as sweet," says Dr. de Araujo. What is it about glucose that makes it so rewarding? Today, the general view is that it is the *energy* in the glucose molecule, not the sweetness, that drives us to consume it repeatedly. This makes sense given that glucose is, like oxygen, a fundamental molecule of life. All our organs, tissues, and cells rely primarily on glucose. There is still, however, debate about where the primary source of glucose sensing in the body occurs. Is it in the mouth, the cells that line our intestine, or the portal vein when blood leaves the liver? What we do know is that fluctuations in glucose signaling to the brain trigger a behavioral response to seek more glucose.

I told Dr. de Araujo about my efforts to minimize my blood glucose fluctuations by controlling what I ate, and that my cravings had been reduced as a result. He explained what I had felt to be true intuitively: "When you avoid these fluctuations, you are minimizing the likelihood that the behavior that caused the increase in dopamine in the first place will be repeated." In other words, the less glucose levels vary, the less behavior is reward-driven.

Dr. Laura Thi Germine, who directs the Laboratory for Brain and Cognitive Health Technology at McLean Hospital, offered a different theory, however, for why cravings are reduced by flattening my glucose curve. She and her colleagues have shown that minimizing glucose fluctuations is linked to optimizing cognitive ability in certain populations. (Whether minimizing glucose fluctuations can increase executive control remains to be studied.) When I asked her if some people might use eating to try to ward off fatigue, she was intrigued. She posited that "fatigue-related decreases in cognitive ability" might make a tired person eat to perk back up again. Intuitively, this rang true for me. During my 10 p.m. cravings, I was trying to fuel my brain to keep working.

We also have evidence that variability in glucose that circulates in the blood affects the brain's addictive circuits and may affect our desire to eat.

Dr. Patrick Wyatt, formerly an advisor to the health science company ZOE, recorded glucose levels in 1,070 subjects after they had ingested standardized meals. The participants with larger average glucose dips two to three hours after a meal reported higher hunger levels, shorter time until the next meal, and greater energy intake at three to four hours and twenty-four hours after the meal compared to participants with smaller glucose dips. When comparing the same person eating the same meal on two different occasions, glucose dips were still associated with time until the next meal, energy intake at three to four hours, and energy intake at twenty-four hours. While glucose dips are a signal for hunger, the correlation among dips, hunger, and meal intake shows that glucose explains only a relatively small part of when people eat.

Other studies show glucose variability affects hunger and caloric intake, especially in people with obesity. Dr. Renata Belfort De Aguiar at Yale found that glucose drops before meals predict hunger, causing higher food intake in obese individuals compared to nonobese. Using CGM systems, data from thirty-one nondiabetic subjects revealed that lower glucose levels led to increased hunger and calorie consumption. Dr. Belfort De Aguiar notes the trend in glucose levels, not the absolute value, signals hunger, and there may be differences in how the brain perceives glucose in people with obesity, diabetes, and prediabetes.

Dr. Elizabeth Parks, a professor of medicine in the Department of Nutrition and Exercise Physiology at the University of Missouri, showed that flattening blood glucose levels using short-term low-carbohydrate diets effectively reduced food cravings. According to Dr. Parks, "Changes in sweet cravings were significantly positively related to the changes in blood glucose concentrations, such that those who exhibited the greatest reductions in blood glucose had the greatest reductions in cravings for sweets."

Beyond the scientific data, there is also clinical support for the notion that blood glucose variability adds to people's struggles with weight. At a meeting of the Obesity Medicine Association, I asked a group of clinicians who had gathered to discuss the use of CGMs whether we could reduce the food noise that many patients experience by getting their glucose readings into a flat and narrow range. All of them thought that, while doing so wouldn't stop overeating entirely, it would certainly help decrease the struggle.

Although blood glucose itself may not be an addictive trigger, it could be that glucose in the intestine triggers intestinal cells that send signals through the vagus nerve to the brain's reward system. For example, Dr. Stephanie Kullmann at the University of Tübingen, in Germany, has shown that high insulin levels can respond to high glucose levels: "Chronically altered insulin levels are associated with persistent consumption of simple sugars and overeating." Tighter blood glucose curves could reflect better behavioral control of the urge to overeat.

Regardless of the source of the glucose signal, whether it originates from the taste receptors, the gastrointestinal tract, or blood, the takeaway from all this research is that avoiding marked variability in glucose may help balance the brain's addictive circuits, which can decrease cravings and overeating. But glucose is just one of many factors that trigger the reward system. It is part of a very complex milieu of hormones and nutrient signals; our individual sensitivities make this exponentially more complicated.

4

· · · ·

Sensitivity and Susceptibility

Everyone has their own story. Mine begins in childhood. When I started to put on weight as a kid, I didn't realize that I was launching an inevitable cycle—*up, down, up, down*—that would play out for the rest of my life. No mere two pounds a year for me, which is the typical trajectory for weight gain into middle age. Instead, throughout childhood, into midlife, and still today, I could gain a considerable amount of weight, somewhere between twenty and forty pounds, over a relatively short period of time, and then painstakingly lose it, only to start the process all over again.

Food was my reward for hard work. It reassured me; it lifted me out of the trenches of everyday life. In college and medical school, I was only able to work late into the night, studying, researching, and writing, if I knew that the refrigerator in my room was full of Sara Lee chocolate cake and Entenmann's donuts. I could keep going as long as these consolations were just an arm's length away. If I needed a more substantial break in the middle of the night, I would prowl for subs, pizza, or wings. To this day, I can still taste the salty roast beef and fresh baked rolls from the Hungry I in Amherst that I devoured late at night. I vividly recall the tangy dressing on the special sandwiches at Elsie's Sandwich Shop in Cambridge and the greasy takeout fries from Busy Bee on Beacon Street in Brookline. In every city I lived in during my medical training, I was on a first-name basis with the owner of the neighborhood Chinese restaurant. Deeply woven into these recollections is another sense memory: my anxiety melting away as I slid headlong into the numb pleasure of overindulgence. That's the tricky thing about food. It's necessary, but it can also be dangerous. And if you're not careful, you lose all sight of the bigger picture.

When I am at my heaviest, I look physically different, of course. My chest strains against my shirt; my waist rolls like an accordion over my pants; my cheeks become visible at the bottom of my line of sight. But there is an emotional component to this state too. It is as if there is another path I can and, more often than I'd like, *do* take that leads me to another existence. I become an alternate version of myself. This person is impelled to eat without any sense of control, even as he knows it will leave him in a state of merciless self-consciousness, even as he profoundly understands it is damaging his health. I have two advanced degrees. I attended my third year of medical school and my third year of law school at the same time. I have been dean of two medical schools. I've run the FDA. No one would ever accuse me of not having discipline and determination. And yet, throughout my life, I have perpetually taken the path back to this other realm, despite how miserable I know I will be when I get there.

Most people who battle weight aren't focused on the addictive circuits that are quietly at play in their brains. For them, as for me, all we see is a daily struggle with eating. Usually, this relationship develops over time. Exposure to ultraformulated food and the consequent food addiction or obesity often begin early in childhood, but the profound ramifications can take decades to be fully seen. That is the case with smokers too: 90% of them had picked up the habit in adolescence, only to find out later that they couldn't quit. "I liked it, but now I hate it," admitted one preteen boy who was part of a focus group conducted for a report called Project 16, commissioned by Imperial Tobacco in the 1970s to study youth smoking. "We all said we'd do it for a few years and then quit, and we really meant it," another adolescent remarked. "Now it's, what, five years later and I'm not so sure." Still another lamented, "You never think you'll do any damage to yourself. You'll know how to control it." But, as this report concluded with sinister clarity, "[A]ddicted they do become."

Today, similar voices of despair are emerging from a population that didn't realize they'd become addicted to ultraformulated food until too late. In 2014, I published a study, along with a team of other doctors, called *The Reward-Based Eating Drive Scale*. In it, we reported that many people struggling with obesity didn't discover that they were unable to give up ultraformulated food until they tried to take weight off. As we concluded in the study: "They lose less weight than desired, gain much of it back within a year, and often undergo repeated cycles of weight loss and gain."

Although there is less known about addictive eating in children and adolescents than in adults, it isn't difficult to conclude that recent generations are made more susceptible to this cycle given the increasing prevalence of ultraformulated food. Additionally, over the last forty years, "the prevalence of childhood obesity has more than doubled in children and tripled in adolescents" (twelve to nineteen years of age). It is also widely recognized that eating behaviors formed in childhood carry over to the adult years.

Dr. McArthur, one of the pediatricians I interviewed about her own food addiction, also has a particular vantage point on a generation of kids growing up with ultraformulated foods surrounding them. "When you look at what so many kids are eating, there's not a vegetable in their entire day," she says. "They start with cereal, and then they go to Lunchables, and then they're having pizza for dinner. There's no real food. Whether you have that genetic predisposition or not, we are laying down these pathways of dopamine reward and deficit in these kids early and often, and I really worry about what their lives are going to be like." Creating addictive pathways in children's brains almost guarantees that they will have to battle them over a lifetime.

Not only does daily consumption of ultraformulated foods increase our future preference for these foods, but as my colleague Dr. Small has shown, it also "reduces preference for low-fat food, rewiring brain reward circuits to enhance response to palatable foods." That consumption creates new learning that further drives desire for ultraformulated foods. We also know that energy density, hyperpalatability, and eating rate, or how fast we consume food, are consistently related to how much food we eat and overeat.

Dysregulated appetite is at the center of the disease of obesity. Psychologists who study appetite detail the components of it as: hunger, wanting (desire), liking (pleasure), satiety (between-meal satisfaction), and satiation (within-meal satisfaction). Accordingly, people who are highly susceptible to food stimuli tend to report loss of control in the face of it, lack of feeling satisfied when eating ultraformulated foods, and a preoccupation with thinking about these foods. Evidence also suggests that, in many people, salient food cues not only activate areas of the brain that trigger desire, but those areas, once activated, also don't readily shut off, so they keep wanting to eat more. Similarly, I found, along with my colleagues Dr. Small and Dr. Elissa Epel, professor and vice chair in the Department of Psychiatry at the University of California, San Francisco, and director of the Aging, Metabolism and Emotion Center, that people who struggle with their weight experience persistent activation of the brain's addictive circuits compared to those who do not struggle with their weight.

Dr. Carl A. Roberts, a professor in the psychology department at the University of Liverpool, argues that people living with obesity have "a biological vulnerability for weight gain which is manifested in eating behaviors that lead to overconsumption. Individuals with obesity tend to demonstrate less regulatory control of eating behavior. Moreover, appetite regulation is more likely to be overwhelmed by environmental cues to overconsume."

Dr. Roberts suggests that appetite control is the interplay between three behavioral phenomena: satiety, reward, and inhibitory control.

Regarding satiety, or between-meal satisfaction, Dr. Roberts states that there is often inadequate impact of the food eaten, accompanied by an increase in eating rate, a failure to develop satiation during a meal, and increased hunger.

Regarding feelings of reward, specifically wanting and liking, Dr. Roberts confirms that this is expressed in greater responsiveness to food cues, craving, eating for pleasure, and eating to relieve negative affect, including stress and mood. He also sees more episodes of loss of control, experiences of uncontrolled hunger, and greater disinhibition in eating behavior.

In essence, Dr. Roberts observes one fundamental phenomenon: We all to varying extents have our efforts to control weight undermined by reward and satiety vulnerabilities.

Most of us know this struggle all too well. To me, the compelling mystery is not who is susceptible to ultraformulated foods, but what protects people who are *not* sensitive to them? Dr. Daniel Bessesen, professor of medicine at the University of Colorado, has spent his entire career trying to understand the biological systems that control human energy balance, weight, and eating behavior. In one study, he overfed both people who were lean and people who had obesity with the aim of seeing how their systems would each adapt. He discovered that lean people had marked reductions in appetite when fed excess calories. He also demonstrated that overeating was correlated with increases in satiety hormones that send signals of fullness from the gastrointestinal tract to the brain. He and his colleagues then conducted another study that similarly shows that hunger in nonobese people drops quickly when they are overfed. By comparison, when he overfed people with obesity who had lost weight, he found that there was no evidence of a decrease in their appetites, nor that their brains sensed the excess calories.

In his lean patients, highly palatable foods such as chocolate cake and pizza elicited a strong response on MRI neuroimaging. But when he overfed these patients, that strong response which signaled desire went away. Their neural responses shut down. But the brain response in people with obesity who had lost weight did *not* shut off. That continued brain activation is why they kept on eating.

The Role of Genes

Although the rise in obesity over the last four decades is not attributable to genes, susceptibility to weight gain, at least to some extent, is genetic in origin. The amount of fat we carry as a population is distributed like a bell-shaped curve. That curve has shifted so that the average amount of fat that people carry has steadily increased, for some more than others. And genetics influences where we sit on that curve. We are only beginning to recognize, not to mention understand, how genes make us susceptible to gaining weight. There are some rare mutations that increase the chance that a person will be obese, but they do not explain much about the overall genetics of body weight. Furthermore, no one gene can explain much of obesity; many genes are involved because body weight is the result of many physiological processes, ranging from metabolism to food intake.

Still, there is no doubt that there *are* forces beyond our control that affect our weight. Numerous studies have shown that identical twins who share an identical genetic makeup are more alike than fraternal twins, who are non-identical but related as siblings. Specifically, identical twins raised apart show similarity in their weight distribution. From these studies, geneticists calculate a heritability index of 40 to 60% for body mass. By comparison, height has a heritability of 80%. Heritability is highly context dependent, however, and decreases twofold with age. And here is where it gets interesting: When identical twins are over- or underfed, there is *still* a higher degree of correlation in weight and body composition changes compared to fraternal twins. Some scientists speculate that the genes we inherited evolved in an environment where there was great variability in the amount of food available over the course of a year, and as a consequence, many of our genes favor putting on weight even in an environment of food abundance. "We are organisms that were developed, designed, if you will, selected for, in an environment of low energy intake or restricted energy intake and high energy output, and we are living in an environment which is exactly the reciprocal," says Dr. Rudolph Leibel, a professor of pediatrics and medicine at Columbia University's medical school. Or, as my colleague Dr. Tamas Horvath, chair of the Department of Comparative Medicine at the Yale School of Medicine, succinctly puts it: "Our default is to put on weight."

Putting together a genetic test to predict who will become obese based on that person's genetics is still developing. When I sent off my own DNA to be queried against selected genes, my polygenic risk score assessing many genes came back with a score of 75 out of 100, with the company telling me I was at increased risk for increased appetite due to low satiety. When I showed it to a geneticist friend, he said that three of five genes on my report looked totally benign. The other two probably have a very modest effect on weight in the order of one or two pounds.

The polygenic score was meaningless. This genetics test did not help me understand why I have a difficult time controlling my weight. Could a different genetics test help me better understand why I have a difficult time controlling my weight? Maybe. We know that genetic variation across individuals plays a role in obesity. However, while our genes may set the stage, it is our environment that choreographs our weight.

5

· · · ·

The Legacy of Obesity

In general, the idea that obesity is "genetic" is largely misunderstood. When most people hear "genetic," what they take that to mean is that a parent who is obese has a gene that causes obesity, which is then passed down to their child. But the actuality is much more complex than this, as discovered by Dr. Michael Rosenbaum, who specializes in pediatric obesity and has worked in the field for over forty years.

In fact, one idea about how a parent's weight might impact a child has to do with a mother's prepartum weight: A woman who is obese before she becomes pregnant can gain the same amount of weight over the course of her pregnancy as a woman who becomes pregnant at a healthy weight, but the baby born to the woman with obesity has a much greater risk of becoming obese later in life. And yet this isn't about the mother's genetic code. Studies suggest that the risk is epigenetic (indicating it is due to biology but not specifically DNA). So when we consider the influence of environment, we're not just talking about a child growing up in a house stocked with ultraformulated foods; we're also talking about the very first moments of development in the womb. "You're laying the metabolic groundwork and the behavioral groundwork for all the metabolic diseases of adulthood really from the moment of conception," Dr. Rosenbaum said. What a mother eats impacts fetal development in a profound way: "The intrauterine environment is a boot camp for life, so if you're in this environment where there's tons of sweets, lots of food, lots of insulin, your brain and other organ systems develop expecting that that's what the world is going to be like when you get out." And indeed, the outside world, in many ways, *does* encourage obesity. As a result, we have set up a generation of children, and beyond, for a legacy of obesity.

For instance, as a fifteen-year-old boy, George (not his real name) always carried some extra weight. His father, Jack (also a pseudonym), had been classified as obese but after he began seeing a nutritionist in 2017, he overhauled the family's kitchen, stocking it with healthy fare like lean protein and vegetables. Jack lost weight, but George, although he liked the taste of much of the healthy new food, did not. When he arrived at a weight-loss clinic in 2024, the physicians there did a full medical workup and uncovered no chronic mental or physical health conditions. (A family member had thyroid disease and Jack wondered if George did as well, but tests revealed normal thyroid function.) George described feeling like he needed a huge amount of food to feel full. He discussed his tendency toward emotional eating and eating out of boredom, and that he craved and thought about food often. He told the doctors he didn't exercise, and he didn't binge eat or have episodes where he felt out of control while eating. He was almost 5 feet 11 inches tall and weighed 290 pounds. Drs. Aaron Kelly and Claudia Fox, codirectors of the Center for Pediatric Obesity Medicine at the University of Minnesota, used a similar case in their lecture at the 2024 Columbia Cornell conference on the etiology of obesity.

George's experience of hunger—that it crept into his mind often, that it was not only a physiological state but an emotional one, that it was, when he was experiencing it, all-consuming—has been echoed by other children with obesity. In 2023, reporter Lisa Miller described shadowing a teenager living with obesity whose mother had noticed that her daughter was "insatiable" from a young age, often having dinner at a friend's house before returning home to have a second dinner with her family. "I tried to stop eating as much as I did, but I couldn't," the teenager told Miller. "I would get hungry if I tried." In another story, the mother of a four-year-old who was the biggest child in her preschool class had struggled to control her daughter's appetite. "She eats very slowly and deliberately and finishes everything on her plate," the mother said. "At a birthday party, she is usually the last one off the table from eating pizza or birthday cake, and she always asks for seconds." The mother used the word many doctors shy away from when talking about kids in this age range: Her daughter, she said, was a carbohydrate *addict*.

The conversation about pediatric obesity exploded in January 2023, when the American Academy of Pediatrics released new guidelines for the treatment of obesity. The seventy-three-page document opened by declaring obesity "one of the most common pediatric chronic diseases" resulting from "a multifactorial set of socioecological, environmental, and genetic influences that act on children and families." It also highlighted the grim statistics, including that while only 5% of children were obese in 1963, that number rose to 19% in 2017, and that obesity prevalence "increases with increasing age," demonstrating that once children develop obesity, it often stays that way. "A predictive epidemiologic model estimates that if 2017 obesity trends hold," the report states, "57% of children aged two to nineteen years will have obesity by the time they are thirty-five years of age, in 2050." Along with this scourge, of course, comes its attendant health problems: Children with obesity are at greater risk of developing type 2 diabetes, elevated blood lipids, and fatty liver disease, conditions once virtually unheard of in children.

How can we start paying attention to the genesis of the problem rather than focus our money and efforts on its end results? Dr. Rosenbaum shared an idea: to study people living with obesity who want to conceive a child who would take medication to reduce their weight, then spend time off the drugs preparing for a pregnancy (weight-loss medications are unsafe during pregnancy) and see if the lower weight had a protective effect for the fetus. If the results confirmed his suspicions, we could shift the paradigm slightly to provide extra treatment for women planning to start a family in hopes that we could prevent obesity before a child is even conceived.

As research continues to investigate the effects of obesity on a developing fetus, pediatricians and other family clinicians can focus on addressing excess weight and its associated health complications as early as possible. "Primary care gets a bad rap," Dr. Eugene Dinkevich, a pediatrician in Brooklyn, New York, explains. "I see many studies where the conclusion is: Primary care does not prevent obesity. I think it couldn't be further from the truth." Dr. Dinkevich says the fact that pediatricians see children so frequently in their early years (the recommendation is for eleven visits in the first two years of life) makes them uniquely suited to address early issues that can arise around food and weight. A strong bond between the family and physician would help to mitigate against a sense of stigma, and the family would come to trust the physician and value their guidance. Advice can be tailored for each stage of development: The parents can be counseled about picky eating and healthy growth during a child's infancy, while a middle school–aged child can be counseled on the fundamentals of healthy eating. Losing sight of lifestyle management in the chatter around drugs—even though obesity medicine doctors themselves almost always concede that an adult on weight-loss drugs still must adjust their diet and exercise habits for optimal health results—would be a grave mistake, because such shifts encouraged by a pediatrician can make a significant and lasting difference. One study showed, for example, that a child who was overweight at age eight but had normalized their BMI by the onset of puberty, around age thirteen, significantly reduced the risk of developing type 2 diabetes in adulthood. Recent research from a sweeping study comparing children conceived and born during or after rationing during World War II in England showed that those who consumed less sugar early in life had a significantly lower chance of developing diabetes and high blood pressure in middle age. Though the full implications of this study are yet to be determined, many scientists suspect that it offers evidence for how taste preferences are developed in early years, as well as the addictive nature of sugar.

In March 1995, I stood in front of an audience at Columbia Law School and declared tobacco "a pediatric disease." Once people understood their children were the targets of predatory marketing tactics, the conversation about consumer choice and freedom seemed to dissipate. Now let me say: Obesity is a pediatric disease. It is a pediatric disease not only because children suffer from it, but also because it has been foisted upon them by the architects of our obesogenic environment, who have ensnared us for their own profit. While we cannot deny treatment to young people already affected, we equally cannot allow the medical and pharmaceutical communities to convince us that the best way—the *only* way—out of this crisis is their way. We need a multifaceted approach to deal with this catastrophe—one that potentially involves medications but with a view toward a future of maintaining our children's health without them—an approach that doesn't shame people for their choices, and that doesn't lose sight of larger systemic issues at play that desperately need to be addressed.

6

. . . .

Regain as Relapse

Weight regain is one of the great unsolved medical mysteries of our modern era. "The minute you reduce treatment or stop doing what you're doing to lose weight, the weight starts coming back," says Dr. Arya Sharma, the Canadian obesity expert who has confessed that powerful biological drivers almost guarantee that his patients cannot maintain weight loss. Few people who treat obesity are as honest and direct as Dr. Sharma. "I've been doing this for thirty years. I haven't cured a single case of obesity. I've had lots of patients that have lost weight and kept that weight off, and their health has improved, their quality of life has improved, but none of these people I would consider to be 'cured,'" he confided at a recent meeting of the European Congress on Obesity. "And I think that is still something that most people don't realize. Once you develop obesity, you're pretty much dealing with this problem for life. You want to run marathons, be my guest, but when you stop running, guess what, the weight is going to come back."

This is true for any of the possible interventions: diet, drugs, and surgery. A meta-analysis of the propensity to regain weight shows that by year three, more than 60% of the lost weight has been regained, with further regain in years four and five. "A lot of the weight comes back early on," adds Dr. Paul MacLean of the University of Colorado School of Medicine. Even after liposuction, the weight still often finds its way back. "There is no article in the plastic surgery literature that shows that people who have had liposuction keep the weight off better than anyone else," explained Dr. Michael

Rosenbaum of Columbia University. Even the new anti-obesity drugs don't have a lasting effect once you go off them. "Weight regain following weight loss is the biggest challenge in obesity management," says Dr. Cátia Martins, associate professor in the Department of Nutrition Sciences at the University of Alabama at Birmingham. "The majority of individuals regain weight in the long term. And this happens regardless of the intervention that is used to induce weight loss. After the acute weight-loss phase is over, what follows is weight regain."

As Dr. Rosenbaum states, if coupling between energy expenditure and appetite existed such that if you ate more, you burned more and if you ate less, you burned less, it should be easy to keep weight off because your body would want to stay weight stable. "There would be no forces to make you regain it," he says. "Unfortunately, it doesn't work that way."

Dr. Rosenbaum has been studying weight-loss maintenance for thirty years. "Losing weight is only the start of the battle," he says. "What's important is finding out how to keep weight off and how to get our bodies to work with us rather than against us in doing it."

What is responsible for this inevitable cycle? There are two parts to this answer: metabolic adaptation—the reduction in the amount of energy the body uses to survive in the face of weight loss—and the brain's addictive circuits.

In 2014, an NIH committee charged with studying this phenomenon concluded that increased appetite and decreased metabolism were the causes of weight regain. "It's the difference between what the body wants to eat and what the body is expending that is the biological pressure driving weight regain," explained Dr. MacLean. And while the view is somewhat controversial, many scientists believe these effects do not resolve over time. In other words, according to these researchers, metabolic adaptation is not a transient state; increased hunger and slowed metabolism persist after initial weight loss.

Another contributor, according to Dr. MacLean, is the predictable decline in adherence to behavioral programs, which happens gradually over time. In a seminal study, first at Rockefeller University and then at Columbia University Medical Center's in-patient clinical research unit, Dr. Rosenbaum and his colleagues fed people of varying body weights a relatively poor-tasting liquid diet of 800 calories a day until they lost 10% of their weight. Some patients with obesity lost up to 50% of their weight. Researchers found that, as people lost weight, energy expenditure decreased, meaning their metabolism

slowed. Indeed, matching for body composition, people who lost weight reduced their energy expenditure by 300 to 400 calories a day. In other words,
if they wanted to maintain their weight, or stay in energy balance and *not*
regain weight, they would have to eat 300 to 400 fewer calories a day or exercise to burn 300 to 400 calories more than someone at their equivalent body
composition who did not have to lose weight to get there. Not only did these
participants have to eat less than before because they were now smaller (with
less muscle mass to burn energy), but also, additional changes in metabolism,
the endocrine system, and the nervous system further reduced the amount
of food that they could consume without gaining weight.

Although Dr. Rosenbaum is careful to point out that not everybody reduces their energy expenditure as they lose weight, metabolic adaptation
isn't the only challenge. This is where the addictive circuits come into play.
"The primary driver of weight regain is the increase in appetite," he says.
"The decrease in energy expenditure is important, but it's the increase in
appetite that really drives it."

Dr. Kevin Hall, the NIH researcher who studies environment and eating, for instance, has modeled that for every kilogram of body weight lost,
appetite increases by 95 calories per day while expenditure decreases by 25
calories per day.

Additionally, Dr. Rosenbaum, along with pioneering obesity researcher
Dr. Jules Hirsch, showed that, after weight loss, an increased reward expectation where you anticipate food will taste better, as well as the sense that
it *does* taste better, occurs alongside decreased restraint because areas of the
brain meant to inhibit the dopamine response are affected. After weight
loss, Dr. Rosenbaum found increased activity in the addictive reward centers of the brain, including the insula and ventral striatum; decrease in the
areas of the brain responsible for restraint; and delayed satiation. In other
words, "After you have lost weight, you have lower energy expenditure and
higher drive to eat," he says. "The perfect storm for weight regain."

Food addiction does not, however, only involve the reward circuits that
trigger "wanting." "You have the devil [in the addictive reward centers] telling you to eat," as Dr. Rosenbaum puts it, "and the angel [in the prefrontal
cortex] telling you not to eat."

The weight regain documented in these studies is evidence of relapse,
and it is the consequence of the physiological shifts we have made in the
face of so much ultraformulated food. Similarly, cue-induced cravings and
negative mood are known to trigger relapse in other addictions, such as

smoking. In the case of smoking, pronounced spikes in negative mood, rather than more gradual daily ups and downs, seem to trigger relapse. It may come as no surprise then that weight regain often occurs after significant life events. Dr. George Koob cites the work of the addictionologist Dr. Alan Marlatt when discussing weight regain. "Marlatt argued years ago, and it's been confirmed within the alcohol field, that most relapse is triggered by unease, by dysphoria, by negative emotional states," he says. "And that's what the term 'hyperkatifeia' is supposed to represent. Dopamine has a key role in that because a dopamine deficit can drive that. It's that negative emotional state that has the most powerful effect. And it's the cues that then facilitate the actual engagement."

Relatedly, in an earlier conversation, Dr. Sami Schiff made an important observation about what happens when people attempt to lose weight. There are, he said, alternating periods where people don't pay attention to their food-related behaviors and times where they renew their motivation to lose weight. This cycling can lead to low self-esteem, depressive symptoms, and feeling unable to reach the goal of losing weight and maintaining a healthy lifestyle. Without explicitly saying it, Dr. Schiff had perfectly described the essence of relapse.

7

· · · ·

Body Positivity, Health Positivity

"I invite you to explore what your life would look like without body neg-
ativity and objectification. What would the freedom from body worry
feel like for you?" writes Evelyn Tribole, MS, RDN, who, along with Elyse
Resch, is cofounder of Intuitive Eating and champion of the body positivity
movement. "What new changes could take place in your life?"

Over the last decade, the body positivity movement—the origins of
which can be traced back to both the fat acceptance movement that began
in the 1960s and the fat positivity movement—has gained new traction on
social media with a proliferation of posts tagged with #bodypositive and
#bodypositivity, meant to subvert the inappropriate and dangerous expec-
tations of bodies as portrayed in social media and advertising. The idea
behind these hashtags is to create a space where people of any size can feel
at home in their bodies and accepted by a supportive and nonjudgmental
community. It has recently given rise to a heated debate about who belongs
in such a space.

The question within the controversy centers on who is authentically accepting their body; this has been fueled in part by the recent rise of anti-
obesity medications. The advent of these drugs has been like a lightning
bolt striking the landscape of this movement, sharply dividing its population into two groups: those who take them and those who don't. Some
celebrities and influencers who've struggled with weight have become suddenly lithe, leaving many of their followers feeling abandoned; others in the
body positivity movement feel an old shame being resurrected by friends

and colleagues who are now shedding weight quickly. And then there's the question of diet raised anew, haunting those of us who are conscious of our weight, of how to maintain a sense of pleasure or, at the very least, a little peace when we eat.

That last challenge beats at the heart of the intuitive eating movement.

Tribole and Resch, both dietitian-nutritionists, created the practice of intuitive eating to take the focus off diets and weight loss and encourage instead listening to one's own internal cues, such as hunger and fullness. This practice offers ten principles—such as "Reject Diet Culture," "Feel Your Fullness," and "Cope with Your Emotions with Kindness"—to help people make choices guided by this innate knowledge. "Think about what steps you can take to begin respecting your here-and-now body," Tribole advises. "I suggest getting rid of the scale."

Clearly, accepting and embracing your body shape is a worthy goal. The body positivity movement has offered meaningful gains toward destigmatizing body size and prompting us, as a culture, to rethink how we understand and talk about weight and well-being. I wholeheartedly agree with Tribole that diets are ineffective in the long run, that the deprivation from dieting can increase the risk of developing eating disorders, and that health should be the focus of any weight-loss program.

But our views diverged when I pointed out to her that randomized controlled trials show that losing adipose fat reduces serious cardiovascular disease. When I asked how we accomplish this without losing weight, she pointed out that there is a growing body of research that shows that yo-yo dieting is harmful. In fact, there are studies that both support and do not support the harms that can arise from yo-yo dieting.

"You are making a huge assumption, *if* you get weight off and keep it off," she added. "There is a huge body of research showing it's been an utter failure."

Ultimately, Tribole believes that for the vast majority, weight is not modifiable.

"Isn't that a bit like throwing in the towel?" I asked her, pushing back, perhaps a bit strongly.

Tribole pushed right back. "If we looked at the association of being male and heart disease," she said, "it would be like saying we should castrate all the men so there'd be no more heart disease. It's the way we look at it."

For decades, those who cared for eating disorder patients, including those with binge eating disorders, anorexia, and bulimia, have adopted the core tenet that dieting can contribute to eating disorders. And most reject the notion of food addiction for fear that it might endorse abstinence, which loops right back into one of the drivers of disordered eating. Some experts don't support the idea of food addiction, ironically, because it shifts responsibility away from the person. "It's an interesting way of moving the focus of blame from the individual to the food," said University of Leeds professor Dr. Andrew Hill. The essence of Tribole's concern, however, is that addiction is often accentuated by dieting and restricted eating. "Food restricted rats show problems with this loss of control," she pointed out. While craving ultraformulated foods and stimulation of the dopamine circuits *can* occur in a sated sate, she is right that signs of addiction appear more readily when you limit access to the addictive substance. Indeed, this is covered by one of the ten Intuitive Eating principles: Make Peace with Food. "If you tell yourself that you can't or shouldn't have a particular food," the dietitian-nutritionists explain on their website, "it can lead to intense feelings of deprivation that build into uncontrollable cravings and, often, bingeing." Tribole argues that we should not engage in dieting or restricting foods, and if this is what is necessary for weight loss, let's not engage in weight loss.

"Reducing weight is not something you would support?" I asked her.

"No, it's not," she replied. "From a weight stigma standpoint, even the concept of intuitive eating, it's about cultivating a healthy relationship with your body—it's not about changing the body. And one of three things can happen with intuitive eating: your weight can stay the same, weight can go up, or weight can go down."

The origin of the theory that dieting is responsible for overeating and can give rise to eating disorders dates to the 1970s. The late Columbia professor of psychology Stanley Schachter theorized that nonobese individuals responded more to "internal" body cues—hunger and satiety levels—while individuals with obesity responded more to external cues, including the type of food and the time of day. Underlying this theory was the thought that the hypothalamus—the part of the brain that controls the homeostatic system—functioned differently in people with obesity.

Another observation at the time was social psychologist Richard Nisbett's finding that people who were overweight tended to eat either very large or very small amounts of food, suggesting they engaged in two extremes of eating, either highly restrained or excessive. This led Peter Herman and Deborah Mack, Northwestern University psychologists, to hypothesize that the cultural pressures of dieting resulted in "restrained eating," which meant that when presented with ultraformulated food, people would overeat, causing weight gain. The theories grew more complex over time, but the upshot was that dieting and restrained eating would cause paradoxical *increases* in eating—periods of "disinhibition" or "loss of control"—that would give rise to weight gain. According to these researchers, the culprit was not ultraformulated food but rather the restraint of dieting. Subsequently, many studies of "restrained" and "unrestrained" eating patterns were conducted, resulting in a proliferation of research and theories that repetitive dieting, or weight cycling, had psychological and metabolically detrimental effects.

Although early cross-sectional studies suggested a correlation between dietary restraint and either overeating or eating disorders, other research raised more questions. These studies investigated whether restrained eating caused overeating or the other way around. A variety of randomized controlled trials were conducted to try to sort this chicken or the egg problem. The most definitive one, called CALERIE (Comprehensive Assessment of Long-term Effects of Reducing Intake of Energy), compared a group of diet-induced, calorie-restricted, restrained nonobese eaters versus a control group, and it did *not* show an increase of binge eating, overeating, or the development of eating disorders in the restrained group.

In 2023, University of Michigan's Drs. Julia Rios and Ashley Gearhardt, attempting to sort out the pathways between restraint and, more specifically, food addiction, studied adolescents and demonstrated that "food addiction significantly predicted future dietary restraint," but not vice versa. That is, "dietary restraint did *not* significantly predict future food addiction."

And yet none of these findings mean that deprivation, food restriction, and body weight loss *don't* play a role in overeating and eating disorders. I think, more importantly, what the research reveals is that the constant accessibility of and exposure to ultraformulated foods sensitizes our addictive circuits. There is evidence too that food restriction and weight loss can *enhance* reward sensitivity and response to rewards. We know, for instance, that food deprivation can increase the reward value of drugs such as cocaine and amphetamines, and deprivation, in general, boosts sensitivity to rewarding substances. Certainly, deprivation of rewarding substances leads to withdrawal and helps perpetuate the cycle of addiction.

Of course dieting is going to induce cravings, and attempts to manage those cravings result in disordered eating. Tribole is right: Deprivation and dieting can trigger overeating. But I believe that overeating behavior is driven by food addiction. I asked Dr. Kim Dennis to tell me how she viewed the differences between binge eating and food addiction. "Binge eating disorder has a lot of cognitive distortions and overvaluation of body shape and size to your self-worth. Many people with binge eating disorder will binge on a whole range of foods," she explained. "People with food addiction oftentimes don't have the eating disorder cognitions and don't have body image distortions and are able to identify certain foods or combinations that either always set them off, or there's a very high chance that they're going to be set off into an out of control eating episode." There are people in the food addiction world, she said, "who talk about different phenotypes of addiction. It's not always binge eating. It could look like grazing, where people are eating every twenty to thirty minutes throughout the day."

While eating disorders may involve many aspects of a person's mental health, it is the addictive circuits that wreak havoc on the mind and body. The fields of eating disorder treatment, obesity medicine, addiction, and endocrinology all grew from different traditions and schools of thought, and they have largely remained siloed from one another, which makes it difficult to identify the connections among them. But addiction to ultraformulated food is a through line for patients seeking treatment in all of these specialties.

Eating disorder professionals have traditionally focused on "impulsivity" and "emotional dysregulation" as being at the core of both eating disorders and obesity. They recognize that, as Dr. Ferdinand Fernández-Aranda, an eating disorders specialist, puts it, "Eating disorders and obesity share neurobiological and environmental vulnerabilities," and there is "evidence of alterations in [brain function] in individuals with obesity and binge diseases."

Additionally, the similarities between obesity and eating disorders are explainable by understanding the central role of the brain's addictive circuits. I asked Dr. Sami Schiff about the relationship between food addiction and eating disorders. He replied, "The mesolimbic dopaminergic system is involved in both eating disorders and obesity and is involved in many psychopathological conditions."

Understanding that the addictive brain circuits and metabolic signals sustain excess body fat, how should we reconceive of losing or resetting weight to improve health? We have to keep in mind that visceral adiposity is a real problem that causes cardiovascular disease and diabetes.

Sick Fat

If excess weight were a mere cosmetic issue, I would not care about obesity the way I do. If obesity caused only one complication, we could treat that condition. The problem is that obesity is the root cause for major cardiovascular and metabolic diseases; it increases the risk of stroke and thirteen different types of cancer; it contributes to nearly one in every five deaths among Americans between the ages of forty and eighty-five.

One of the complicated consequences of the current body positivity movement is that, in our attempt to right our cultural wrongs, we have also managed to obscure the health consequences of toxic fat, or what some experts refer to as "sick fat." Despite its medical urgency, weight remains one of the most challenging subjects to discuss. It is personal, highly sensitive, and can trigger feelings of shame, regret, and self-blame. It's also true that many people, including doctors, still unfairly view struggles with excess weight as a personal failing. These views stem from the misguided belief that weight is entirely under our control. The answer to this falsehood, however, is not to shut down, but rather to engage in the difficult conversations that will shine a light on the best path forward toward self-acceptance *and* long-term health. Two things can be true at once, of course: One can love their body at any size *and* be proactive about health concerns. The aim is to allow these ideas to peacefully coexist.

Perhaps we have also not yet been able to embrace this duality because both notions are relatively new—the resurgence of the body positivity movement has only occurred over the last decade, and the research showing that excess visceral adiposity is a cause of cardiovascular disease and diabetes is also relatively new.

In 1988, the late Dr. Gerald Reaven, an endocrinologist and professor emeritus in medicine at the Stanford University School of Medicine, as well as a pioneer of insulin resistance, introduced the idea of metabolic syndrome, a conglomeration of abnormalities—including high insulin levels, glucose intolerance, hypertension, and abnormal lipid levels—that increase the risk of cardiovascular disease and diabetes. Dr. Reaven did not include obesity as part of the syndrome because he had found people with obesity and increased fat mass who did not have the same metabolic abnormalities. And yet, at about the same time, a group of researchers at the University of Gothenburg, in Sweden, reported that the accumulation of abdominal or visceral fat was associated with metabolic disease. Thirty years earlier, the French physician Dr. Jean Vague had identified two different shapes of fat distribution: apple and pear. The apple shape, or what he called "android obesity," reflected a wider waist circumference. The pear shape, or "gynoid obesity," reflected increased fat in the legs and gluteal muscles. What Dr. Reaven initially missed was that it was the visceral abdominal fat, or apple shape, that was associated with the constellation of cardiovascular disease and diabetes. Dr. Jean-Pierre Després at the Université Laval, in Québec City, built on the work of the Swedish group, noting that it was specifically the visceral fat, not total fat mass, that posed the metabolic danger.

In its simplest form, when someone ingests excess calories, that energy gets stored in adipose tissue. There is a limit to how many excess calories, or fat, these adipose tissues can hold before they start spilling out as free fatty acids. In the ideal situation, the liver holds excess energy and releases it when other organs need it, such as during exercise or an overnight fast. But as Dr. Anthony Ferrante of Columbia University Medical Center says, "We know that efficiency is in fact not true, no biological system is." When these sites can't hold any more fat, the fatty acids overflow; these are precursors for the increased fat that gets deposited in various non-fat organs, including the liver, brain, pancreas, and arteries, disrupting the workings of those organs, and possibly increasing immune cell activity and inflammation. Fat in the liver has become the largest driver of chronic liver disease; so-called "silent liver" disease, caused by obesity, has become the second most common reason for liver transplantation due to liver inflammation, fibrosis, cirrhosis, and failure. The fat that gets stored in the liver also ends up in the circulation as triglycerides, high levels of which increase the risk of heart disease and stroke. Fat that collects in the pancreas affects how its beta cells make insulin. According to work by diabetologist Dr. Roy Taylor, type 2 diabetes is, in its simplest terms, more fat inside the liver and pancreas than those organs can handle.

Lose 15% of total body fat and pancreas function returns. In fact, there is a linear relationship between the amount of weight lost and diabetes remission rate. Remission increases around 5% for every 1% of total body weight loss early in the disease.

The same mechanism is at work when fat infiltrates cardiac cells. Systemically, fat cells produce hormones that, in excess amounts, contribute to arthritis, cancer, blood clots, type 2 diabetes, hypertension, increased blood lipids, atherosclerotic heart disease, and stroke. These hormones contribute to inflammation that affects local immune cell activity. The damage is not just from its body-wide metabolic effects; it can also occur because of its location, mass, and mechanical forces. Fat around the neck causes sleep apnea. Weight on joints can cause osteoarthritis. Fat around the heart affects its function and puts stress on it, causing it to work harder. Fat around the kidneys affects blood pressure. Excess fat has a role in at least two hundred other diseases.

"As you carry more weight, you carry more fluid and that affects your pumps and excess nutrients that get into cells and damage them," says Dr. Naveed Sattar, a professor of metabolic medicine at the University of Glasgow. "One of the strongest influences between obesity and COVID-19 was thrombosis [a blood clot], because when you carry too much weight you are making too many clotting factors."

Hemodynamics (the dynamics of blood flow), cellular nutrition, and inflammation, or a combination of these things are all at play when it comes to kidney disease and heart failure. "What the relative weightings of those things are, I don't think we understand," says Dr. Sattar.

There is also research that attempts to put a finer point on these findings. Dr. Katherine Flegal, an epidemiologist and senior scientist at CDC for many years, showed that when all-cause mortality—meaning death from any cause—is examined, significant obesity carries significant health risks, but the same is not true for those in the overweight category. Her study also showed, however, that grade 1 obesity, classified by a BMI, or body mass index, of 30 to not more than 35, was *not* statistically linked with higher mortality, and overweight was also correlated with lower all-cause mortality. Some of my colleagues challenged these findings because they did not exclude participants with chronic or preexisting disease at baseline, or people who smoked. I myself am not persuaded by studies that measure what is called all-cause mortality, which includes any cause of death, be it a car crash or lightning, as opposed to specifically from non-weight-related conditions, because such a broad category adds too much noise to the analysis. And subsequent meta-analyses by the Global BMI Mortality Collaboration, a study of the correlation between BMI and all-cause mortality, showed the opposite of Dr. Flegal's results. They found that across overweight and obese BMI categories, all-cause mortality is increased. This result has been confirmed across multiple continents.

Here, then, are some meaningful statistics about the relationship between weight—admittedly, visceral fat studies would be better—and specific health conditions. For every five units above a BMI of 25, there is a

29% increase in cardiovascular disease. There is a fivefold risk of developing type 2 diabetes for every BMI unit above 25. Thirteen types of cancer have between a 1.1- and 7.1-fold increased risk with obesity. A man with a BMI greater than 40 gets 9 years shaved off his life; 7.7 years are lost for females. The following chart shows additional conditions and their increased risk.

Heart Failure	Each unit increment in BMI above normal increases the risk by **5%**.
Sudden Cardiac Death	A five-unit increase in BMI correlates with a **16%** increase in risk.
Atrial Fibrillation	A five-unit increase in BMI also results in a **29%** increase in the risk.
Dilated Cardiomyopathy	A BMI of 40 in young women is associated with a **sixteen-fold** increase.
Hypertension	The risk increases by **2.0 to 3.7-fold**.
Coronary Artery Disease	There is a **twofold increase** in the risk.
Stroke	The risk increases by **1.4 to 2.7-fold**.
Peripheral Artery Disease	The risk increases by **1.2 to 4.8-fold**.
Childhood Obesity/ Diabetes	Children aged seven to early adulthood with obesity have a **threefold risk** of developing diabetes.
Adolescent Obesity/ Diabetes	Adolescents aged thirteen to early adulthood with obesity face a **fivefold risk** of developing diabetes.
Long-term risks	A seventeen-year-old with obesity, followed for ten years, **has double** the risk of dying from cardiovascular disease.
Respiratory and Inflammatory Diseases	There is a **twofold increase** in the risk of developing sarcoidosis, restricted lung disease, and pulmonary emboli. Additionally, the risk of asthma increases by **1.4 to 1.9-fold**.
Influenza Complications	There is a **1.7-fold risk**.
COVID-19 Complications	The risk of serious complications increases by **2.0 to 3.1-fold**.
Infections	There is a **2.0 to 4.3-fold** increase in hospital-acquired and postoperative infections.
Rheumatoid Arthritis	The risk of developing rheumatoid arthritis increases by **2.2-fold**.
Multiple Sclerosis	There is a **1.6-fold** increase in the risk.
Infertility	Elevated BMI is linked to a **1.3 to 2.7-fold** risk of infertility.

Indeed, the role that toxic fat plays in longevity is critical. Ten years ago, researchers identified several key characteristics of aging. These hallmarks encompass a range of biological phenomena, including mitochondrial dysfunction, stem cell exhaustion, genomic instability, and dysregulated nutrient sensing. But look around, and you will see that another noticeable change that comes with aging is the increase in abdominal fat among many elderly people, even those who had not previously struggled with weight. As Dr. Després has shown, visceral obesity is directly related to nutritional quality and physical activity. If we look at waist circumference, not BMI, we can see a link between waist size and longevity.

And yet the medical profession is just waking up to the extensive damage that excessive weight causes. For over four decades, diabetes expert Dr. Ralph DeFronzo focused on a triumvirate of three major defects as the causes of the disease: impaired insulin secretion, increased liver glucose production, and decreased muscle glucose uptake. Now he is more direct in saying that these effects are the result of excessive fat. "The epidemic of diabetes is secondary to the epidemic of obesity," he declares. "Obesity represents a state of tissue fat overload. Accumulation of fat within cells is toxic, incites inflammation, causes insulin resistance, and impairs insulin secretion." Toxic fat, or lipotoxicity, is, he says, at "the heart of what's driving the diabetes and cardiovascular epidemic."

Endocrinologist Dr. Harold Bays, medical director and president of the Louisville Metabolic and Atherosclerosis Research Center, uses the term "sick fat." Others call it "dysfunctional fat." No matter what you call it, the harm results from the release of reactive lipids that impair vital cell function. Chronic inflammation of adipose cells is increasingly seen as a component of metabolic disease. This is a marked shift from when the medical profession not long ago thought adipose tissue was simply a benign structure of connective tissue comprising adipocytes, or fat cells.

We are beginning to recognize toxic fat as a root cause of disease that needs to be treated early in life. "We have lots of people on statins and blood pressure medications. We have reduced smoking . . . but that means more people are living longer with obesity. Aggregated exposure to excess weight is going up and up, and therefore people are developing the second or third complications from obesity. We are facing an epidemic of people facing multiple conditions," says Dr. Sattar. "The average clinic in a hospital is full of people in their seventies and eighties on fifteen to twenty tablets with five or six conditions. High BMI is a major driver. It's a bloody mess. Treating chronic disease without tackling excess adiposity promotes multimorbidity." The medical profession needs to shift to a weight-centered approach to diabetes and cardiovascular and liver disease.

While evidence shows that obesity increases the risk of disease considerably, proving that weight loss decreases risk has been less straightforward. In one of the largest and longest medical trials following five thousand people with overweight or obesity and type 2 diabetes, weight loss averaging around 6% of body weight through reduced dietary intake and increased exercise was not shown to reduce cardiovascular events. On the other hand, greater weight loss after bariatric surgery has shown a 38% reduced incidence of heart attack, stroke, and cardiovascular death, and a 62% reduction in heart failure. There was a 24% reduction in cardiovascular events after weight loss from a new anti-obesity medication in people with type 2 diabetes and obesity. This shows cardiovascular risk can be reversed. And evidence shows that every 10% decrease in BMI decreases risk of heart failure by 21%; for every 10% decrease in waist circumference, there is a 32% lower risk of heart failure.

An even larger 2023 trial studied whether weight loss due to one of the new anti-obesity medications reduces cardiovascular events in nondiabetic obese and overweight patients. The outcome showed a dramatic 20% reduction in death from cardiovascular disease. These results are of great significance. Up until this study, cardiologists did not, as a group, overwhelmingly believe the causal link between obesity and cardiovascular disease. But now that the evidence is clear and we know, in addition, that the longer obesity is present, the greater the cardiovascular risk, it is imperative that we find a way to focus on weight as a root cause of disease.

This is true even for those who may not yet have any evidence of metabolic or cardiovascular complications. The degree to which body fat causes significant disease varies dramatically among individuals. People can be overweight and live to be one hundred. People can be lean and die at age forty. Many factors impact health and longevity, including genetics. One school of thought asserts that moderate overweight can be healthier, in certain instances, for some people. At any point in time, about 15 to 20% of patients with obesity do not have any evidence of metabolic or cardiovascular complications. There is no elevation of blood glucose, abnormal lipid profiles, hypertension, or evidence of cardiovascular disease. The percentage of men who have "metabolically healthy obesity" and no risk factors runs from 2 to 17%, while, for women, it ranges from 7 to 28%.

How do we make sense of these people who are obese but metabolically healthy?

The distribution of "sick fat" is the key to understanding its accompanying health risks. "If you store fat in the lower part of your body, that is relatively protective against cardiovascular disease and diabetes when BMI is the same as someone with abdominal obesity," says Dr. Gijs Goossens of Maastricht University Medical Centre in the Netherlands. A higher waist to hip ratio, a measurement of fat distribution, rather than BMI, *does* predict an increase in the risk of cardiovascular disease. Dr. Goossens also points out that some people with a high BMI (for example between 40 and 50) can have high insulin sensitivity, which dictates how well your body regulates blood sugar levels and is associated with a lower risk of diabetes. As Dr. Goossens puts it, "The outside does not tell everything."

Fat accumulates in the body through two different mechanisms. One is by increasing the number of fat cells. The other is by putting more fat into existing cells. The former is more common in childhood and adolescence, according to Dr. Goossens; the latter is more common in adulthood. "In people with obesity, these fat cells are already overloaded with dietary lipids, which means that dietary lipids will remain in the circulation at higher levels for prolonged periods of time after meal intake and that will cause an excessive flux into other tissues like the liver, the muscle, the pancreas, and the heart, as well as the visceral fat." (Dietary lipids, or fats, are those that are eaten.)

The critical finding is that people with obesity without hypertension, abnormal lipids, or diabetes have smaller fat cells or no enlarged fat cells, less toxic fat, less liver fat, less muscle fat, and, most importantly, lower amounts of visceral fat. And yet, according to Dr. Goossens, that only contributes to normal insulin sensitivity in approximately 10 to 20% of people with obesity with fairly normal metabolic health at a certain moment in time.

This is especially characteristic of premenopausal women, who tend to store fat in the subcutaneous tissue (located between the skin and muscles) in the lower body. "These premenopausal women have greater insulin sensitivity, lower fasting glucose, lower type 2 diabetes incidence, and a more protective lipid profile, which together contribute to less cardiometabolic disease risk," Dr. Goossens says.

However, he cautions that these metabolically healthy women are more likely to develop unhealthy obesity with increased cardiovascular risk when they go through menopause, as there seems to be a redistribution of lipids from the lower part of the body to the upper part. The lower body and subcutaneous depots can hold fat more easily without triggering inflammation. Over time, though, there is a shift in fat storage from these less risky locations to the body's midsection, where both inflammation and mechanical pressures of the increased fat mass have a more toxic effect on organs, including the kidney, heart, and pancreas.

The bottom line is that the more toxic fat a person has, the greater the risk of cardiovascular disease. In the famous Framingham Heart Study, a long-term, ongoing cardiovascular cohort study, metabolically healthy obese people had a greater risk for diabetes and hypertension than metabolically unhealthy lean individuals. In other words, it's the excess fat mass that causes metabolic and cardiovascular risks. Therefore, metabolically healthy obesity is likely to be a transition phase on the road to ill health. For many people who struggle with excess weight, it's only a matter of time before more serious disease sets in.

Part II

· · · · · ·

THE NEW
UNDERSTANDING
OF ENERGY
AND WEIGHT

8

· · · ·

The Journey

We know that ultraformulated foods trigger the addictive circuits of our brains, causing so many of us to struggle with our weight. And we know that excess visceral fat is an underlying condition for many deadly diseases. Given these realities, it is essential that we develop realistic strategies to help us manage weight. Successfully countering the addictive circuits, or our reward system in our brain—quieting the food noise— requires stimulating a feeling of fullness that will inhibit hunger. Therefore, any effective treatment requires both understanding what triggers reward and what triggers satiation.

One way to conceptualize the wide array of influences that drive food addiction and the actions we can take to offset them is to think of a seesaw balancing these opposing forces.

On one side are the forces that instigate eating by stimulating the brain's addictive circuits and increasing our responsiveness to cues that make us crave food. Here, of course, are the ultraformulated foods, with their super-normal combinations of fat and sugar, fat and salt, and carbs and salt, that are always within reach. Changes in blood glucose and insulin also play a role. Fatigue and lack of sleep, stress and depression, fasting and hunger, as well as medications that cause weight gain can also drive the reward circuits to increase the desire for and seeking of food. Crucially, these forces don't make us like food more; they make us *want* it more.

On the other side of the seesaw are the forces that can increase satiation and quiet the reward circuitry. These include the new GLP-1 (glucagon-like

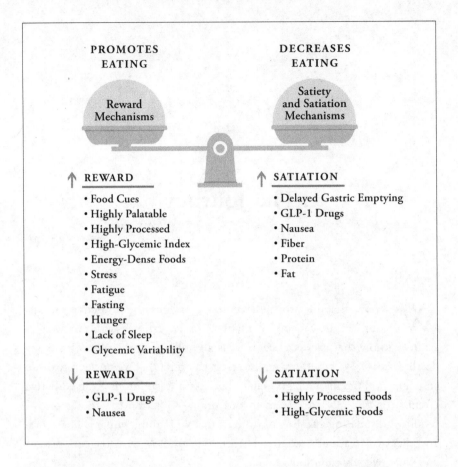

peptide-1) anti-obesity medications. These drugs work by decreasing gastric emptying time—the time it takes for food to move out of the stomach and into the small intestine—increasing nausea and dampening the brain's reward response. In other words: These anti-obesity drugs often make people feel too sick to eat. In addition to these powerful drugs, there are also specific foods and macronutrients that can increase satiation, or a feeling of fullness, by, among other things, stimulating the release of the endogenous gut hormone GLP-1. Not all of these forces are equal, of course. In the upcoming chapters, we will explore how certain brain mechanisms work in connection with weight, and the variety of ways in which we can tip the balance—straightening the seesaw—by diminishing reward sensitivity and increasing satiation.

Addiction is a chronic, often relapsing disease; the same is true of obesity and weight gain. Given this, weight loss is inevitably a winding journey.

There is no single solution; there is no turning the corner "for good." And because both addiction and obesity are influenced by a wide variety of biological, psychological, and social factors—from a person's weight to susceptibility to food reward to the environment each of us lives in—the journey is not only unpredictable, but unique for every one of us.

As I have shared, I'm intimately familiar with this experience, having been engaged in a battle with my weight since I was young. And yet, until recently, I never viewed my own difficulties as a lifelong journey, despite their familiar cycle: lose weight, get new clothes, believe I'd triumphed, gain the weight back again. Perhaps it was too daunting to think that I would always struggle. Life events would change my focus, redirect my vigilance, impose new roadblocks and barriers. But no tool or strategy was ever foolproof; nothing could guarantee there wouldn't be a relapse.

In early 2023, I left government service, two years to the day after I'd been asked to co-lead Operation Warp Speed for the Biden administration, responsible for all vaccines and drugs used during the COVID-19 pandemic. For two years, I'd been strapped to my desk for about eighteen hours a day, seven days a week. The long, hard-driving days had been worth it: We'd defanged the virus and gotten the country back to work. Through vaccines and infection, most of the population had acquired the immunity to be protected from becoming seriously ill from COVID. By and large, the country was in good shape. And yet, personally, all I could think about was that the circumference of my waist was as large as it had ever been. I'd gained forty pounds.

So I began my familiar trudge, this time taking the path in the opposite direction, back to my leaner self. In the past, I'd reliably been able to do this with a low-carb, high-protein diet as well as exercise. This time, however, after a few months of dieting, I'd only lost about six pounds, and I was growing impatient. At around the same time, I developed a kidney stone that landed me in the emergency room. This led to a referral to an endocrinologist for what, in the end, turned out to be a spurious lab result. I mentioned to this doctor that I was trying to lose weight, but it was going very slowly and I was frustrated. By chance, he told me that he was doing a clinical trial on some of the new weight-loss drugs I, too, had been studying. Was I interested in trying one of them, he asked. Under his direction, I injected myself right then and there in his office.

I was as surprised as anyone about this. For most of my career, from my medical school days in the 1970s to my time at the FDA in the 1990s and beyond, I doubted that there would ever be a highly effective drug for controlling weight. Eating is a complex biological activity deeply wired into the human nervous system, including the brain's learning, memory, motivation, addiction, energy, and executive control circuits. Any drug that reduces appetite would have to work on those circuits. It seemed unlikely to me that a drug could be targeted enough to be able to single out appetite without triggering serious adverse side effects. But the GLP-1 drugs are able to target appetite.

In my defense, history was very much on my side. People have been searching for drugs to reduce body weight at least since the time of the Greek physician Soranus of Ephesus, who lived in the second century CE. He recommended a treatment of laxative medicines, perhaps accompanied by massage and heat. The *Sushruta Samhita*, a founding text of India's Ayurvedic medicine that might be even older, identified obesity as a serious health problem and proposed combating it with enemas, massage, and pea flour. Jump forward nearly two millennia to the eighteenth century and the influential Scottish physician Malcolm Flemyng was still struggling to understand the physiology of obesity, and still recommending laxatives and diuretics as antidotes for patients.

The misses kept coming in modern times. The FDA has withdrawn more than two dozen other weight-loss drugs from the market because they were shown to trigger severe adverse events. Dinitrophenol was removed in the 1930s because it could lead to cataracts and nerve damage. Amphetamines were removed in the 1970s because of the risk of addiction. Fenfluramine (combined with phentermine and popularly known as fen-phen) was highly effective for weight loss but it was withdrawn in 1997 due to the dangers of cardiac valve disease and pulmonary hypertension. Phenylpropanolamine, sold as Dexedrine or Acutrim, was withdrawn in 2000 because it elevated the risk of stroke. Sibutramine was removed in 2010 because of risk of heart attack and stroke. In 2020, lorcaserin was withdrawn due to a slight increase in the risk of cancer.

In the mid-2000s, a colleague asked what I thought about rimonabant, a new drug marketed in Europe for weight loss. I was skeptical. Rimonabant is what's known as a CB1 antagonist: a chemical that switches off, or *antagonizes*, the brain circuits that respond to cannabis. When those CB1 circuits are stimulated by cannabis, the result is hunger and weight gain. This effect is probably why marijuana use is associated with "the munchies." Marijuana is not the only thing that triggers the CB1 circuits; the cannabis-response system has also been shown to be highly activated in obese individuals. Rimonabant inhibits those circuits. In clinical trials, the drug resulted in an 8% weight loss. I worried about what else the drug was doing, however.

I told my colleague that in the case of drugs that worked primarily on the brain it was only a matter of time before serious adverse side effects would appear. When the FDA refused to approve rimonabant in 2007 because early trials in Europe showed an increased risk of suicide, I looked prescient. I knew that it is hard for a drug to target weight loss without also hitting other essential brain functions, such as learning and memory. That is one reason why the FDA looks closely for risks of depression and suicide in weight-loss drugs that affect the brain.

Even the drugs currently approved for weight loss before the current GLP-1s came with significant drawbacks. Phentermine was cleared by the FDA in 1959, the first weight-loss drug to receive such approval, and until recently it was one of the most commonly prescribed weight-loss medications. It is currently approved for short-term use (up to three months), it is cheap, and it can produce weight loss in the range of 5 to 10% of body weight. Phentermine is far from ideal, however. The drug works by stimulating the sympathetic nervous system, which decreases hunger. In the process, phentermine also causes insomnia if taken late in the day, and it can lead to tremors, increased heart rate and blood pressure, restlessness, and a number of other adverse side effects.

Recognizing that phentermine tends to elevate a user's heart rate and blood pressure, FDA researchers worried that it could also increase the risk of cardiovascular disease. One retrospective study found no increased cardiac risk after two years of taking phentermine, and many obesity medicine specialists prescribe it. Still, concerns about the poorly understood long-term effects persist. Doctors are uneasy about potential liability and about running afoul of state regulations. Phentermine has never been subjected to thorough long-term randomized controlled trials, which means that there is no definitive evidence regarding the drug's side effects.

To increase the effectiveness of weight-loss drugs and to counterbalance side effects, pharmaceutical companies have developed combination drug therapies, again with limited effect. For instance, phentermine has been paired with topiramate, a drug used to treat seizure disorders. Topiramate can cause fetal harm, however, so women of childbearing age need to be sure they are not pregnant before or while taking the drug. It also causes kidney stones, among a host of other side effects, including increased heart rate, suicidal behavior, and mood and sleep disorders. On top of all that, topiramate may cause cognitive deficits in up to 40% of people taking the drug. At any rate, the combination of phentermine and topiramate results in an average 10.5% weight loss, but they are difficult drugs to take, and their risks have concerned me. The combination therapy is not available in Europe due to safety concerns.

Another combination therapy mixes two drugs to suppress the addictive nature of ultraformulated foods. Bupropion is used to help people stop smoking; naltrexone is used to treat opioid and alcohol addiction. Both drugs affect the reward center of the brain. In combination, they are sold under the name Contrave. The FDA has placed a special warning box on Contrave packaging to alert users about the possibility of suicidal thinking and behavior in children and adults. Other potential effects include nausea, vomiting, dizziness, insomnia, dry mouth, and diarrhea. Average weight loss is 5 to 6% of body weight.

Weight-loss drugs that target other systems in the body have their own poor track records. One of the most notorious examples is orlistat, initially approved in the 1990s, which inhibits the absorption of fat. It blocks an enzyme that breaks down fat, so that around 30% of fat that a person eats is not absorbed by the body. The drug was widely promoted and received considerable media attention, especially after it was approved for over-the-counter purchase in 2007.

Orlistat works mainly within the gastrointestinal tract, commonly leading to unpleasant, oily stools. A weight-loss drug that causes significant diarrhea, anal leakage, flatulence, and deficiencies in fat-soluble vitamins never made sense to me. At least those side effects would certainly help condition people taking the drug not to eat a diet high in fat. There have also been reports that the drug can lead to pancreatitis and severe liver injury. Orlistat is still on the market, but it is not widely used.

Even beyond their unpleasant or dangerous side effects, all of the anti-obesity drugs on the market before the GLP-1s were meant to be used only in conjunction with behavioral modification; they were not standalone solutions for weight loss. Yet, we know from extensive research and personal experience that behavioral modification is hard to stick with and is not very effective. By design, diets put the dieter in a state of caloric deficit—the body expending more energy than it is taking in—which triggers symptoms of deprivation.

The job of any anti-obesity medication is to help induce caloric deficit while minimizing the hunger associated with deprivation, without causing significant side effects. Unfortunately, all the anti-obesity weight-loss medications prior to GLP-1s were simply not very good at their job.

The secret to a successful anti-obesity drug, researchers finally recognize, is targeting the gastrointestinal hormones. That approach can tip the equilibrium seesaw between reward and satiety, the yin-yang biological states that control the amount and types of food we eat. By directly influencing reward and satiety, GLP-1 drugs can enable users to drastically reduce their caloric intake while largely sidestepping the feelings of deprivation. In short, GLP-1s come close to the anti-obesity drug that I didn't expect I would ever see.

Like many seemingly sudden breakthroughs, GLP-1 drugs are actually the result of decades of scientific work, replete with setbacks, detours, and failures. That story extends back at least to 1982, when Dr. Joel Habener at Harvard Medical School discovered a gene in anglerfish that codes for proglucagon, a protein that helps raise levels of sugar and fatty acids in the bloodstream, and for other small molecules called peptides. Proglucagon-like molecules perform similar functions in other animals, including humans, so this work offered a glimpse into a whole world of biology. Canadian endocrinologist Dr. Daniel Drucker explored the regulation of the proglucagon gene to learn more about how it operates. Different tissues carrying that gene can produce different peptides, he found. The pancreas produced glucagon, whereas the gastrointestinal tract produced what scientists called "glucagon-like peptides," dubbed GLP-1 and GLP-2. Although GLP-1 molecules are produced naturally in the brain and the lower intestine, Dr. Drucker and his colleagues discovered that the molecules could also be chemically synthesized and injected into an organism to artificially manipulate its blood sugar levels.

In 1996, a number of researchers discovered GLP-1 receptors throughout the brain and in other organs: the lungs, heart, pancreas, kidneys, and the gastrointestinal tract, including the stomach. Further studies showed that GLP-1 stimulates insulin production in the pancreas when glucose concentrations are high. At this point, GLP-1 started to look promising as a treatment for diabetes.

Dr. Jeffrey Flier, another professor at Harvard Medical School, teamed up with Dr. Habener and the Massachusetts General Hospital (which owned the patent for the pharmaceutical form of GLP-1) and with Pfizer's research team in Groton, Connecticut, to explore this possibility. The collaborators began GLP-1 infusions on test subjects with type 2 diabetes. The GLP-1 infusions successfully enhanced insulin secretion and lowered glucose levels, but with a half-life of just a few minutes, the drug broke down quickly in the body, which rendered it impractical for medical use. Pfizer pulled its support for the program. As Dr. Flier told me, the company believed "there would never be another insulin." For a moment, it seemed that GLP-1 research had hit a dead end.

The idea of using GLP-1s to treat obesity was almost an afterthought compared to the strategy of pursuing it for its insulin-enhancing effects. Dr. Stephen Woods at the University of Cincinnati demonstrated that brain injections of a GLP-1 agonist in lab animals significantly affected their feeding behavior, but other researchers doubted the importance of his result. "We all know that there are hundreds of peptides and chemicals and biologically reactive species that, when administered into the brain of a mouse or a rat, can inhibit food intake. A lot of them produce aversive responses: The animal is not well," Dr. Drucker says. "In fact, when you give GLP-1 into an animal in my lab, depending on how much GLP-1 you give, the animal might not move for hours. It can't even walk over to the part of the cage that has the food because it's so unwell. I was quite skeptical that this had any real clinical relevance, and I was wrong."

Around the same time, "an internal research group was working with a rat model that had a tumor that produced a lot of GLP-1, and these rats starved themselves. That kind of went into my motivation to say we should pursue [anti-obesity applications] for our molecules," said Dr. Lotte Bjerre Knudsen, who was studying GLP-1 compounds at the Danish pharmaceutical company Novo Nordisk. She had difficulty persuading her colleagues to pursue the compound, however. A GLP-1 mimic could not survive the digestive tract, so it had to be injected rather than given as a pill, and it did not readily get into the brain, so it seemingly could not produce a significant effect there.

Also in 1996, Drs. Mads Tang-Christensen and Philip Larsen confirmed that GLP-1 could reach areas of the brain that are not protected by the blood-brain barrier in laboratory animals, affecting how much water they drank. Then, in 1998, Dr. Arne Astrup and Dr. Jens Holst at the University of Copenhagen completed a randomized, placebo-controlled trial in humans showing that an infusion of GLP-1 drug promoted feelings of satiety and decreased food intake by 12%. "The key finding is that the day when [the test subjects] received the GLP-1 infusion, their satiety ratings were enhanced throughout the infusion," Dr. Astrup said. In 2002, Drs. Astrup and Holst further demonstrated a small but statistically significant reduction in body weight among human test subjects who had received doses of GLP-1. "We had two different observations showing that GLP-1 is not just enhancing satiety, but it's also translating into a reduction in food intake," said Dr. Astrup.

Finally, twenty years after Dr. Habener's discovery of the proglucagon gene, researchers had solid evidence that GLP-1 agonists could be useful as anti-obesity drugs. Even then, it took a lot of further development to transform GLP-1 drugs into a stable, safe, manageable drug. Developers working for the pharmaceutical industry had to chemically modify the molecule so it does not degrade in the body, lasting days instead of minutes, and increase the dose to levels that would amplify the effects of the naturally occurring GLP-1 molecules. They also had to find a way to reduce side effects, most notably nausea and vomiting. (Even GLP-1 drugs are not perfect.) New formulations of GLP-1 helped. So did a controlled regimen for users, starting at low doses and building up slowly as the body adjusts to the drug.

The payoff has been remarkable. People taking GLP-1 drugs can often lose 25% of their body mass, a significant improvement over most previous weight-loss drugs. Along with the reduction in body mass comes a variety of health benefits from GLP-1s: reduced risk of heart disease, kidney disease, and fatty liver disease; lower blood pressure; reduced severity of lipid disorders; and reduced risk of type 2 diabetes and perhaps diabetes-related nephropathy.

At my first Obesity Medicine Association meeting after the height of the COVID-19 pandemic, doctors were giddy about the effectiveness of the new anti-obesity medications. They were witnessing profound degrees of weight loss accompanied by notable improvements in the traditional markers of health. "What I'm trying to get across, at least from my perspective as an endocrinologist and clinical researcher: It's an entirely different age. It's light-years from where we have been," said Dr. Harold Bays, the Obesity Medicine Association's chief science officer. And then, in a burst of enthusiasm, he added: "Remember this day, tell your grandkids, 'I was at the Obesity Medicine Association back then.'"

A recent finding showed that 65% of patients in a clinical trial with the GLP-1 drug tirzepatide had lost greater than 20% of their body weight. Nearly a quarter of participants had lost more than 30% of their body weight. That is almost the same amount as with bariatric surgery. Only 3.7%

of the patients had lost less than 5%. How much weight could a high responder lose? "When you look at the data from the SURMOUNT-1 clinical trial, the highest responder to tirzepatide lost 56% of body weight," says Dr. Jesse Richards from the University of Oklahoma Health Sciences Center. "Okay, that is one out of one thousand people. But even if your patient loses two-thirds of that, that is a radically life-changing amount." Compared to a 5 to 7% weight loss with lifestyle interventions, which include both intensive behavioral treatment and dieting, 56.6% of patients on tirzepatide lost 25% of their weight.

It was a stunning turn of events. I imagined people *excited* to get on the scale because their weight was dropping so quickly. I imagined people walking over to a well-stocked refrigerator, as I have done at least fifty thousand times before, pulling open the door, looking inside, and, instead of mindlessly grabbing something to eat, saying, "Eh, I don't want anything." I imagined *that* becoming the norm someday in the near future.

For a former skeptic like me, the new GLP-1 drugs are an important development in taming obesity and navigating a healthier path through our modern landscape of ultraformulated foods. The drugs have become a cultural phenomenon as well as a medical one. Sales of GLP-1 drugs are expected to be over $40 billion annually by the end of 2024. According to a recent poll, roughly one in eight Americans now says they have tried one of the new GLP-1 drugs.

With the advent of anti-obesity drugs, for the first time in medical history we have the capability to specifically tamp down the addictive neural pathways, allowing us to significantly reset our body weight. It's not simple or easy, nor can it be done overnight. Still, a lower weight is now eminently more achievable with the appropriate medical support and the right tools. The drugs are not for everyone, and they are not without substantial risks. In part, this is because they work only while they are being taken; there's no known method for stopping them without weight gain. Their efficacy is also highly variable and individual. People lose different amounts of weight; some don't lose weight; some have even *gained* weight taking GLP-1s. These drugs make food almost irrelevant for some people. There are known and unknown side effects. The fact that the anti-obesity medications are considered "forever drugs," that people are meant to take for the rest of their lives, is particularly concerning given that we may not yet know all the longer-term adverse health consequences. But there are also significant physical and mental health benefits for many of us.

As I came to learn, losing weight, and maintaining weight loss, is still a complex journey. While the anti-obesity drugs offer a powerful wind at our backs, pushing us in the right direction and making the way easier than it was just a few years ago, we still must address food addiction, in a variety of ways. Anti-obesity drugs are the shiny new tool, but the other tools have been there all along: diet, exercise, and behavioral therapies. The difference now, however, is that, in this new era of food addiction and with the rise of anti-obesity medications, these tools are no longer useful in the same ways.

"The self-control theory which undergirds the treatment of obesity has outlived its usefulness as the change agent in behavioral treatment," Professor Michael Lowe, a psychologist who has studied behavioral treatment for obesity for forty years, declared during a webinar hosted by the United Kingdom's Association for the Study of Obesity in 2021. For decades, Dr. Lowe was a consultant to WeightWatchers International, whose program, at its core, relies on behavioral changes. But here he was indirectly admitting that these and other programs were no longer adequate to deal with the rising incidence of obesity.

Dr. Steven Nissen, professor of medicine at the Cleveland Clinic, is even more direct about the long-term ineffectiveness of counseling patients about diet and exercise. The NIH-funded 2013 Look AHEAD clinical study was the longest and largest randomized controlled trial of lifestyle interventions of diet and exercise on cardiovascular health. According to Dr. Nissen, the results were "an unmitigated disaster."

The NIH spent $100 million. "They had coaches. They decreased caloric intake and increased physical activity," says Dr. Nissen. "They followed [people] for a maximum of 13.5 years, a median of 9.6 years. They followed them for cardiovascular death, nonfatal myocardial infarctions, nonfatal stroke, or hospitalization for angina. It did not work. The intervention produced no benefit."

It's true, few diets or other weight-loss interventions work in the long run. We know that people have a hard time maintaining nutrition-based or behavior-based diets. People lose patience or they persevere, but they still don't lose enough weight or, as Evelyn Tribole and Elyse Resch address with their Intuitive Eating program, they feel dieting creates an unhealthy, antagonistic relationship with one's own body. We need to view these options differently. People still need to pay attention to proper nutrition. They still need to be able to regulate their behavior. And none of these techniques, not even the anti-obesity medications, work for all people at all times. Realistically, then,

the journey requires choosing what is best for you among these choices—
drugs, nutrition, physical activity, and behavioral therapy—and understanding how to combine them or switch emphasis if one approach begins
to wane in its effectiveness. Because while each of these methods individually may not work forever on their own, they are important parts of a
collaborative system.

It will always take a certain amount of diligence to walk the beam of
healthy weight, but if you understand the neural and biological forces at
work, as well as the most productive ways to address weight loss in this new
landscape, it *is* possible to keep your balance throughout.

9

· · · ·

The Biological Forces That Oppose
Weight Loss

In addition to addiction, there are certain operating principles about body weight that need to be understood to grasp why it is so difficult to lose toxic fat. Part of what makes it so hard is that we are not only treating an addiction, but we are doing so while also dealing with the complex physiology of weight. All diets, drugs, and surgery work by creating an energy deficit. If I eat less and exercise more, that can create an energy deficit. For instance, if I consume 1,000 calories a day but I burn 1,700 calories a day, I expect to lose weight. But the crucial truth is it's not as simple as just creating an energy deficit. Because when the body senses an energy deficit, the homeostatic system increases appetite and decreases the amount of energy the body burns. At a certain point, our bodies are designed to fight *against* weight loss. And yet no one ever says that. The mantra is simply: eat less, exercise more. Nobody ever offers the more accurate axiom: eat less, exercise more, and your body's counterregulatory systems will work against your efforts.

It follows then that if I continue to eat fewer calories than I burn, my weight will eventually plateau; the body becomes a smaller furnace and burns fewer calories. Put simply, as I eat less, my body will burn less. "Basically what we have is a pair of negative feedback loops such that changes in body weight give rise to compensatory changes in calorie expenditure and appetite that *resist* changes in body weight," Dr. Kevin Hall of the NIH explains. "It's almost like the system is trying to maintain whatever the baseline body weight is before you intervene."

Dr. Hall's research lab—where he also studied how environment influences people's eating habits—has built mathematical models to quantify the strength of these feedback loops. He has shown that for every kilogram of body weight loss, our bodies, on average, decrease the amount we burn by 25 calories a day. So, for instance, if a person loses 22 pounds, they will burn 250 fewer calories daily than they burned before that weight loss. And the feedback loop that controls appetite is even stronger. For every kilogram of body weight loss, appetite increases by 95 extra calories per day. As Hall sums it up: "That is a huge feedback control that is resisting maintaining those lifestyle interventions."

This harkens back to Dr. Rosenbaum's seminal study, in which patients with obesity lost between 10 and 50% of their weight and, as a result, slowed their metabolism, reducing their energy expenditure by 300 to 400 calories a day. At the same time, their appetites increased.

The combination of reduced metabolism and increased hunger makes it very easy to regain weight. Consequently, treating the counterregulatory forces—the homeostatic system, our addictive circuitry, and an increase in appetite hormones as well as a decrease in satiety hormones—is our only hope to support sustained weight loss. The telltale signs of these forces winning out include excess hunger and decreased fullness. Any approach to weight loss that does not reduce those two key symptoms will not be effective in the long run. As Dr. Carel le Roux has said, you can always tell if a treatment will be successful if the person who is losing or has lost weight says, "I don't feel hungry, I feel fuller, and I am not thinking about food all the time." In addition to a reduced appetite and increased fullness, a shift in food preferences, including a desire for smaller portions and fewer high-fat, high-sugar foods, benefits weight-loss efforts.

Therefore, to unlock weight loss and sustain it, we must affect not only the addictive circuits, but also the body's underlying energy biology.

What It Takes to Achieve and Sustain Weight Loss

The number of calories that can be consumed daily to lose a significant amount of weight—meaning 10% or more of body weight—is the same across the board, whether a person is using diets, drugs, or surgery. While there's a great deal of individual variability, and it depends on energy expenditure, people can generally achieve that degree of weight loss by consuming around 1,000 calories a day, with a range of 500 to 1,500 calories a day. Those numbers aren't surprising. What *is* surprising, however, is that, according to research done by Dr. Thomas Wadden, the inaugural Albert J. Stunkard Professor of Psychology in Psychiatry at the University of Pennsylvania, to successfully *maintain* weight loss, women must consume, on average, 1,550 calories, or somewhere between 1,200 and 1,800 calories per day. This number rises slightly for men, who must consume an average of 1,770 calories a day. These, too, apply whether the weight loss is due to diet, drugs, or surgery.

When I asked several scientists who work at or with the companies that make the new anti-obesity drugs how many calories people consume while losing weight on these medications, they agreed that, on average, it may be less than 1,000 calories a day. For people who'd reached a plateau after achieving their lowest weight, they estimated maintenance would require somewhere in the range of 1,500 calories a day. More specifically, they stated that people who'd successfully lost weight on anti-obesity drugs reduced their caloric intake by about 50% from their baseline while losing weight and by about 25% while maintaining their weight.

At the Columbia University Seminar on Appetitive Behavior, I asked Dr. Louis Aronne, professor of metabolic research at Weill Cornell Medical College, and one of the most skilled clinicians when it comes to the use of anti-obesity medications, "How many calories are people eating during weight loss, and how many calories are they eating to maintain it? What is the range of what they are consuming?" Citing other scientists' work, he estimated a reduction of about 1,000 calories during weight loss and about 400 calories during weight maintenance for people on anti-obesity drugs. For a female, that would translate to around a 1,000-calorie-a-day intake during weight loss and 1,600 calories during weight maintenance. Eat more than that and weight will return. When I pressed further, inquiring whether people could realistically sustain weight reduction for life, Dr. Aronne responded, "I don't know. We are going to find out."

Dr. Holly Wyatt, a leading clinician and expert in weight management at the University of Alabama at Birmingham, estimates that successful weight maintenance requires a reduction of between 300 and 500 calories daily. Of course, the less weight a person wants to lose, the less they need to reduce their intake.

The Body Weight Planner on the NIH website allows people to enter their height, weight, sex, and level of physical activity to receive an estimate of how much to reduce caloric intake, as well as how much to increase levels of physical activity to reach their goal weight. I entered the data for a five-foot-two-inch, fifty-year-old female who weighs 165 pounds and wants to reach a weight of 125, which would put her at a healthy BMI. According to the calculator, she could eat approximately 2,100 calories daily to maintain her 165 pounds. To reach her goal weight in 180 days, however, she would need to eat 1,051 calories. And, according to the NIH's calculations, once she reached her goal, she would need to eat 1,744 calories daily to maintain it.

A thousand calories a day is considered a low-calorie diet. Very low-calorie diets get down to between 600 and 800 calories a day. The key is that people usually only need to stay on these diets for three to six months. And, during that period, the active weight loss serves as positive reinforcement. By contrast, sustaining weight loss on 1,600 or 1,700 calories forever—without losing weight as an incentive—seems daunting.

In the face of both the addictive circuits and the energy circuits, it's no wonder people tend to gain back weight. What generally has not been said is that this level of long-term caloric reduction is often only achievable with help from medication or specific eating patterns.

10

. . . .

How to Determine Your Healthy
Weight Goal

Given that every weight-loss journey is unique, I wanted to pin down the specifics about my own physiological needs, as well as the latest findings on body mass index and what amount of weight loss actually decreases future risk of disease. To do this, I put myself forth as my own guinea pig, isolating in a sealed room and allowing clamps and tubes to be placed on me to ascertain my resting metabolic rate (RMR), the rate at which one's body burns calories at rest.

Metabolic Rate

A healthy metabolism should adjust to both an excess and a deficit in energy. For example, in one well-known study conducted in 1967—which would surely be considered unethical if it took place today—inmates in a Vermont prison were paid to overeat. They were all lean to begin with and then they consumed 8,000 calories a day. The prisoners gained weight, but not enough to account for all the extra calories they were eating. Instead, researchers observed that their metabolisms adjusted and burned off many of the excess calories as heat. As soon as the study ended and the prisoners were no longer paid to overeat, they went back to their old diet, and they lost whatever excess weight they had put on. Their metabolisms worked to keep their weight in a healthy range.

If you have ever tried unsuccessfully to lose weight, or lost weight only to regain it, these findings might seem surprising. That's because our biology doesn't treat weight gain and loss equally. In people with obesity, something happens to interfere with or dysregulate this homeostatic balance.

One way we measure metabolism is by testing for resting metabolic rate. Put simply, this is the number of calories the body burns in a day just to sustain itself. People with obesity who have lost drastic amounts of weight have marked drops in their RMR.

For example, researchers led by Darcy L. Johannsen of the Pennington Biomedical Research Center studied the contestants on the popular reality television show *The Biggest Loser*, which first aired in 2004. On the show, obese contestants agreed to eat a very restricted diet while engaging in a program of strenuous exercise—ninety minutes per day, six days per week. Under that regimen, most of the contestants experienced a dramatic reduction in weight. But the data also showed another more troubling reduction: Their resting metabolic rates decreased significantly, from an average of 2,600 calories a day to about 1,750. Yet going merely by the loss of lean tissue, which reduces calorie needs, the contestants should have had RMRs of around 2,280 calories a day, meaning that their metabolism had slowed by as much as an extra 500 calories a day. As a result, they would have had to eat 500 fewer calories just to maintain the same weight. Indeed, many of the show's contestants who lost enormous amounts of weight eventually gained much of it back.

I wanted to know my own resting metabolic rate. One method for assessing RMR is to measure the amount of heat the body generates. This is technically challenging but scientists and engineers have pioneered indirect ways to measure the amount of energy generated over different periods of time, from minutes to hours to days, and when the body is in different states—at rest, during exercise, while fasting, and fed.

Soon, I found myself sitting in a chair at Composition ID, a body composition establishment in Washington, DC. They measure body fat, lean mass, and bone mineral density, no prescription needed. I was told not to eat or exercise for eight hours before my appointment, and I'd followed these instructions. The test, called an "indirect calorimeter," measured my resting energy expenditure. The amount of heat I produced was calculated from the amount of oxygen I consumed and carbon dioxide I produced. I applied a nose clamp so no air would be lost through my nostrils and a tube was inserted into my mouth, with a mouth guard, to capture all gases I would exhale.

To my surprise, my RMR was only 1,152 calories. This was classified as "slow" compared to people of the same sex, age, height, and weight as me. I repeated the test several times to make certain that I had sealed my mouth around the mouth guard and that no gases had escaped from my nose. In addition to the 1,152 calories that made up my RMR, the test suggested that "lifestyle, exercise, and activity" generated another 462 calories a day, for a total energy output of 1,614. Sure, I can exercise more and increase that number, but as it was, what that measurement told me was that if I eat about 1,600 calories a day, my weight should be stable. If I eat more, I should gain weight; if I eat less, I should lose weight.

It was a blow: 1,614 calories are *not* a lot of calories. At the FDA, I'd been responsible for the modern food label, and we'd used an average of 2,000 calories for women in calculating daily nutrient food values. With a total energy expenditure of 1,614 calories a day, it was hard for me to see how I would not gain weight.

I went to New York City to have my energy expenditure measured by other methods by my friend and colleague Dr. Michael Rosenbaum, a professor of pediatrics, and Dr. Kathryn Whyte, both at Columbia University's medical school, which has one of the major obesity research centers in the world, the New York Nutrition and Obesity Research Center. There, they have constructed a tightly sealed room where they were able to measure all my respiratory gases. I was again instructed not to eat, drink, or exercise for eight hours and then to lie resting in bed in this sealed room for an hour, but not to fall asleep. After a while, there was a knock on the window of the room, stirring me from my non-compliant dozing. My colleagues had calculated that my resting metabolic rate was 1,270, a bit higher but still relatively low, even if you added to that the number of calories burned from exercise.

I tried a third method, which was a bit more complicated, called the "doubly labeled water" (DLW) method. Some scientists refer to it as the current gold standard for measuring energy expenditure. For this, I had to drink "non-radioactive isotopes" and collect urine samples that were sent off to a lab. The test calculated not my resting metabolic rate, but a total daily energy burn of 2,111 calories. The reason they found a number that was substantially higher is that my exercise level for that week had been particularly high.

According to Dr. Eric Ravussin of the Pennington Biomedical Research Center in Louisiana, several studies—but not all studies—have shown that a relatively low energy expenditure is a predictor of weight gain. In one of his most important studies, Dr. Ravussin showed that in the Pima, a Native American tribe currently living in Arizona and Mexico, those with the lowest energy expenditure levels among three groups studied also had the highest incidence of weight gain after four years. He believes this holds true in groups that have a predisposition to obesity. However, several factors make it difficult to sort out the specific role metabolic rate plays in this, including when the data are collected and at what point the patient is along their weight journey at the time of the study.

The equation seems straightforward: If I burn 2,111 calories a day, I can consume that same number of calories without gaining weight. By eating more than that amount, I will gain weight, and if I eat less than that amount, I will lose weight. So why is it so hard for me to control my weight? This is the question that many of us grapple with on a daily basis. Is it that most of us don't know how many calories we burn in a day, or how many calories we eat in a day, or even know how many calories we should be eating, or is it simply too difficult to keep the number of calories we consume within that limit?

The Truth About BMI

When it comes to health, it doesn't matter whether somebody is tall or short or big or small; what matters is how much visceral fat they are carrying. This is true for cardiometabolic disease, coronary disease, elevated blood lipids, and type 2 diabetes.

And yet, typically, BMI (body mass index) is the tool that is used in healthcare to measure total body mass relative to height. This is found by taking one's weight (in kilograms) and dividing it by the square of one's height (in meters). The resulting number places a person on a scale of classifications ranging from underweight to "normal" to overweight to obese. But, while BMI corrects for height, it doesn't differentiate between muscle and fat. This means that a professional athlete with a very high muscle mass and low body fat percentage may fall within the "obese" range of BMI, despite showing none of the health risks associated with obesity. BMI also provides no information whatsoever on the distribution of fat—as body composition measurements do—which is much more important than total body fat in understanding the risk of health complications. More specifically, numerous studies have shown that total body fat is a relatively poor predictor of cardiovascular complications, which are highly correlated with toxic fat. Ultimately, BMI is not a reliable tool in the clinical diagnosis and impact of obesity in individuals.

In fact, BMI was never meant to serve as a diagnostic or treatment cutoff for health. This measurement was first suggested by the Belgian polymath Adolphe Quetelet in 1832, in an attempt to use mathematics to explore the physical characteristics of humans. As part of this work, Quetelet sought to develop an equation representing the "average man." In an effort to apply a curve to a large set of data he'd collected on the height and weight of men at different ages, Quetelet determined that the relationship could best be approximated by the proportion of body weight in kilograms to the square of height in meters. Originally, then, this measurement was developed as an indicator of population-level trends, not for the diagnosis of individuals. It wasn't until 1972, however, when physiologist Ancel Keys suggested using this measurement in an analysis of his Seven Countries Study, that it was first referred to as "body mass index." Keys, recognizing the challenge of direct measurements of body fat, claimed incorrectly that Quetelet's formula was an effective index of relative body weight that accounted for both human build and the amount of fat in the body.

Even in the earliest work touching on BMI, it was evident that it was far from a perfect representation of all humans. For instance, Quetelet realized from the outset that the ratio between weight and height was variable in children and adolescents and therefore the equation, W/H^2, could only apply after both weight and height had stabilized in adulthood. Additionally, the data both Quetelet and Keys used was from a male-only population. Therefore, the ratio is most relevant to adult European men and is less accurate for other demographics, especially women, who generally have better cardiovascular health than men at higher body fat levels, particularly before menopause. "BMI, if we look at its origins, is quite racist," says Dr. Fatima Stanford, pointing to its derivation in white men and how it was used to stigmatize and discriminate. Dr. Katherine Flegal has traced how a BMI of 30 and above became the definition of obesity to a group of doctors in the late 1990s who were funded by the pharmaceutical industry.

Using waist-to-height ratio and body mass index together seems to be the best predictor of future risk from the major complications of obesity. (Simply put, waist circumference should be half or less than half one's height.) According to research by Dr. Luca Busetto, associate professor of internal medicine at the University of Padova, "Waist-to-height ratios were more strongly associated with lowering the risk of type 2 diabetes than BMI reductions. Only changes in the waist-to-height ratio were associated with reduced atherosclerotic coronary vascular disease, and only changes in BMI were associated with reduced hypertension and hip osteoarthritis risk." It's better to use both measurements together. A BMI of less than 27 and a waist-to-height ratio of less than 0.53 puts one in the low-risk group. Waist circumference on its own is not a bad measure, but to correct globally for various heights and weights, the waist-to-height ratio is optimal.

There *are* other methods, such as DEXA (dual-energy X-ray absorptiometry) and visceral adiposity scans, that can provide considerably more accurate information in this regard. When available directly to the consumer—as it is becoming increasingly so in many countries—DEXA is a good measure both of visceral fat and fat free mass. But currently, these technologies are expensive and difficult to access. Given that an easier, less expensive measurement is necessary for monitoring health on a regular basis, many experts endorse waist circumference or waist-to-height ratio as an alternative measure. Some also now recommend that the waist-to-height ratio be considered in conjunction with BMI.

No simple measurement, however, is a substitute for a thorough clinical assessment that focuses on all the cardiometabolic, physical, and mental conditions caused by excess visceral fat. Still, improving on the BMI will allow us to make strides toward the change we urgently need to make in medicine: focus on obesity first, rather than on its variety of resulting diseases.

Weight Loss to Combat Metabolic Disease

Another way to determine a healthy weight goal is to consider the research that has determined percentages of body weight loss that instigates positive physiological changes. "Progressive amounts of weight loss cause progressive benefits in metabolic health," says Dr. Samuel Klein, a professor at Washington University School of Medicine and expert on metabolic health. "When you lose 2 to 4% of your body weight, you reduce blood glucose concentration. When you lose 15% of your body weight, you get even lower glucose concentrations." Blood pressure, lipids, triglycerides, and cholesterol all follow the same trend, including improvements in insulin sensitivity.

When discussing how much weight loss a person should target, Dr. Klein says even 2 to 5% is impactful for someone who is relatively healthy. But for people who have type 2 diabetes, he adds, "You need a significant amount of weight loss to achieve remission." According to the United Kingdom's Diabetes Remission Clinical Trial, also known as DiRECT, which used medically supervised diet interventions, 86% of patients with diabetes achieved remission with 15% weight loss. "Fifteen percent weight loss is a pretty good target to get near maximal benefits for those who are obese with type 2 diabetes," Dr. Klein agrees. Data from surgical-weight-loss clinical trials show that there is increased benefit with up to 20% weight loss, but that benefit plateaus at 20%. And Dr. Klein emphasizes that only people with metabolic dysfunction will show these benefits.

For cardiovascular health, the most important recent clinical trial, the SELECT trial, demonstrates that an average weight loss of 8.5% with one of the newer anti-obesity medications for overweight and obese patients without diabetes who were at high risk for cardiovascular disease was associated with a 20% reduction in cardiovascular events. What is particularly noteworthy about these results is that reduction in cardiovascular events was associated with weight loss not only in people with obesity but also in high-risk overweight individuals with a BMI of less than 30. There was also a marked reduction in evidence of inflammation in both groups.

Given what we now know to be the limitations of BMI, is it possible to determine a broad optimal number? Research by Dr. Frank Hu at the Harvard T. H. Chan School of Public Health shows that beginning at a BMI of 20, there is a variety of increased health risks. "Epidemiological studies provide overwhelming evidence that above a BMI of 20–21," Dr. Hu writes, "a strong and linear association exists between BMI and the risk of developing type 2 diabetes, hypertension, cardiovascular disease, cholelithiasis [the presence of gallstones in the gallbladder], and other chronic diseases in both men and women." In contrast, other research suggests a target BMI of less than 27 and a waist-to-height ratio of less than 0.53.

While scales are problematic for many reasons, Professor David Levitsky from Cornell has shown that daily weighing is a highly effective tool for maintaining weight. Research shows that setting a goal weight does increase the likelihood of achieving clinically significant weight loss, although degree of engagement is even more key to achieving that.

When my doctor asked me about my weight-loss goal, and I proposed a BMI of 22 to 23, what I should have suggested instead was a weight at which my blood pressure, glucose, and lipid levels would all be within normal ranges. In some cases, as we've seen, it may not even be possible to achieve a specific goal, because weight loss levels off, or plateaus, at a certain point. And this is true across the board: Dietary intervention, medications, and surgery each plateau after varying periods of time and at different amounts of weight loss. The prime determinant is the degree to which each therapy shuts down appetite. Given that our own biological forces can counter our weight-loss efforts, increasing appetite and decreasing energy expenditure, it is critical to learn how to create satiety as a way of battling our addictive drive to eat.

11

· · · ·

Toxic Fat

Even the strongest advocates for specific weight-loss plans—for example, low-carb diets—recognize that a caloric deficit is essential to lose body weight. "It has always been about the calories," says Dr. Eric Westman, associate professor of medicine at Duke University and founder of the Duke Keto Medicine Clinic. "In our early studies, we found that people on a low-carb diet, even though we didn't tell them to restrict calories, were restricting calories. So, it became a low-calorie diet without talking about calories." Additionally, in a review of overfeeding studies—in which participants intentionally consume more calories than they need to maintain their weight—Dr. George Bray, an obesity researcher and professor emeritus at the Pennington Biomedical Research Center, found a close to 90% correlation between excess calories and weight.

And yet, calorie consumption isn't everything. Body composition analysis, which measures the mass of different parts of the body such as fat and bone and muscle to give a better sense of fat distribution throughout, offers a more complete picture of cardiometabolic health. As we know, higher amounts of visceral, or toxic, fat are associated with greater risk of disease. Indeed, having one pound or less of toxic fat is associated with less risk of cardiometabolic disease. It's important to consider, then, how to lose this fat to shift body composition for better overall health.

Toxic fat is more metabolically active than subcutaneous fat, which accumulates under the skin. Dr. Darcy Kahn of the University of Colorado spent five years studying changes associated with visceral fat that occur with excess weight gain. According to Dr. Kahn, with increasing obesity, visceral adipose tissue (VAT) becomes more inflamed due to the buildup of inflammatory cells, while anti-inflammatory cells decrease.

"As metabolic diseases develop," Dr. Kahn writes, "the composition of healthy adipose tissue changes significantly. Initially, it contains anti-inflammatory cells. However, with obesity and insulin resistance, there's an increase in endothelial cells [which act as a barrier between the bloodstream and surrounding tissues and play a role in inflammation] and a decrease in anti-inflammatory cells, replaced by proinflammatory cells. This shift leads to more inflammation and negatively affects insulin sensitivity."

Dr. Kahn and her colleagues took secretions from both subcutaneous and visceral adipose tissue in people with obesity. They demonstrated that the visceral adipose tissue released more inflammatory molecules and negatively affected insulin action. The molecules secreted by these cells also "disrupt insulin sensitivity, signaling, and glucose regulation in metabolic tissues."

Living with obesity means living in a state of chronic inflammation, a condition Harvard Medical School's Dr. Peter Libby has characterized as "a fire within." Inflammation affects many parts of the body, including the brain. Recent evidence demonstrates that inflammation impacts both the supporting cellular architecture and the number of neurons in the area of the brain's hypothalamus responsible for sending signals to reduce hunger. It is hypothesized that the inflammatory changes make neurons less responsive to the hormone signals responsible for satiety. In animal models, these changes start before the onset of obesity.

Furthermore, there is a direct causal link between ultraformulated foods and visceral fat. "What is needed to lose visceral adiposity or, more specifically, liver fat?" I asked Dr. Jeffrey Browning of the University of Texas Southwestern Medical Center. Visceral adiposity, as I mentioned, is the fat that is found deep within the abdominal walls, surrounding your stomach and other organs, whereas liver fat is fat buildup in only the liver. Metabolic-associated fatty liver disease affects about 25% of the US population.

By way of illustrating the effects of different diets on visceral fat, in particular the fat surrounding the liver, Dr. Browning explained the difference between eating bacon—a high-fat, low-carb food—and a piece of toast—a high-carb snack.

When a piece of bacon journeys through our body, he explains, it's absorbed through the intestines, packaged up into particles that go through the lymph system, entering the bloodstream, which means that your fat tissues get first dibs on the fat in those particles. And then whatever's left over ends up circulating back to the liver, repackaged as blood lipid particles, or very low density lipoprotein (VLDL), which is shipped back to the periphery to be reloaded back up into fat tissue, or wherever else the body wants to put them.

Put more simply, the fat of bacon, and dietary fat in general, contributes very little fat to the liver.

Dr. Browning adds, "Those on a low-carb (high-fat) diet are quite capable of reducing liver fat content despite an enormous increase in dietary fat intake." Essentially, caloric restriction will help a person lose weight, but a low-carb, high-fat diet will help a person clear out the liver fat, or the toxic fat.

But when you eat a piece of toast, he explains, "your body breaks the carbohydrates down into glucose."

In muscle, the glucose is broken down and used up as energy, Dr. Browning told me. In people with insulin resistance, however, things can get a bit off track. When there is too much of those breakdown products from glucose, instead of using them for energy, the body uses them for fat production. The body then adds more carbon molecules to those breakdown products, eventually forming fatty acids.

"If I'm overweight, insulin resistant, and constantly in an overfed state," I ask Dr. Browning, "what is the number one culprit causing liver fat?"

"I would say carbs are definitely a source of problems for the onset and maintenance of a fatty liver," he responds. "In healthy people, fat production ramps up immediately after a meal because of the insulin burst, and then it just shuts off and goes away. But in folks with fatty liver, it's up and it stays up and it really doesn't show any variation at all over time."

"Fats are not the primary culprit?" I ask.

"I think it's dietary glucose," he says.

Dr. Browning believes, therefore, that a low-carb diet is the most effective way to decrease visceral fat. "In my experience, altering macronutrient content (i.e., low-carb) has an immediate effect on liver fat/visceral fat that occurs over the first few weeks of the diet (50% reduction in liver fat at two weeks on low-carb versus 30% reduction on low-calorie). Both low-carb and low-calorie groups had a 5% reduction in weight," he tells me.

I asked him to explain the phenomenon of people experiencing similar weight loss but different reductions in liver fat. "It has to do with the size of the depot of fat in liver," he says. "The average liver weighs 1,500 grams. If the liver fat content to begin with is, say, 50%, then there is 750 grams of fat that can be theoretically reduced. A 50% reduction of this amount would be 375 grams and a 30% reduction would be 225 grams. This is only a difference of 150 grams and is tiny in comparison to a 5% reduction in total body weight." While reduction in liver fat is unlikely to cause a significant drop in overall weight, it will make an outsized contribution to metabolic health. In essence, the loss of toxic liver fat is relatively small in terms of overall weight, but enormously beneficial to your health.

And yet when I asked Dr. Browning if those with toxic fat or increased waistline and insulin resistance should be on a low-carb diet, his reply surprised me.

"The answer is no," he said. "I think people should choose the diet they are most likely to stick with. However, I think achieving ketosis"—a state in which your body burns fat, as opposed to glucose, for energy—"is critically important. This can be done to a lesser degree with calorie restriction (much lower level of ketosis but higher than those who are weight stable after an overnight fast). The other options are low-carb, timed feeding, or some form of intermittent fasting. I do not believe humans were designed to stay in a prandial or postprandial state their entire lives. This is not how we lived as a species on the plains of the Serengeti. There were times of feasting, fasting, and starvation."

Dr. Barbara Gower at the University of Alabama at Birmingham has shown that carbohydrate restriction without reducing calories improves pancreatic beta cell function (which makes insulin) and decreases liver fat independent of weight loss. Eating fewer carbohydrates, she explains, changes the effect of hormones on the liver. Specifically, insulin levels drop, and glucagon—also a pancreatic hormone that raises blood glucose—levels rise, whether you're fasting or have just eaten; these hormone changes significantly affect how the liver metabolizes glucose and fats. When insulin is high, the body focuses on making glucose and fat, which can lead to fatty liver and type 2 diabetes. However, when glucagon is high, the body uses some of its resources to make ketones instead of storing fat, which helps keep the liver healthy and free of fat.

Ultimately, the *kind* of fat you lose can make a crucial difference in overall health.

The Challenges of Toxic Fat in Menopause

Most women know all too well the changes that announce they're moving into menopause, including weight gain that occurs seemingly out of nowhere, even if they are eating and exercising exactly as they always have. But rarely are they told that this transition alters body composition and redistributes fat in ways that dramatically increase the risk of metabolic dysfunction and cardiovascular disease. In 2020, the American Heart Association recognized menopause as a risk factor for cardiovascular disease, independent of aging, and urged physicians to counsel patients on ways to counteract the damage of estrogen loss. The statement was significant, and some experts say overdue, given that all women experience menopause and can expect to live in this estrogen-depleted state for about thirty to forty years afterward.

The hormonal changes of menopause start during perimenopause, which can occur anytime between a woman's mid-thirties to her mid-fifties and continue for three to four years afterward, though the transition can be as short as a year or as long as a decade. Research has shown that 60 to 70% of women gain an average of 1.5 pounds per year from age fifty to sixty. But weight gain may be even more common than the data suggest, because some studies exclude women who have a healthy BMI and a healthy waistline when menopause begins, even though they, too, often gain weight in the years that follow. As the scale ticks up, health risks mount. One longitudinal study, for instance, found that an increase of eight to twenty pounds in women elevated the risk of cardiovascular disease by 27%.

Because menopause and aging coincide, the medical community has long debated which is responsible for the weight gain. Mayo Clinic endocrinologist Dr. Maria Daniela Hurtado Andrade believes "it has been well established that the main root cause for weight gain is age."

While estrogen regulates hunger hormones, and its decline intensifies hunger and food cravings, men experience the same effect as they lose testosterone, and they put on weight in midlife, too. As people age, metabolism slows, muscle mass decreases, fat mass increases, and we tend to become more sedentary and burn fewer calories.

What's different for women, however, are the physical, biochemical, and metabolic changes that menopause sets in motion. While menopause is a normal part of aging, these alterations can have serious health consequences, especially for women who are overweight or obese. As progesterone and estrogen wane, the loss of muscle mass and the increase in fat mass accelerate, even among women who do not gain weight. Fat stores also shift from beneath the skin, predominantly in the thighs, hips, and buttocks, to accumulate deep inside the midsection, in cavities that house the liver, pancreas, kidney, lungs, heart, and other organs.

Scientists have theorized that the positioning of fat is an evolutionary response to the energy and mechanical requirements of childbearing. Subcutaneous fat, especially in the lower limbs and gluteal region, offsets the load of carrying a pregnancy and then a baby. These areas can store more fat without causing inflammation or other problems.

But when generous fat stores are no longer needed, fat amasses inside the abdomen wall and deep inside the abdominal cavity. Visceral fat accounts for 5 to 8% of total body fat before menopause but 15 to 20% afterward. Abdominal fat is the telltale sign: Waist circumference expands by about two inches, on average, in the six years following menopause.

Why is this a problem? As we've discussed, excess visceral fat elevates levels of "bad" low-density lipoprotein cholesterol, releases inflammatory proteins perilously close to vital organs, and exerts physical pressure on them. This fat is also less sensitive to insulin, and insulin resistance, in turn, promotes the storage of visceral fat, a cycle that can impair blood sugar control. An increase in waistline signals danger even for women of normal weight and BMI. In fact, women with BMI in the healthy range but abdominal obesity may have a higher risk of cardiovascular disease than those who have obesity-level BMI but without abdominal obesity.

One place where menopause spurs fat buildup is in tissue surrounding the pericardium, the sac that encloses the heart. This fatty buildup is associated with calcium buildup in the heart's blood vessels, a prime indicator of coronary artery disease. And, notes the American Heart Association, having fatty tissue release inflammatory proteins just outside the heart muscle may be "particularly deleterious." Scientists are coming to see changes like this—and there are many—as an important reason why the risk of cardiovascular disease increases precipitously after menopause, especially when BMI is high, to become the leading cause of death in women.

"What people often don't realize is that postmenopausal women with obesity often have a risk of cardiovascular disease equivalent to that of a male. And it's frequently missed," says Dr. Rekha Kumar, an associate professor of clinical medicine at Weill Cornell Medical College. "I can tell you stories from practice where it's been missed many times."

And the heart isn't the only organ at risk. The prevalence of metabolic dysfunction-associated steatotic liver disease (previously called nonalcoholic fatty liver disease; to simplify, I will use the term "fatty liver disease" throughout), the leading cause of chronic liver disease, cirrhosis, and liver cancer, doubles in postmenopausal women. Men aged fifty and older show no such upswing.

"In women, we should explain the pathological changes that occur because of aging and menopause *before* they occur," warns Dr. Ada Cuevas, director of the Center for Advanced Metabolic Medicine and Nutrition in Santiago, Chile. But that message has been slow to break through. Relatedly, Drs. Tara K. Iyer and Heather Hirsch reviewed the clinical impact of the 2020 American Heart Association's statement on cardiovascular disease risk for women entering or experiencing menopause and concluded, "Currently, there is a widespread missed opportunity to educate women about the health risks associated with menopause."

And yet, as science has revealed more about the effects of estrogen loss and other hormonal changes of menopause, women's knowledge about the associated health risks has fallen. In 2009, 65% of women who responded to an online survey recognized that cardiovascular disease is the leading cause of death in women. By 2019, awareness had dropped to 44%. The decline showed up in every age group except women aged sixty-five and older, and across race and ethnicity, though it was most pronounced among Hispanic and Black women. Similarly, the subject seems to be a challenge for doctors. In a nationwide survey, only 22% of primary care physicians and 42% of heart specialists said they feel extremely well prepared to assess cardiovascular risk in women.

Studies have found that women rely largely on friends and online resources for menopause information. Physician education about menopause-related health needs would help to bridge this knowledge gap. In a survey of medical residents at a large, prestigious academic medical center, 70% said they received little, if any, education about gender-specific medical concepts in clinical training or the classroom.

The general guidance on weight and abdominal fat for women of menopause age is the same as the advice given for all adults. Dr. Hurtado Andrade also urges women to avoid weight-promoting medications such as gabapentin, which is typically prescribed to control seizures or chronic nerve pain but can also reduce menopausal hot flashes, and clonidine, a medication that lowers blood pressure in addition to decreasing the frequency of hot flashes, to manage menopause symptoms.

Hormone therapy relieves menopausal symptoms as well. Estrogen treatment alone or in combination with progestin also protects against menopausal changes in body composition, including the accumulation of visceral fat, abdominal obesity, and impaired glucose metabolism. The use of hormone therapy plunged from 1999 to 2020, after the initial results of a major federal study, the Women's Health Initiative, suggested that the therapy increased the risks of heart attack, stroke, and breast cancer. But subsequent research has found that when hormone therapy is started before age sixty and/or within ten years of the final menstrual period—earlier than it used to be prescribed—the risks are low and can be outweighed by the benefits, as long as women have no history of cardiovascular disease, certain cancers, and other contraindications.

Although randomized clinical trials have shown that hormone therapy mitigates heart risk factors, the studies have not found that it reduces coronary heart disease itself. But many clinicians find compelling evidence of the benefits of hormone therapy from more than forty observational studies, research that tracks health metrics of people over time without intervening to affect outcomes. These studies have shown a 30 to 50% reduction in heart disease in hormone therapy users compared to nonusers.

Although hormone therapy doesn't cause weight loss, research by Dr. Hurtado Andrade suggests it may strengthen the response to anti-obesity medication. She followed 106 women who took semaglutide. Sixteen of them, who were also on estrogen or estrogen-progestin patches or pills, were more likely to experience significant weight loss. This was the first study to look at the effects of combining a GLP-1 medication and hormone therapy, and, as Dr. Hurtado Andrade noted, it's too early to attribute the weight-loss boost to hormone therapy's effects on body composition. Hormone therapy is indicated primarily for the treatment of uncomfortable menopause symptoms, and can improve sleep, physical activity, and quality of life—benefits that can help someone stick to a weight-loss regimen. Given the growing acceptance of hormone therapy and the soaring use of GLP-1 drugs, the combination is sure to become more common. Larger studies are needed to investigate the upsides and potential risks.

12

· · · ·

Resetting Body Weight

D r. Randy Seeley is a professor of surgery and director of the Michigan Nutrition Obesity Research Center at the University of Michigan. In my estimation, he knows more about weight loss than anyone in the field. I went to Boston to attend his lecture focused on how pharmaceutical and surgical interventions can effectively change body weight set point.

I have never believed in the concept of a set point. As I've said, my view has always been that body weight "settles" within a range where many opposing forces come into equilibrium and, as a result, has the appearance of a set point. I also recognize that neither the set point nor settling point or alternative theoretical models account for all the data. In his talk, Dr. Seeley made clear that he was using the term "set point" to mean that the body defends against weight loss, which is the role of the homeostatic system. He showed us a picture of a bathtub and compared the water level to the amount of fat in our bodies. The faucet was for input, the drain for output; it was also an illustration of energy in (faucet) and energy out (drain). Another example of set point is body temperature. Our bodies actively regulate temperature; we constrict and dilate our blood vessels, sweat, and shiver to keep body temperature in an acceptable range. But we know that 98.6 is not really "set," as temperature fluctuates based on the inputs the body receives. When we are fighting infection, our temperature goes up. While we sleep, our temperature goes down. Temperatures are variable based on time of day and other circumstances.

Consistent with this analogy to temperature, Dr. Seeley argued that weight set point is not, in fact, set. He suggested that what we eat, the accessibility of food, genetics, and age can all affect this set point. So, whether we call it a set point, settling point, or resulting homeostasis from opposing pressures or forces, the evidence suggests the level is malleable. And *that* is what is important.

Dr. Seeley's second point was that the brain is the major controller of this set point. He has overfed and underfed animals and subjected them to different drugs and surgeries, and what he has found repeatedly is that animals naturally get to the weight they were intended to be at—that is, based on their natural weight trajectory. When pushed on where this set point occurs, Dr. Seeley says it is the property of neural circuits to defend against weight loss. Here, in alignment with Dr. Kevin Hall's research, he is referring to the counterregulatory forces of increased appetite and decreased resting metabolic rates that occur when we lose weight.

If there *is* such a set point, can it be altered? Dr. Seeley explains that you can choose to push that circuit around, but this takes focus and effort. "If I told you to hold a life preserver below water, you could do it as long as you were strong enough or paying attention," he explains. "As soon as you get bored or aren't strong enough, the life preserver goes back to its buoyancy, to the top of the water. Pressure to go back is there all the time, so in just one weak moment, it goes back to where it was." When you take drugs or have bariatric surgery, you change inputs in the system, and the body will begin to defend a different weight than before. But once you remove those inputs—if you stop taking drugs or watching what you eat—the system goes back to what it was before.

I asked Dr. Seeley what it would take to reset the system after weight loss so that the body would defend this lower weight permanently. "Consider seeing a light," he explained. "Each time you see it, your brain responds the same way: neurons fire, the signal travels down the optic nerve, and other neurons activate. This process doesn't change the brain's wiring. But if you pair that light with a shock, you start associating the light with fear. Now, seeing the light triggers anxiety because your brain circuits have been altered to remember this fear. So, we can either input something that the sensory system responds to consistently, or we can create lasting changes in the brain's circuitry."

In other words, if we change our "input" (for example, by dramatically restricting calories) enough that we are able to change our neural circuits, we have to keep the pressure up by continuing to limit what we eat in order for the system to work at that lower weight. "Take away that pressure, and the system reverts back," Dr. Seeley says. "To change it permanently, I have to change the circuit so that once the signal or pressure is taken away, there's more permanent change." The goal is to identify factors, such as reducing calorie intake or increasing muscle mass, that not only encourage the body to maintain a lower weight but also make it easier to sustain that weight without continuous effort. Dr. Seeley concluded by saying that "effective therapies for obesity target the brain *and* alter the set point."

The addictive and satiety circuits influence our desire to eat, but there are additional forces at play that contribute to the amount of energy we consume and expend. Some of them, including age, height, genetic sex, and genetic disorders, are out of our control. Dr. Harold Bays points to the ones that are often alterable—nutrition and exercise habits, behavior, and environmental factors, along with physical and mental health—as the ones we can work on. Among these, he also lists the satiety and hunger hormones.

The key to sustaining a lower weight is to eat in such a way that we feel full and satisfied, which will diminish the emotional appeal of food and decrease its reward value.

Satiety Is the Key

The introduction of GLP-1 weight-loss drugs has changed our understanding of appetite. For decades, scientists have distinguished between two regulatory systems that influence weight: the homeostatic, or the energy/hunger circuitry, and hedonic, or reward/addictive circuitry. But, in truth, we should have been viewing them in tandem with a third system: satiety. It took four decades of scientific research, but we now understand that the gastrointestinal hormones, or gut hormones, including the glucagon-like peptide, or GLP-1, play a crucial role in regulating appetite. And the pharmacological form of GLP-1 is uniquely capable of tipping that seesaw from reward to satiety.

"I think the simplest conceptualization would be to say there are three highly integrated systems of general circuits that are referred to as homeostatic, satiety, and reward," says Dr. Jeffrey Friedman, a molecular geneticist at Rockefeller University who discovered leptin, another gastrointestinal hormone that helps to regulate energy by suppressing hunger.

I believe that, in our modern food environment, our addictive circuitry has come to overpower our homeostatic system—leaving it to vie with the satiety system for control over how much we eat. Unfortunately, the modern food environment has given our addictive circuits the advantage here too: Ultraformulated foods that are made of rapidly absorbable carbohydrates leave us with little satiety. One of the major opportunities for controlling weight, then, is to strengthen the satiety system so that it can overpower the addictive circuitry of the brain.

The gastrointestinal tract is a major endocrine organ. Hormones, referred to as metabolic messengers, produced in the gut play key roles in appetite, satiety, and regulating glucose. Some hormones, such as ghrelin, form in the stomach and can stimulate eating and addictive circuits. (Indeed, ghrelin is widely known as the "hunger hormone.") Hormones that originate in the gastrointestinal system, such as naturally occurring GLP-1s, may enhance the satiety system. The concentration of these hormones relative to the others determines whether the body's physiological balance tips toward or against eating. (Which is why pharmaceutical companies have modified the naturally occurring GLP-1 hormones for the anti-obesity medications so that they may be administered in mega-doses exceeding the level that is normally found in the body.) The satiety hormones are constantly communicating with the reward system. They provide information regarding the body's physiological status—hungry or sated; fasted or fed—that is essential for the brain's motivational circuits. These circuits focus on stimuli that the body needs on a moment-by-moment basis, creating demands that range from "Do I need to escape a predator?" to "Does my body need fuel?" These signals, or goals, help the brain to prioritize what the reward system should focus on. Such goals are "dynamic and subject to change," says Dr. Mitchell Roitman of the University of Illinois, Chicago; they can change based on learning, but also based on our physiological state.

As such, hunger arises due to an ever shifting, and relating, set of forces. "All these hormones influence the classic homeostatic system, but they also influence the positive hedonic system," Dr. Roitman says. "As you get further away from your last meal, you start to have higher levels of one of the gastrointestinal hormones, ghrelin; you're tuning up the dopamine mesolimbic circuits even if you need those calories. Even if your body is in energy homeostasis, a hint of ghrelin, changes in cues, they all interact with one another."

In a study published in *The New England Journal of Medicine* in 2011, overweight and obese participants were put on a very low energy diet. Consequently, they lost 14% of their body weight over ten weeks. For the first time, investigators could study all the known hormones regulating body weight in these participants. At the Obesity Medicine Association's 2023 spring summit, Dr. Louis Aronne, who is also an attending physician at New York Presbyterian Hospital, cited this study to discuss what he thought were the key hormones involved in body weight regulation.

He put up a slide with two columns. The first column listed the hormones that had decreased because of this weight loss; this included leptin, the hormone signaling satiation, which had dropped by a dramatic 65%. The second column listed the hormones that had increased. Ghrelin, the hunger hormone, appeared here. Indeed, the study suggested that a 10% weight loss produces changes in eight hormones that encourage weight to be regained.

To better understand how these hormones correlated to appetite, I called Dr. Priya Sumithran at Monash University in Australia, who was the lead investigator on the study Dr. Aronne referred to in his talk. She mentioned that the study did not clarify how and to what extent these hormone changes were correlated to changes in appetite. "I think I'm less sure now than I was then how related these hormones are to appetite and satiety," she confided. "We're just measuring these things in the circulation, and we have no idea exactly what the ratios are and how they're acting in the brain individually that's then contributing to the appetite, etcetera. Clearly, they are related to appetite in the sense that that's what they do in the body, but I'm less convinced about the fact that you can measure a level in the blood and know what that means for that person's appetite."

So, the role of the natural gastrointestinal hormones remains unclear. That's not surprising given the variety, and complexity, of the counterregulatory forces. Am I hungry because of a drop in my satiety hormones or is it that I'm addicted to ultraformulated food? Professor Tamas Horvath at Yale has suggested that the "fundamental flaw" of all our biological circuits, the "default wiring and default drive, is to promote hunger." Said differently, our bodies are basically always telling us, "When in doubt, eat."

And yet, that this remains a mystery should not obscure the fact that if we can increase satiety—by drugs, diet, or exercise—we can disrupt our addiction to ultraformulated food and create the space for sustainable weight loss.

Part III

· · · · · ·

THE PATH
TO SUSTAINABLE
WEIGHT LOSS

13

· · · ·

A New Era

The first time I injected myself with a GLP-1 drug, sitting in my endocrinologist's office in the spring of 2023, the effects kicked in within a few days. I lost my appetite. I also felt bloated. Within twenty-four hours of injecting myself with the next few doses, I experienced intense chills and had to wrap myself in an electric blanket while I worked. I wasn't ill; it was more like a persistent malaise, a feeling of weakness and discomfort. On more than one occasion, I felt a mysterious, sharp abdominal pain. And then my relationship to food and eating began to change.

A particular moment from my experience stands out to me as emblematic of the key shift that occurs while taking the weight-loss drug. I was having dinner with my family. There was a ricotta-stuffed organic roasted chicken breast with sage and brown butter polenta on the table. Under any other circumstances, I would have happily dug in, and likely would have gone for seconds. But that night, I could hardly eat a bite. I almost had to fake eating altogether, because I was so uninterested in the food sitting in front of me.

It wasn't just that my appetite was drastically changed. My cravings had changed too. I no longer wanted salt, fat, sugar; I ate simple foods instead. Sometimes, I would take only a little bread with butter. I began eating vegetables on a regular basis for the first time in my life. I finally felt a freedom from a near-constant yearning, a break from the clamoring "food noise" of daily existence.

There is something unique about GLP-1 drugs, something that makes them different from any of the anti-obesity drugs that came before. Dr. John Blundell of the University of Leeds, who has done several studies with the new anti-obesity drugs, explains that they profoundly change how people respond to food. "People don't stop eating completely," he tells me. "They still do eat, but they eat small amounts of food, and these small amounts of food now have the same satiating capacity as formerly was the case with a much larger amount of food," he continues. "The whole system has been amplified, or you can say it's been curtailed, but these people are now showing a pattern of eating based on small meals with very high satiating capacity. I don't think you need any specific change in palatability."

When food stays in the stomach longer, satiety signals intensify: You feel full, so you lose the desire to eat more. Dr. Blundell suggests that small meals consumed by people on GLP-1 drugs, which once would have left them unsatisfied, have gained a new ability to suppress hunger. It's as if the entire system of appetite has been rewired. These smaller meals provide the same level of satisfaction as larger meals used to provide. These results offer a new perspective on the long-running debate about a weight set point. GLP-1 drugs may be teaching us that we should begin to think instead about whether there is an *"appetite* set point" that can be adjusted using targeted therapies.

The dramatic consequences of taking GLP-1s, including those that I experienced firsthand, made me want to know more about the precise physiological effects of the drugs. At the most general level, the drugs work by reducing caloric intake, the same as diets and bariatric surgery, but the way they accomplish this is totally different. Dr. Blundell and I have discussed whether the changes caused by GLP-1s are due primarily to delayed gastric emptying—the movement of food out of the stomach into the small intestine—leaving the stomach full for a longer period. We know that when food lingers in the stomach, it sends prolonged satiety signals to the brain, but that is unlikely the whole picture.

"There's no doubt that people still enjoy food, but something fundamental has shifted," Dr. Blundell says. "When you measure the appetite sensations like hunger, fullness, desire to eat, and so on, they all change. It's a consequence of feeling satiated, which makes food less attractive. With GLP-1s, because the levels are high twenty-four hours a day, people have this sensation all of the time, feeling full, or fuller, and having no disposition to eat. What GLP-1s do in the long term is decrease any craving for food, to take away that constant feeling that people are stimulated by food, and it increases their sense of control over eating. It allows them to control their hunger drive."

In personal testimonials, people who take GLP-1 drugs report eating smaller meals with longer intervals between them, suppressing hunger more effectively. Users describe a transformed relationship with food: an indifference, a lack of desire, a state in which food no longer holds its usual allure. It is as if their internal dialog around meals has changed. Evidently, GLP-1 drugs impact both gut and brain mechanisms. They reset how we eat. Food still seems pleasant, but it no longer commands our attention. There is an absence of wanting and craving—at least, while we are taking the drugs.

The Anti–Obesity Medicine Cabinet

In the United States, there are currently two major GLP-1 drugs approved for weight loss: Novo Nordisk's semaglutide and Eli Lilly's tirzepatide, both of which are weekly injectable drugs. (There is also liraglutide, an older GLP-1 drug developed by Novo Nordisk that requires daily injections.) In a head-to-head clinical trial, patients taking Lilly's tirzepatide lost an average 20.2% body weight compared with 13.7% among those taking Novo's semaglutide. Tirzepatide patients lost an average of 50.3 pounds compared to 33.1 pounds for patients taking semaglutide. Overall, tirzepatide is a more potent drug for weight loss than semaglutide.

Tirzepatide pairs GLP-1 with another molecule called GIP (gastric inhibitory polypeptide), which also stimulates the release of insulin; semaglutide targets GLP-1 alone. Dr. Matthew Hayes and Dr. Tito Borner, who have studied the action of these drugs, believe that GIP masks some of the gastrointestinal effects of the GLP-1 molecules, allowing higher doses and greater weight loss.

In all obesity interventions, there is significant variation in individual responses. GLP-1s don't change that reality. Dr. Scott Kahan, an obesity medicine doctor in Washington, DC, emphasizes that the averages given for weight loss are amalgamations of dozens, hundreds, or even thousands of people who were studied. "Essentially no one is average, no one has an average outcome. There are people [on these drugs] that lose no weight or even gain weight. There are other people that lose more weight from medication than bariatric surgery," Dr. Kahan says. "There's essentially a

bell curve of outcomes around the average. So when drug companies report that 50% of patients lost more than 25% of their total body weight,
you should be aware that not everyone reached even a loss of 15%," he
concludes. The studies also don't indicate how many calories people were
consuming during both the weight-loss and weight-maintenance phases of
their trial.

Dr. Deborah Horn at the University of Texas Health Houston Center for
Obesity Medicine and Metabolic Performance has investigated why some
individuals on GLP-1s lose significantly more weight than others. Looking across clinical trials with tirzepatide, Dr. Horn notes that people with
higher BMIs do not necessarily lose a different percentage of body weight
than those with lower BMIs, but individuals who lose more than 5% of
their weight in the first eight weeks are likely to have shed more pounds by
the end of the trial. People with type 2 diabetes lose less weight than nondi-
abetics. We don't know why that is the case.

Higher drug doses correlate with achieving greater than 15% total body
weight loss. People who lose a lot of weight (around 18 to 19%) by week
twenty-four typically go on to lose more weight. "Early response predicts
how people are going to do in the long run," says Dr. Horn. Women lose
more weight than men, overall, but women also experience more side effects, whether on tirzepatide or semaglutide.

When people go on GLP-1s, the average rate of weight loss is greater
during the initial twelve weeks than it is in later stages. By week twelve,
weight loss plateaus in 20% of people taking the drug. By week twenty-four,
it plateaus in 40%. By week forty-eight, it plateaus in 80%. According to
Dr. Horn, younger people, women, and people taking higher doses of tirzepatide experience a longer period of weight loss before they plateau.

The pharmaceutical industry is now racing to develop newer, even more
potent anti-obesity medications. They're striving for weight-loss targets
that are comparable to those produced by bariatric surgery, which can lead
to total weight loss in the 20 to 30% range. The next round of anti-obesity
medications after semaglutide and tirzepatide looks likely to come very
close to this goal. Eli Lilly has completed phase II clinical trials (used to
establish the effectiveness of a treatment) for a new drug called retatrutide.
It combines three hormones: molecules that bind with the body's GLP-1,
GIP, and glucagon receptors. The phase II results indicate up to a 24.2%
change in body weight after forty-eight weeks on the trial. Patients with a

BMI greater than 35 lost a mean of 26.5% of body weight after forty-eight weeks taking retatrutide.

With the great power of these new GLP-1 drugs comes great responsibility to understand their benefits as well as their risks.

Feelings of Aversion

The GLP-1 medications are remarkably effective for weight loss because they are strong enough to overcome the reward system, triggering a feeling of satiety even in the absence of significant eating; at the same time, the drugs are specific enough to food that they do not interfere negatively with learning, memory, and other vital brain circuits. The primary mechanism by which these compounds produce satiety is delayed gastric emptying, a slowing of the movement of food from the stomach to the small intestine. GLP-1 drugs target the aversive system that steers us away from unpleasant or dangerous stimuli, and delayed gastric emptying is part of an aversive response.

Aversion is crucial to survival. To survive, organisms must avoid environmental toxins and learn which foods cause illness. Our appetite decreases if we eat something that upsets our gastrointestinal tract, which is why we generally lose our appetite during infections or food poisoning. Before the discovery of GLP-1s, targeting the aversive circuit as a way to reduce weight was not on anyone's radar. It was not an intentional part of the development of the drugs, but it is an important part of what makes the GLP-1 drugs both powerful and sometimes unpleasant, or worse.

Early on during the drug-discovery process, researchers became aware that the GLP-1 molecules caused visceral illness and malaise. Some of the test animals injected with these molecules did not move after treatment. As I've mentioned, in 2018, Dr. Daniel Drucker, the Canadian endocrinologist who did much of the early work on these compounds, reported that when he administered GLP-1 to animals in his lab, they became so unwell that they could not walk over to their food. In 2024, I followed up with Dr. Drucker about human impacts. "For a long time, we had seen nausea and vomiting, and the GI effects were limiting. We always saw people getting sick," he says.

Unsurprisingly, a drug that triggers nausea or vomiting will also decrease appetite. Pharmaceutical companies are reluctant to admit that their GLP-1 drugs work, at least in part, for some people, by making them sick. In addition to their effects on the brain's reward centers, these drugs stimulate the hindbrain, which contains the brain's nausea and vomiting center. "There is no question that these drugs are characterized by the side effects, and it is fair to say that a component of the suppression of eating is mediated in part by inducing an aversive state," says Dr. Tito Borner, an expert in the aversive system at the University of Southern California. "Whether we want to call it aversive, malaise, malaise state, it plays a role."

GLP-1s specifically seem to stimulate toxin-detecting receptors in a region of the brain called the area postrema. Dr. Thomas Lutz, who studies the neurocircuitry of the hindbrain at the University of Zurich, says, "There is very clear evidence that GLP-1 molecules are aversive according to a multitude of tests."

Dr. Amber Alhadeff became interested in the specific ways that GLP-1s can trigger an aversive response. "These drugs work great for weight loss, but it's not all flowers and rainbows," she says. "There are a host of side effects associated with them, and at the top of the list are the gastrointestinal side effects." She notes that almost two-thirds of participants in a clinical trial with one of the new anti-obesity medications experienced nausea.

Dr. Alhadeff, whose work at the Monell Chemical Senses Center focuses on the gut-brain connection, investigated to see if the therapeutic effects of the GLP-1 drugs could be separated from the side effects at the level of the neural circuits. When she suppressed activity in the area postrema, her test animals exhibited signs of nausea, avoidance of food, and decreased food intake, suggesting that the aversive system was responsible for part of the drug's mechanism. When she activated another aversive part of the brain, the nucleus tractus solitarius, the animals still decreased their food intake but did not exhibit nausea, indicating that the aversive system was not the only system responsible for the drug's action. I asked Dr. Alhadeff which circuit in the hindbrain she thought was more responsible for reducing food intake. She suggested that both seemed equally involved. Therefore, it is probable that GLP-1s also affect brain regions beyond the aversive circuits.

Drs. Borner and Hayes explain that aversive symptoms exist on a spectrum. GLP-1 medications tend to drive the system toward the intense end, eventually leading to nausea and vomiting. To make the drugs effective for weight loss, pharmaceutical companies had to set the doses as high as patients could tolerate. The companies recognized that they needed to increase the dose slowly, over weeks, to manage the side effects. Even so, common symptoms range from outright nausea and vomiting to more tolerable queasiness, low-grade feelings of nausea, and gastrointestinal "unsettling."

"Hunger, satiety, and nausea are all interconnected elements of our eating behavior," Dr. Hayes notes, so the desirable effects of increasing satiety are intertwined with the unwanted nausea, forming a continuum of responses. "When we start a meal in a state of hunger, it has negative associations," he continues. "As we start eating and the meal is enjoyable, hunger diminishes and we experience a positive response that drives us to consume more. Our body's internal feedback from the digestive system will eventually lead to satiation and meal termination. But we can override this system. For example, during Thanksgiving dinner, even when we are not hungry, social and cultural expectations may lead us to eat pumpkin pie, pushing us beyond fullness and into an uncomfortable feeling of fullness and even nausea. Our body's internal regulation is disrupted, resulting in discomfort and causing the body to reject overconsumption through vomiting." By enhancing the satiety response, making individuals feel full sooner and eat less, GLP-1 drugs inevitably have the ability to initiate nausea and vomiting as well.

Perception of the side effects of GLP-1s varies widely among people taking the drug. Some people who experience significant weight loss do not report any nausea. I asked Dr. Rachel Batterham, an obesity researcher at University College London, now at Eli Lilly, what is different about the users who seem to sidestep the drugs' more unpleasant effects. "These people never feel full. It's how their brain responds," she told me.

"So that subclinical nausea is there, but they are not perceiving it?" I asked.

"Absolutely," she said. For those who do experience nausea, the sensation seems to be more than a side effect; it is part of how GLP-1s work. Users feel sick if they consume excessive amounts of food. To avoid that feeling, they learn to eat smaller portions.

The companies selling GLP-1 drugs argue that the rate of gastrointestinal adverse events decreases over time. That appears to be true, but they don't disappear altogether. Moreover, Dr. Borner points out that the time when these adverse events start to taper off is about the same time when weight loss stops. I studied the clinical trials of the GLP-1 drugs. Sure enough, the curves for weight loss and reports of nausea over time seemed to match: Weight loss tapered off when the amount of nausea decreased. "You develop tolerance to nausea, and because of that, the drugs are less effective," Dr. Borner says. The temporal relationship should not be taken as evidence of causality, but it is not credible to deny that the adverse GI events are, in fact, part of the mechanism.

I've wondered if GLP-1s also induce a conditioned taste response, changing the ways that foods taste to us. I put the question to Dr. Harvey Grill, an obesity expert at the University of Pennsylvania. He explained to me how taste aversion conditioning works with laboratory animals, where an animal is conditioned to associate a pleasant stimulus, like sugar, with something unpleasant, such as lithium chloride (an intense salt). The resulting association then alters the animal's reaction, so that it will develop an aversion to something that was previously perceived as pleasant. Dr. Grill confirmed my suspicion: "If you associate a novel taste with GLP-1 injection, animals develop an aversion." He explained that the new GLP-1 drugs could condition people both to eat less (avoidance) and to recoil from certain foods (aversion).

I asked Dr. Grill, "If you create this visceral discomfort during the first three days of taking GLP-1s, what potential effect might it have on reduced food intake leading to weight loss? Is it possible that you are conditioning a long-lasting aversion?"

"In animals, I have, and other people have," Dr. Grill responded.

People taking these drugs must eat smaller portions to avoid feeling ill. Once again, the negative aversive effect seems inseparable from the positive anti-obesity effects of GLP-1s. Foods that cause nausea for individuals on these medications are ones that are high in fat and sugar, fat and salt, or a combination of all three—that is, the foods that are linked to weight gain. Learning to avoid foods that lead to nausea and malaise is a key to changing food choices and behaviors. By increasing a sense of fullness, especially with high-fat, energy-dense foods, GLP-1 drugs can help people understand the body's interoceptive signals and learn to eat and stop eating without feeling nauseous. Put simply, the drugs can help rewire eating behavior.

All of these thoughts were going through my mind as I monitored my own progress on a GLP-1 drug. Originally, I'd set a goal of reducing my weight to 175 pounds, considerably lighter than my starting weight. I reached that point more quickly than I'd expected, and I soon shifted my goal to 155 pounds. When I reached that, I decided to adjust my target once again, this time to a BMI of 20, which for my height was 137 pounds.

With the help of GLP-1s, I reached a BMI I never thought I would achieve. More importantly—and what felt like a life transformation—my relationship with food had changed completely.

Putting Satiety to Work

In his research, Dr. Arne Astrup and his colleagues have shown that satiety increases when protein replaces carbohydrates in the diet, in a dose-dependent way: more protein leads to higher levels of satiety. "We saw exactly the same dose response stimulation of [natural] GLP-1s," he says. "The more protein in the meal, the higher GLP-1 and their gastrointestinal hormone response." High-protein (and high-fat) foods tend to delay gastric emptying, which would explain this relationship. Taking GLP-1 drugs simulates the natural effect of a high-protein diet. The slowing of the initial digestive process also matches common reports of bloating from people taking GLP-1 drugs.

A delay in the movement of food out of the stomach is apparently responsible for another significant effect of the GLP-1 hormones: They reduce blood glucose and insulin levels. When GLP-1s were discovered, Dr. Jens Holst showed that they stimulate the pancreas to increase insulin production. However, when Dr. Astrup infused GLP-1 drugs into human test subjects and then gave them a meal, he found that *both* glucose and insulin levels were reduced compared to the control.

Dr. Astrup has conjectured that delayed gastric emptying due to GLP-1s slows the passage of glucose into the small intestine, which in turn results in slower absorption of glucose through the gastrointestinal system, lower peak glucose levels in the blood, and a lower rise in insulin levels. "By slowing down gastric emptying, all the carbohydrate digestion and absorption is significantly reduced or prolonged, so you get a much lower glucose response, which results in a much lower insulin response," he says. "If you talk to patients after five weeks of treatment, they still have this sensation that gastric emptying is slowed down."

The glucose-lowering effect of GLP-1s has an intriguing similarity to the effect of switching to a low-carb diet, Dr. Astrup notes: "These GLP-1 molecules mimic the effect of low-glycemic-load diets. When glucose excursion is reduced, inflammation goes down, and this reduced inflammation, together with the weight-loss effect and reduced insulin resistance, could easily explain the impact on cardiovascular effects." He concludes that GLP-1 works in part indirectly through slowing gastric emptying and reducing insulin secretion. "Reducing circulating insulin might reduce insulin resistance, and cause weight loss and reduced inflammation," he says. But he points out that GLP-1 also seems to work directly by affecting the brain. We still don't fully understand how these drugs do what they do.

A number of studies indicate that the drugs not only influence the *satiety* side of the equation, but also modulate the *reward* side. Researchers have found preliminary physiological evidence that there are GLP-1 receptors in the ventral tegmental area and the nucleus accumbens, two parts of the brain that are closely associated with the body's reward-response system. The presence of GLP-1 receptors there strongly indicates that GLP-1 drugs could affect the reward system and its associated influence over urges and cravings. Animal tests support that conclusion. Injecting a GLP-1 agonist into the animals' brains reduces their pursuit of food, particularly for "high responders," those individuals that work the hardest for food rewards.

It stands to reason that if GLP-1 can affect eating behavior through the reward system, then it might also affect other reward-related behaviors— for instance, the consumption of drugs or alcohol. Animal experiments show this to be the case. Dr. Lorenzo Leggio, a senior investigator with the NIH Intramural Research Program, has been searching for effective therapies to treat alcohol use for several decades. Intrigued by the evidence that the GLP-1 drugs can disrupt powerful reward effects, he and others have conducted studies showing that GLP-1s reduce alcohol-conditioned place preference in rodents and nonhuman primates. In addition, they have demonstrated that the drugs reduce self-administration of alcohol in laboratory animals.

Dr. Leggio has shown that semaglutide reduces alcohol drinking and modulates brain chemistry involved in alcohol addiction. In their animal models, he and his collaborators have demonstrated that GLP-1 drugs reduce binge alcohol drinking in a dose-dependent manner. Interestingly, the researchers also found that GLP-1 drug effects are not just limited to alcohol, but also extend to corn oil, saccharin, and maltodextrin. Dr. Leggio sees evidence that the impact of GLP-1s extends to opioids, cocaine, amphetamine, and nicotine as well. A study by researcher Cajsa Aranäs and colleagues in Sweden showed that the GLP-1 drugs significantly reduced alcohol intake in both male and female rats, with higher doses showing a more prominent effect. The drugs reduced the ability of alcohol to elevate dopamine levels in the brain's nucleus accumbens, which is part of the reward circuitry.

In addition, several recent cohort studies indicate that people taking GLP-1 drugs have a lower incidence of opioid addiction and alcohol intoxication or hospitalization than similar people who are not taking the drugs. Such preliminary findings bolster the case that the GLP-1 drugs have lasting effects not only in taming food noise, but in taming addictive noise in general. A number of researchers, including Dr. Sue Grigson-Kennedy and Dr. Scott Bunce at Penn State College of Medicine, are now investigating whether GLP-1s can be used to treat opioid addiction and to reduce alcohol use disorder.

Dr. Christos Triantos, a gastroenterologist in Greece, has reviewed a number of recent studies on digestive hormones. Summing them up, he writes, "These naturally occurring hormones, including PYY [a hormone also known as peptide YY] and GLP-1, have been associated with the decreased activation of brain reward areas in response to food- and alcohol-related cues in healthy controls and obese and diabetic patients and patients with alcohol-use disorder." He concludes that GLP-1 and its companion molecules "modulate the way the brain attributes incentive values to a variety of different stimuli, thus shaping pleasure-seeking behaviors."

Dr. Triantos's comments clarify how the pharmaceutical form of GLP-1s exert a powerful push on the all-important equilibrium seesaw—the body's delicate balance between satiation and sensitivity to reward. The key to controlling the addictive circuits is to rebalance that seesaw, increasing satiety and reducing reward responsiveness. That is precisely what the GLP-1 hormones do. They decrease gastric emptying, induce nausea, suppress reward sensitivity, and reduce blood glucose variability. Taken together, those effects make the GLP-1 drugs very powerful in quieting the addictive circuits and, ultimately, in controlling appetite.

Dr. Jens Holst is concerned that nausea and other aversive responses that are essential to the operation of the GLP-1s will ultimately limit their long-term effectiveness, however. "Why do you lose weight? Why do you stop eating?" he asks. "It's because you've lost your appetite and the joy of eating. The pleasure of a great meal is gone. How long can you endure that?" That question will become increasingly relevant for next-generation drugs like retatrutide. Judging from the early trials, it reduces appetite even more than the currently available GLP-1 drugs, semaglutide and tirzepatide, and comes close to the appetite reduction achieved in bariatric surgery. I've seen people consuming just around 1,000 calories a day during the active weight-loss stages while on tirzepatide. The number of calories has to be even lower for retatrutide to achieve the greater weight loss seen in its clinical trial.

"Semaglutide does not cause as profound an effect as tirzepatide in terms of people having shut down their appetite. The one to watch out for is retatrutide. That's where we're going to start seeing problems with people losing weight too fast," said Dr. Donna Ryan, a leading clinical investigator. "People need to be monitored for their caloric intake, their protein intake, and their water intake," she says.

I pointed out to Dr. Ryan that patients with bariatric surgery are losing even more weight, so they must be eating even less than with drugs like retatrutide. Why isn't that equally concerning? "With bariatric surgery, there is a regimented diet," Dr. Ryan responded. "With some of these newer drugs, people just stop eating. They stop eating and they stop drinking [water], and they don't know it's not good for them. They have no appetite. They're happy. They are losing weight. I think the appetite effect of retatrutide is profound. Not eating enough and not drinking enough, that is what I really worry about."

After talking with Dr. Ryan, I went back to look at the adverse effects reported with retatrutide during its phase II trial. There was an increased number of cardiac arrhythmias in the treatment group at the highest dose, as well as a rise in average heart rate by ten beats per minute at twenty-four weeks of treatment compared to the placebo. For now, we don't know whether this signal is indicative of a serious problem. But these drugs are so potent that it seems likely that many potential areas of concern will arise. These are some of the reasons why GLP-1s require careful monitoring.

Loss of Desire and Want

A notable effect of the new anti-obesity drugs is what's clinically known as *avolition*, broadly defined as a lack of desire or want. Like so many aspects of the GLP-1s, avolition is a double-edged sword: It is both an effective mechanism for weight loss and a potentially undesirable side effect. Avolition is a less extreme symptom than anhedonia, often seen in patients with depressive symptoms, which is characterized by a marked decrease in enjoyment of activities one previously found pleasurable. With avolition, people may discover that the things they used to like, such as taking a walk in the park with a friend, are still pleasant, but it feels harder to summon the motivation to do them.

Avolition illustrates the downside of the sudden cessation of food cravings that comes with the GLP-1 medications. The disappearance of wanting can feel like the snuffing of a flame, perhaps even like the loss of something essential to the human experience. Dr. Manejwala, the addiction psychiatrist, says that a similar phenomenon occurs among people who are in the early recovery stages from drug and alcohol addiction "because their dopaminergic tone is so crappy that nothing is enjoyable, and they may feel like during that time period, that it's always going to be miserable." He adds that "reliable data is not yet available on how many patients experience avolition as a side effect of taking anti-obesity drugs. Anecdotally, people report everything from a manageable but still noticeable sense of blah-ness all the way through diagnosable depression, but studies have generally not shown a connection between GLP-1s and severe depression."

No one is entirely clear on why avolition often arises in users of the new anti-obesity drugs. One theory relates to how closely interconnected our reward pathways are with our hunger-satiety systems, Dr. Kent Berridge tells me. "Evolutionarily, this might be because food was the original high-priority reward that mesolimbic systems evolved to seek," he explains. In modern times, "The system expanded its target range to apply to lots of other rewards, too." We are primed to want, in other words. Even now, when there is less immediate pressure on most individuals to procure food and secure a mating partner, our reward system will still find a way to exert itself. And when that system is tampered with, as it is with GLP-1s, the changes could have a dampening effect on all desires.

Journalist Shayla Love interviewed numerous researchers to hear their concerns about avolition produced by the new anti-obesity drugs. Some of them posited that the avolition response could simply be related to a person's energy level dropping due to their reduced calorie intake. The Penn State neuroscientist Dr. Karolina Skibicka told Love that for a person accustomed to strong cravings, their sudden absence might register as a more existential loss: "All of a sudden, that [feeling] goes away, and you have to reestablish what your behavioral drivers should be."

And yet, that loss is also what makes the GLP-1s seem almost magical in their effectiveness. If you choose to take these drugs, your cravings—

both the ones that peak in intensity and the low-grade static of food noise so many people describe—will likely disappear. With your cravings eliminated, or at least strongly reduced, you might then find it easier to change your eating patterns and lifestyle behaviors.

A Serious Side Effect

One of my major medical concerns about GLP-1s centers on delayed gastric emptying, the mechanism that is responsible for so much of the drugs' effectiveness. By slowing the passage of food out of the stomach and into the small intestine, GLP-1s induce feelings of fullness. One of the critical drivers of overeating is not feeling full or satiated. Without feeling full, ultraformulated foods will keep delivering reward signals to the brain with no end. GLP-1s help break this pernicious addictive process. But they may also create their own medical condition.

Doctors have a name for delayed gastric emptying: *gastroparesis*, meaning gastric palsy. Delayed gastric emptying in the absence of an obstruction is traditionally considered a chronic disease. It is seen in diabetic patients and is thought to result from a dysfunction of nerves, muscles, and intestinal cells in the gastrointestinal tract. Symptoms include nausea, vomiting, bloating, belching, abdominal discomfort, malnutrition, and pain. It is treated with metoclopramide, and sometimes other drugs that target specific brain areas. Doctors may have patients consume food containing a radioactive tracer to see how fast food moves from the stomach into the intestine. If more than a certain percentage of food remains in the stomach after specific points of time, it can point to a diagnosis of gastroparesis.

Framed this way, the use of the GLP-1s seems strange, if not outright perverse: Induce a medical condition in people who are obese, and we have a solution for obesity?

Pharmaceutical companies promoting GLP-1 drugs paint a picture that the gastrointestinal effects are generally mild to moderate, and unsurprising. The companies say that the effects are commonly experienced only during the first weeks during the dose escalation period. In one clinical trial, called SURMOUNT-4, 81% of the patients had an adverse event, with 68% designated as being related to the drug. Companies counter that only 7% of the patients drop out. "Although people complain of side effects, they are loath to discontinue the medicines," said Dr. Louis Aronne. He presented the trial result at a meeting of the European Association for the Study of Diabetes.

In the SELECT trial, 16.6% of the patients on GLP-1s discontinued due to adverse events, with 10% dropping out due to gastrointestinal side effects. Thirty-three percent of patients in that trial reported nausea. In still another trial, SURMOUNT-3, 39.7% of patients reported nausea. "Nothing unexpected," said Dr. Jamy Ard, who presented the results at the Obesity Society meetings. He showed the incidence of patient-reported gastrointestinal-related events over time and noted that the number of reports is concentrated in the first weeks after starting treatment and levels off after twenty-four weeks, tracking with the gradual ramp-up in GLP-1 recommended dosage.

When I asked physicians who conducted the clinical trials about gastric slowing, I was assured that it returned to baseline after a few weeks. "Eighty percent of the patients don't have any side effects," one clinical investigator told me. I knew that wasn't right.

I started digging into the data. Every one of the companies' clinical investigators I talked to said that delayed gastric emptying persists with the GLP-1s only for the first hour after digestion and only for a few weeks after beginning treatment. I contacted Novo Nordisk, manufacturer of one of the leading GLP-1 drugs, who reiterated that clinical trial data showed delayed emptying only for the first hour but there was no statistical difference between GLP-1s and placebo in the overall rate of gastric emptying.

What was going on? A prospective randomized controlled trial of patients without diabetes by Dr. Michael Camilleri showed that at five weeks on GLP-1, more than half (57%) developed significantly delayed gastric emptying. When the trial stopped at sixteen weeks, 30% of the patients still reported having persistent delayed gastric emptying consistent with gastroparesis. Data published in the journal *Obesity* by Dr. Camilleri indicated that most patients experienced delayed gastric emptying during the first five weeks, with some maintaining that delay until the study concluded at week sixteen. Does gastroparesis persist after sixteen weeks? We don't know.

A 2023 study by Dr. Mojca Jensterle Sever at the University of Ljubljana found that patients taking a GLP-1 drug retained 37% of a solid meal in their stomachs four hours after ingestion, compared to no retention in those on a placebo. This prolonged gastric retention can make patients feel sick and reduce their appetite.

A complication in interpreting these results is that gastroparesis is also a general response to a severe shortage of calories. During starvation, the body slows down certain nonessential functions, such as a functioning gastrointestinal tract, to preserve energy for the brain. It's unnecessary for the gastrointestinal tract to expend energy when there is no incoming food. I asked Dr. Jennifer Gaudiani, an eating disorder specialist who has written about starvation and gastroparesis, for her assessment of the connection among GLP-1s, starvation, and gastroparesis. She responded, "Pure calorie restriction, regardless of body size, causes gastroparesis in most cases. GLP-1s independently cause gastroparesis in many. So there may be two sources for gastroparesis, starvation and GLP-1."

Patients need to take gastroparesis seriously. It can lead to dehydration, electrolyte imbalance, and malnutrition. The effect of GLP-1s on intestinal mobility also raises a risk of intestinal obstruction from something as common as constipation. In rare cases, constipation can be deadly. It can cause intestinal obstruction, perforation, and infection, especially if not diagnosed. The prescribing information for the GLP-1 drugs currently omits any warning about gastroparesis. This must be corrected.

There is an important broader message here: Reducing appetite can be dangerous. Drug manufacturers need to fully and clearly disclose all possible risks of taking GLP-1 drugs, and patients should approach this treatment with a thorough understanding of those risks, and do so under professional care.

14

· · · ·

Using the Anti-Obesity Drugs

I made my decision to try the new anti-obesity drugs quickly, but I did not make it lightly. By the time I took my first GLP-1 injection in my doctor's office, I had already thought very carefully about the medical implications and the potential consequences. Nobody should go on such a powerful medication without knowing all the details of how it might impact your health. It doesn't matter if you've spent your career overseeing the pharmaceutical industry or if you started reading this book with no knowledge at all about GLP-1s and the neurobiology of food addiction. Regardless of your background, you want to be careful about starting a medication that can fundamentally alter your relationship with food, shifting your body's whole balance between reward and satiation.

A particularly startling detail emerged during human trials of the GLP-1s: The overall weight-loss results in the SURMOUNT-3 clinical trials, which included intensive lifestyle and behavioral treatment, were the same on average as those in the trial without such interventions. The result sounds like a dieter's fantasy. Is it really possible that obese patients could take a drug and lose 20% of their body weight while otherwise living just the same as before?

Alas, the reality is not so simple. GLP-1 medications, powerful as they are, may not be sufficient for lifelong weight management. Even if patients find the drugs effective, tolerable, and affordable for years upon years (which is hardly a given), relying on pharmaceuticals alone to control weight does not address all the other aspects of human biology. The best way to control weight is to have all of the arrows, including lifestyle, behavior, and diet, pointed in the same direction: toward lower weight, reduced toxic body fat, and better health.

As part of that process, it's important to understand that it is okay to seek medical help for weight loss. Seeking support is a sign of strength, not weakness. There is no easy way to escape the ubiquitous, ultraformulated foods that disrupt our natural eating patterns. And there is no easy way to escape the ways that those foods activate the addictive circuits in the brain, increase our responsiveness to reward, and decrease satiety because our dietary hormones are not powerful enough to shut off appetite in the face of such stimuli. The entire modern food industry is colluding to dysregulate your appetite in ways that have a harmful impact on your health. It's perfectly reasonable for you to seek out a medication that could help you find your way onto a healthier path.

It's important to remember, too, that you are not alone, and you should not be alone, on your journey. Obesity is a chronic disease, similar to hypertension or type 2 diabetes. It will require at least some degree of long-term monitoring and treatment. If you decide to take an anti-obesity drug, it should be part of a long-term commitment to improving your health, developed with professional medical guidance that also includes nutrition changes, lifestyle modifications, and behavior changes. GLP-1 medications should not be the only component of your treatment.

I encourage anyone embarking on this journey to choose a qualified physician who is knowledgeable about treating obesity and is ready to provide comprehensive support over the long term. Treating obesity involves more than just focusing on the numbers. A good shorthand for your strategy is SMART: specific, measurable, achievable, realistic, and timed goals regarding nutrition changes, duration and frequency of exercise, and lifestyle improvements, in addition to your weight-loss targets. Above all, you want to find your own personal solutions for reducing food noise and improving your relationship with food.

There are two major acts in the life of a drug. The first is how it performs in clinical trials. The second is how it performs in real life. Before you decide if GLP-1s should be a part of your journey, there are some important considerations to navigate.

For people who have obesity, liver disease, progressive prediabetes, type 2 diabetes, cardiovascular disease, or some combination of these problems within metabolic syndrome, GLP-1s are especially appealing. The extreme weight loss that's possible with these medications could provide significant reduction in disease risk. Conversely, people with a personal or familial history of medullary thyroid cancer or multiple endocrine neoplasia type 2 are advised to avoid GLP-1s, as should people with chronic kidney disease, pancreatitis, inflammatory bowel diseases, uncontrolled diarrhea or constipation, gastroparesis, or eating disorders. People who are pregnant should not go on the drugs, nor should anyone with an allergy or hypersensitivity to the medications or any of their ingredients. (There are reports of increased fertility with the drugs.)

There are additional reasons to be careful with GLP-1 medications. People taking the drugs can experience hypoglycemia due to decreased food intake (especially carbohydrates) or metabolic changes. Users may experience dehydration due to the significant decrease in appetite, which causes both reduced food and fluid consumption. Dehydration is a very real risk. In rare cases, dehydration may lead to acute kidney failure, particularly among people with chronic kidney disease, who are at a greater risk. GLP-1s raise the likelihood of pancreatitis because they prompt the pancreas to release more insulin in response to high blood sugar levels. That risk is further heightened for people who consume excessive levels of alcohol, so individuals on these medications are advised to either avoid alcohol or limit their intake.

Whether GLP-1s are appropriate for you also depends in part on your body mass index. The FDA originally approved the use of anti-obesity medications for people who have a BMI above 30 (classified as obese) or who have a BMI above 27 and at least one coexisting obesity-related condition. It is debatable whether these medications are the best first-line treatment for people who have a BMI in the overweight range without any related medical problems; they may be better off attempting to lose weight by diet and exercise changes alone. The long list of potential health benefits, contraindications, and body-mass considerations is yet another reason why you need medical guidance before going on anti-obesity drugs. Your doctor can also advise which drug to start with.

The two main available GLP-1 drugs, semaglutide and tirzepatide, are broadly similar in their mechanisms of action, and both are typically administered once a week. Semaglutide is sold commercially for weight loss as Wegovy (Ozempic for diabetes); tirzepatide is sold for weight loss as Zepbound (Mounjaro for diabetes). Ozempic pens hold a month's supply, offering flexibility for "in-between" dosing, which can be advantageous for certain patients. Conversely, Wegovy and tirzepatide pens provide a single predetermined dose per pen. Although the side effects are generally similar, individual responses may vary.

To date, semaglutide has undergone more extensive research than tirzepatide, simply because it has been on the market longer. As I'm writing this, only semaglutide has undergone clinical tests that demonstrate reduced cardiovascular risk. (Tirzepatide's cardiovascular clinical trial results should be completed soon.) As noted earlier, tirzepatide promotes greater weight loss than semaglutide on average in clinical trials, but there are significant variations from person to person. The GLP-1 options are also changing rapidly as pharmaceutical companies are pouring resources into the development of new drugs that will lead to even greater weight-loss effects and improved glycemic control. Retatrutide is just one of what is likely to be a whole family of upcoming triple-action GLP-1-type drugs.

Benefits Beyond Anti-Obesity

With the significant weight loss that is possible with the GLP-1 drugs, we may be able to reverse a portion of the morbidity and mortality associated with aging by focusing on weight management. People are living longer but they are not necessarily living better, especially later in life. From 1960 to 2020, the number of years of expected disability at the end of life also rose from five years to ten years. While lifespan increased by almost a decade for both men and women, *health span* (the number of *healthy* years of life) increased by only three years for men and two years for women.

The main driver of this disability is excessive weight. Obese people live with about three additional years of disability, on average, compared to people who have a healthy weight. As we know, excess weight is cumulative for most people as they age. Think of how many older people we know who suffer from back pain, joint pain, or severe cardiovascular disease who are 40 or 50 pounds overweight, for whom a reduction in that weight can give them back both mobility and improved quality of life.

Healthy weight delays the onset of several diseases across multiple organ systems, according to Dr. Sue Roberts, who studies energy and metabolism at Tufts University. In the musculoskeletal system, a healthy weight decreases the risk of arthritis and loss of muscle. Benefits to the brain include slower cognitive decline and a decrease in dementia risk. (The underlying physiological changes seen in type 2 diabetes and dementia are closely linked, so much so that dementia is sometimes referred to as "insulin resistance of the brain" or "type 3 diabetes.") Vision loss is less common, with fewer cases of central vision loss and cataracts. Hearing loss, type 2 diabetes, and various heart diseases and cancers are less common in people who are at a "healthy" BMI.

Weight loss can delay or prevent the progression of many of these disabling conditions even after the initial symptoms have begun. We need more studies about the effectiveness of the GLP-1s in reversing age-related morbidities in older people. To date, most of the clinical study data is in middle-age, active people. Understanding the risk benefits in the elderly, especially with concerns about the effect of GLP-1s on muscle and bone, is vitally important.

What to Expect When You Inject

Starting a treatment with a GLP-1 drug can bring both excitement and anxiety. People often ask, "What should I expect?" and "How will I feel?"

Generally speaking, both the benefits and side effects may kick in gradually, as drug manufacturers recommend titration—slowly ramping up the dosage—to help patients tolerate the medication. According to the manufacturers' guidelines, the initial doses are 0.25 mg weekly for semaglutide and 2.5 mg weekly for tirzepatide. Even at those low initial doses, some patients may see significant weight loss. The general recommendation is to maintain the low initial dose for one month before increasing the dosage in monthly increments until an effective level is achieved. The guidelines suggest a maximum dose for semaglutide of either 2.4 mg (Wegovy) or 2 mg (Ozempic) weekly and 15 mg for tirzepatide, though many patients will find a suitable effective dose within a lower range. Every obesity medicine recommends that slowly increasing the dose and adjusting it accordingly is very important. As Dr. Judith Korner says regarding dose, "Start low, go slow."

In the clinical trials, patients on semaglutide lost an average of 6%, 11%, and 16% of body weight after three, six, and twelve months of treatment. Patients on tirzepatide lost 8%, 15%, and 22% of body weight after three, six, and twelve months of treatment. Remember, though, that these are average results over large clinical populations. In other studies, patients lost less weight. Age, gender, metabolism, genetics, diet, and diabetes status play a role. About one-third of users on semaglutide lose more than 20% of their body weight and are termed "super responders"; around 15% lose less than 5% of their body weight and are called "non-responders."

Weight plateaus are common while taking GLP-1 medications, just as with weight loss in general. In some cases, people encounter these plateaus fairly frequently at each dose and need to keep adjusting. In other cases, people are able to stay at the same dose of GLP-1 for a long time and continue to experience weight loss. Using GLP-1 medications for weight loss requires ongoing weight monitoring, along with continued adjustment and refining of dosage, diet, and lifestyle until people achieve their weight goals. After that, the key is finding the right dosage for weight maintenance while making adjustments if weight gain recurs.

People who are starting on GLP-1 drugs often ask how much weight loss they can expect per week. The answer again varies among individuals, although losing one pound or more per week is generally considered a typical therapeutic response. Losing two to three pounds per week is not uncommon. Users should be aware that the amount of weekly weight loss almost always fluctuates. They might see a weight loss of four pounds one week, followed by one pound the next week, but with a general downward trend in weight over time. Setting weight-loss goals ahead of treatment is important for managing expectations; for designing a realistic and balanced weight-loss program; and for maintaining motivation, especially on the toughest days.

In terms of what you will feel, everyone's experience is unique. I already touched on the general nature of the adverse reactions that may occur, but as a former FDA official, I feel it's important to be very direct about side effects that patients might experience, and about how to recognize them.

Patients often report fatigue. This is likely due to a significantly reduced daily energy intake. Nutrient shifts and micronutrient deficiencies might also account for some of the reported fatigue. Dehydration may contribute as well. In clinical tests, subjects on these drugs often experience a reduction in thirst in addition to a reduction in appetite. Finally, rapid weight loss itself can cause tiredness. Losing more than two pounds per week concerns me because of the potential for malnutrition. However, some people report feeling *more* energetic due to the weight loss.

Most people on GLP-1 medications will experience some gastrointestinal issues, with nausea being the most common and constipation close behind. About half of users experience nausea. Users tend to shift away from certain foods because of delayed stomach emptying, which results in nausea, vomiting, and heartburn, particularly after large or fatty meals. Vomiting and reflux are less likely to happen if users eat relatively small high-protein, high-fiber meals. Many people adjust their eating habits or condition themselves by eating smaller portions so they don't feel ill from consuming too much food while on GLP-1 medications. Up to 40% of people taking GLP-1s may experience constipation. The drugs reduce gastrointestinal motility; in other words, stool travels more slowly through the gut, decreasing the frequency of bowel movements and increasing the amount of water reabsorption by the colon, which results in harder stools.

One of the most noticeable effects of the GLP-1s is reduced appetite, which is central to the way that they promote a decreased overall calorie intake and lead to weight loss. Appetite suppression and the various side effects are generally strongest in the first one or two days after taking a weekly dose of GLP-1s and when the dosage is increased. Some users prefer taking the medication on Friday to control appetite over the weekend, when people often indulge in big meals. Others prefer not to take it over the weekend to avoid having any side effects. Symptoms typically become less severe over many weeks or months. Some people notice that their appetite suppression and reduced cravings for food completely vanish a few days before their next scheduled dose, indicating that an increase in dosage might be necessary.

New users of GLP-1 drugs are likely to feel bloating due to the sloweddown transfer of stomach contents to the small intestine. In some cases, the effect may be so severe that it results in "stomach paralysis," where the stomach barely empties, leading to persistent nausea, vomiting, heartburn, and other complications. Another potentially serious effect is cholelithiasis (gallstones), which is fairly common in patients with rapid weight loss, whether from these medications, a very-low-calorie diet, or bariatric surgery. Combining obesity with rapid weight loss can lead to a buildup of gallbladder sludge and can prompt preexisting gallstones to cause obstruction and gallbladder inflammation.

One of the most concerning symptoms that GLP-1 users may experience is malnutrition. This is why medical oversight is so important; many people could be harming themselves without even realizing it. Consuming fewer than 1,000 calories a day requires strict medical monitoring. That is not generally happening for most of the people now taking GLP-1s. In my opinion, dispensing the drugs without providing appropriate care is inappropriate.

The truth is that most doctors have little training or expertise in nutrition, and the prescribing information for the drugs does not provide adequate guidance. The onus is on the pharmaceutical companies that are selling

GLP-1s to ensure that doctors and patients have appropriate nutrition information about how to safely use the drugs. Right now, that important detail is missing.

Using the Medications Responsibly

Some people may be tempted to take the new anti-obesity drugs for aesthetic reasons. That is not the clinical purpose of the GLP-1s. If losing weight makes you feel better about yourself, and if you do it in a safe and medically sound way, and it improves your overall health, that is a win. After all, people will change their behavior only if there's a reason that matters to them. But the reason for losing weight that really matters—the reason that motivates me—is to reduce body fat, especially the toxic visceral body fat that causes inflammation and significant disease. If you have an increased waist circumference, losing weight and reducing your visceral fat will provide health benefits, regardless of your motivations.

Now the FDA has changed the indications for prescribing Wegovy and Zepbound to remove specific BMI criteria. The label states the drugs are approved "to reduce excess body weight and maintain weight reduction long term in adults with obesity or adults with overweight in the presence of at least one weight-related comorbid condition." Some doctors have gone beyond these guidelines, however. They prescribe GLP-1 drugs to people who are not obese, who have no comorbidities, and who are experimenting with intermittent use rather than a lifetime of dependence. Some patients treat the GLP-1s not as a lifelong commitment, but as a helpful short-term crutch.

I recently talked with someone who falls close to the border of the prescribing guidelines. At six foot one and 190 pounds, Dr. Jason Atwater did not feel he had a weight problem until his mid-fifties, when he slowly started gaining weight. Eventually, he reached 220 pounds, none of his clothes fit, and he began to feel unhealthy. He tried various diets, but nothing worked. Then the GLP-1 drugs came on the market. Dr. Atwater noticed that Mounjaro was offered at a discount, with the first month free. He contacted his general internist. "Sure, no problem," his internist readily agreed when he asked to start the medication.

"I wasn't obese, but I had a BMI of about 28, and I had some calcification of my arteries," Dr. Atwater told me, so he fell within the eligibility guidelines. He began with a 2.5 mg dose, gradually increasing to 5 mg and then 7.5 mg. Over three months, his weight dropped to approximately 195 pounds and stabilized at that level. Having achieved his goal, Dr. Atwater stopped using Mounjaro, but after five months, his weight began creeping up again. He got another prescription, going right to the 5 mg dose, and within a month, he was back at 195 pounds. Once again, he stopped using the drug. Six months passed with his weight more or less stable, but when it went back to 205 pounds, he used Mounjaro for another month, returning to 195. Over twenty months, he used the drug for a total of six months, starting with an initial treatment over four months and then two "booster" months to help him maintain his weight.

"This kind of intermittent medication utilization has been enormously helpful," he explains, noting that it served as a reminder to control portion sizes and eating habits. "The reduction of appetite is pretty significant. I would say I was not hungry at all. Some days, I had to remind myself to eat." He believes that he has been able to better control his eating habits by remembering the fullness he experienced on the drug, and he reports that he experiences no "rebound" effect when he comes off the drug.

Using the drug intermittently is not unusual. A former president of the Obesity Medicine Association also uses the drug this way. Data suggest that 30% of people who discontinue will restart the medication. But Dr. Atwater goes further. He believes that GLP-1 use should not be restricted to the obese, but should be available to those who are merely overweight and simply want to lose 15 to 20 pounds.

The prevalent viewpoint in the medical community is to stay firmly within the FDA guidelines, but I see many doctors willing to bend the rules. I have spoken with plastic surgeons who will prescribe GLP-1s for any patient who has evidence of abdominal adiposity, whether or not they have accompanying comorbidities. The FDA's recent removal of specific BMI criteria does give doctors and patients more flexibility in determining who should receive these drugs. The problem is that the GLP-1 drugs have not been studied for, say, a patient who wants to lose 15 to 20 pounds. In the end, insurance companies will have a significant influence on who qualifies. There will also be people who want to push their weight down to unhealthy levels for cosmetic reasons, which could lead to eating disorders such as anorexia. Personally, I would not prescribe GLP-1 medications outside the guidelines, out of concern that there are not enough data on such use.

I believe the GLP-1 drugs are major therapeutic advances. The big question for me is how to use them safely. I've been trying to listen to how doctors treat their patients after the initial weight-loss period. Understand that doctors learn primarily from other doctors, but also from pharmaceutical sales representatives. At a recent panel session of the American Society of Plastic Surgeons meeting, a panel of physicians was describing their own unique approaches to dosing the medication. "Instead of dosing four shots a month, we give them enough medication for three shots, and then two shots, and one shot for a while," one panelist said. Another physician at the meeting said she practiced GLP-1 microdosing using her own compounded version of the drugs, an approach which has not been approved and has not been studied in clinical trials.

Many doctors and patients are making up their own rules, and that's a serious problem. On YouTube and social media, there are multiple tutorials describing do-it-yourself approaches to how patients should use GLP-1s, giving their own ideas about dosages and intermittent use. Apparently they have access to doctors who are prescribing the anti-obesity drugs without closely monitoring how they are being used. I have learned that any time physicians are improvising doses, it means there are not enough data out there to ensure optimal care.

This is tantamount to running a national experiment with these potent new drugs. Tens of billions of dollars are being made by the pharmaceutical industry. The FDA has abrogated its responsibility by allowing GLP-1 medications in the marketplace without appropriate data on their longer-term use. The solution is not to abandon the new drugs; they are valuable in breaking the hold of food addiction and improving health. But the medical community needs to do better at helping patients use them effectively and safely.

Concerns About GLP-1 Drugs for Children

Pediatric obesity is a huge and growing problem in the United States. According to statistics from the CDC, nearly one in five young people between the ages of two and nineteen now have obesity. But the idea of administering anti-obesity drugs to children is highly controversial, as evidenced by the outcry in January 2023, when the American Academy of Pediatrics (AAP) released guidelines covering the treatment of pediatric obesity. After a comprehensive review, the AAP concluded that pediatricians "should offer adolescents twelve years and older with obesity weight loss pharmacotherapy, according to medication indications, risks, and benefits . . ." The

AAP also recommended that adolescents thirteen and older with severe obesity be referred for bariatric surgery. ("Severe obesity" is defined as having a BMI that is 120% of the 95th percentile BMI.)

Parent advocates sharply criticized the AAP for relying on flawed measures like BMI, and argued that recommending medical treatment would further stigmatize obese children. The journalist Virginia Sole-Smith called for "a paradigm shift to weight-inclusive approaches, which see weight change as a possible symptom of, or a contributing factor toward, a larger health concern or struggle." Some psychologists worried that focusing too much on a child's weight would put them at risk for developing an eating disorder. The United States Preventive Services Task Force declined to follow in the AAP's footsteps and instead recommended treating pediatric obesity solely with intensive behavioral treatment. "We believe we need more evidence to be able to make a recommendation for or against medications in children and adolescents," Dr. Wanda Nicholson, chair of the task force, said in an interview.

Doctors who treat obesity supported the new AAP guidelines, however. They cited studies showing that children do well on the GLP-1 drugs, and that the reported side effects (mainly gastrointestinal distress, as in adults) are moderate in intensity. "When young patients with obesity use these medications and experience effective weight loss, it has a significant impact on their lives," says Dr. Vibha Singhal, director of Pediatric Obesity at UCLA Mattel Children's Hospital. "They are healthier, can move more quickly, are more motivated to make healthy lifestyle changes." Supporters of the AAP guidelines especially pushed back on concerns about putting a child on long-term medication. What was the difference, they asked, between giving a child a drug that everyone agrees is essential—like insulin for type 1 diabetes—and giving a child a weight-loss drug that could stave off chronic disease? One shouldn't "apply a double standard to practicing obesity medicine," says Dr. Aaron Kelly, an expert in pediatric obesity.

To make sense of this debate, I called my friend Dr. Rosenbaum. He noted that he usually starts children with obesity on metformin, a type 2 diabetes drug that helps lower blood sugar, and that a number of them have "done very well on metformin alone." He also has them see a nutritionist, monitors their vitamins and minerals via blood tests, and discusses lifestyle interventions. Dr. Rosenbaum doesn't refrain from prescribing anti-obesity medications, but he is cautious in doing so. "They're effective tools, but they're much sharper and much riskier," he says. "The bigger the effect you could have on growth and development, the more cautious I would be." He tries to prescribe lower doses if possible, and reduces the use of medication as early as possible.

When I asked for his overall opinion on GLP-1 drugs, he offered a conservative assessment consistent with his medical philosophy. "Before prescribing medication, I like to know as much as I can about how it works and what it's doing," he explained. "And I don't think we know enough about how these drugs work yet."

I share Dr. Rosenbaum's worry that we don't know enough about how targeted the GLP-1 drugs are. We know some of what they do, but we don't know whether they might affect body systems other than the endocrine and gastrointestinal, including the brain. The fact that GLP-1s work both for weight loss and for weight maintenance could mean that the drugs are affecting different systems for each process. Again, we don't know. That information gap is particularly salient when talking about children, whose bodies are still developing and who could be on these medications for decades. Pediatric studies of Wegovy—the only GLP-1 currently approved for children twelve and up—have a two-year follow-up at the maximum, but the deleterious effects of medications can take much longer than that to show up. It took around five years for doctors to realize that fen-phen caused cardiac damage in up to a third of patients.

We should not deny effective treatment to young people who have been harmed by our addictive-food environment. At the same time, we equally should not allow the medical and pharmaceutical communities to convince us that the only way out of this crisis is their way. We need a multifaceted approach to deal with the pediatric obesity crisis, one that leaves room for pharmaceutical intervention, but that also envisions a future of maintaining our children's health without dependence on medication.

The Surgical Alternative

For much of recent medical history, bariatric surgery has been the definitive treatment for people struggling with obesity, particularly if they have disorders such as hypertension or diabetes. Before the approval of the GLP-1 drugs for weight loss, I often wished that certain patients would have availed themselves of these surgical procedures earlier on in their lives. I have referred critically ill patients for heart transplant surgery, only to have them rejected because they were considered too high risk for transplant due to their obesity.

GLP-1s are rapidly changing the medical reality for obese patients. The drugs can't yet match the level of weight loss that's possible with bariatric surgery, although they might get there soon. Then again, bariatric surgery has greatly improved over the last three decades, becoming substantially safer. No longer can a surgeon perform a gastric bypass procedure and leave the patient to fend for themselves. Now, more commonly, it takes an entire team to care for patients undergoing weight-loss surgery. This level of inter-disciplinary care should be available to people taking the new anti-obesity medications as well. Patients who rapidly lose weight, whether from surgery or medication, need careful monitoring.

Today, one of the most pressing questions in obesity medicine is who should be considered for bariatric surgery now that drugs can provide some of the same benefits. In the most recent guidelines published by the American Society for Metabolic and Bariatric Surgery and the International Federation for the Surgery of Obesity and Metabolic Disorders, surgery is recommended for three distinct populations: (1) any individual with a BMI over 35, regardless of any associated metabolic disorders; (2) people with a BMI over 30 who have associated metabolic disorders; and (3) individuals of Asian descent with a BMI of 27.5 or higher, due to their increased incidence of insulin resistance.

Undergoing bariatric surgery causes an energy deficit, resulting in weight loss of up to 30% of body weight and up to 70% of excess body weight. Bariatric surgery has also been proven to produce long-term health gains. In general, 30 to 40% of patients can put their diabetes into remission after a year. There is about a 25% drop in using anti-hypertensive medication, and about a 3–7% drop in lipid-lowering medications. Patients also experience a decrease in liver failure, obstructive sleep apnea, and cancer. These numbers remain fairly stable even many years after surgery, resulting in a decrease in all-cause mortality of about 50% in people who undergo metabolic surgery compared to obese people who do not receive treatment. Because the current generation of GLP-1 drugs cannot match the level of weight loss associated with bariatric surgery, they also cannot match the documented reductions in metabolic dysfunction.

There are several theories on how bariatric surgery yields such extreme weight loss: restriction, malabsorption, and hormonal. There are many types of bariatric surgeries, but they all reduce the size of the stomach, which means that patients can no longer physically eat as much as they did before. Surgically removing part of the stomach also takes away cells that secrete acid and other enzymes that aid in digestion. And after surgery, food passes through the stomach and intestines more quickly, giving the body less time to absorb nutrients and causing malabsorption. Many bariatric surgeries restructure the intestines, resulting in further digestive changes.

After metabolic surgery, some patients report not only a loss in appetite but also a change in the type of food they want to eat. They no longer crave chocolate, perhaps, or now find Chinese food distasteful. This change intriguingly resembles preference shifts that happen to some patients who take GLP-1s, although the cause is probably different. According to Dr. Rachel Batterham, "The patients who report changes in taste have greater weight loss in the long term." Unfortunately, we cannot yet predict who will have these kinds of changes after bariatric surgery, though they are believed to be genetic.

There is a more worrying side to bariatric surgery, however. Approximately 60% of patients who had the most common bariatric procedure (sleeve gastrectomy) end up regaining significant weight by ten years after surgery, according to Dr. Gerhard Prager of the Medical University of Vienna. Here's where my concerns kick in.

At the 2024 International Federation for the Surgery of Obesity and Metabolic Disorders (IFSO) meeting in Melbourne, Australia, a group of doctors debated the causes of post-surgical weight regain. I was interested in their thoughts about the sleeve gastrectomy. About 150,000 such operations are performed every year in the United States. The procedure removes about four-fifths of the stomach, causing a narrow, sleeve-like structure to form. At the meeting in Melbourne, buried on an unpublished slide, I saw the results of a ten-year randomized controlled trial that compared the gastric sleeve to an older gastric bypass surgical procedure called the Roux-en-Y, in which surgeons create a small pouch from the stomach and connect it directly to the latter portion of the small intestine. The sleeve gastrectomy group had significantly higher rates of follow-up surgery, 34.4% versus 6.3%. That's a startlingly high failure rate for a popular surgical procedure.

At a 2023 IFSO meeting in Naples, Italy, Dr. Khaled Gawdat, president of the IFSO Middle East–North Africa chapter, claimed that bariatric surgery has been flawed ever since early procedures using gastric bands. Gastric bands were popular but eventually fell out of favor with patients because of poor long-term weight loss and a high incidence of complications.

Word of mouth, rather than action by the FDA or the surgical community, was the primary reason for declining use of gastric bands. "This was the birth of commercial bariatric surgery. Easy procedure, short-term success, and in the long term, who cares, if the surgery fails, blame the patient," said Dr. Gawdat. "Bariatric procedures give some weight loss in the first eighteen months. All bariatric procedures show weight gain after that, and results at five to ten years will be completely different than your initial results." He further claimed that 50% of sleeve gastrectomy patients have irreversible problems with reflux after surgery.

From 2022 to 2023, there was a 25% drop in the number of bariatric surgeries being performed in the United States, probably due to the rising popularity of GLP-1 drugs. If Dr. Gawdat is right, the move away from gastric-sleeve surgery is good news for patients. While these are still early days, it may turn out that drugs end up being a better option for some patients who had previously turned to surgery.

Going Off the Drugs?

The conventional wisdom among obesity medicine specialists is that the GLP-1 drugs will need to be taken for a lifetime, or there will be weight regain. After I started taking GLP-1 injections and experiencing their powerful effects on eating and weight loss, I began to think about my future. I wasn't sure I wanted to be on these drugs for the rest of my life, especially given the uncertainties about their long-term effects. I also thought about the many other people who have been trying these drugs. Data suggest that people take these medications, on average, for six to eight months but may restart. It's clear that GLP-1s are going to be hugely important in easing people along the journey away from food addiction. It's less clear whether these drugs can deliver a lifelong solution for people who struggle with obesity, even if they genuinely want to stay on them.

Stopping the medication will inevitably lead to weight gain. A year after stopping the medication, patients on semaglutide gain back two-thirds of the weight they lost. In one clinical trial, patients regained 70.6% of their weight by forty-eight weeks off semaglutide. At a medical meeting about long-term weight-loss maintenance, one of the chief clinical investigators told me she was losing sleep over the fact that when patients discontinue the drug, appetite comes back ferociously. An NIH investigator in attendance suggested that such weight rebound might be a sign of a withdrawal response. As of now, the only sure way to avoid rebound is to stay on these medications forever. Then again, the same is true if people stop dietary and lifestyle interventions required for weight loss—as many of us know all too well.

Some obesity researchers believe that weight regain after going off GLP-1s occurs because people revert to old habits, but that reversion may in fact be due to the influence of the addictive circuits and to metabolic changes. When patients stop taking GLP-1 drugs, they lose the increased satiety that is a hallmark property of the drug. Without that increased satiety, and with increased reward responsiveness, many (though not all) people find themselves hungrier than ever before. A survey taken by Dr. Sarah Sorice-Virk, a plastic and reconstructive surgeon with the Stanford Health Care Cancer Center, suggests some wiggle room for people going on a GLP-1 hiatus: In about one-third of the patients, reduced addictive behaviors seem to last for an extended period, up to six months after discontinuation of the drugs.

Why would people go off these medications if they are likely to regain weight? One reason is sheer optimism or just not wanting to be on a medication. We all think we are the ones who can control our eating, only to have to confront the reality of the inaccuracy of that belief. Second, the current cost of these medications in the United States is the equivalent of paying off a car loan or covering tuition at an in-state public university. Third, gastrointestinal adverse events and other side effects can continue even after the initial ramp-up period for drug dosages. Shortages of the drugs, medical contraindications, weight-loss plateaus, and a desire to reduce drug burden are other reasons people stop using anti-obesity medications.

The discontinuation rates are highly variable depending on the drug and the population. In one of the longest clinical trials, 23% of test subjects dropped out by forty-eight months, despite considerable efforts by the investigators to keep people enrolled. Dr. Patrick Gleason, who leads clinical research at Prime Therapeutics in Minnesota, found that less than one-third of insured adults living with obesity who do not have diabetes remained on GLP-1 therapy after one year. For semaglutide, the discontinuation rate was 53% at one year. Dr. David Liss, a research associate professor at Northwestern University's Feinberg School of Medicine, reported a GLP-1 discontinuation rate at one year of 50.3%. A study conducted by Blue Cross Blue Shield revealed that 30% of patients using GLP-1 discontinued the medication within the first four weeks. The newest GLP-1 drugs have been available only for a few years, often with limited supply, so it is too early to make reliable estimates of how many people will continue taking these medications long term.

If the discontinuation rate remains this high, the drugs could turn out to be a real-world failure despite their impressive results in clinical trials. It's remarkable that we even have to seriously consider such a possibility. I am puzzled how my former agency, the FDA, approved GLP-1s for long-term use without an actual understanding of how to use the drugs over the long term.

My obesity medicine colleagues point out that many drugs, such as those for treating blood pressure or high cholesterol, need to be taken indefinitely, and stop delivering benefits if patients ever stop using them. Why should the GLP-1 drugs be any different, they ask. It's a variant of the argument that Dr. Kelly makes in favor of using the drugs to treat pediatric obesity. But this argument misconstrues the continued effect of taking GLP-1 medications.

Leaving aside any continued adverse events, the new anti-obesity drugs work by reducing appetite and increasing satiation, whereas medications for blood pressure and lipid-lowering usually work without any notable side effects. Maintaining a reduced body weight requires eating less than what was being eaten at the old weight. The GLP-1 drugs make it easier to resist increased appetite and to maintain the reduced caloric load, but people then need to live at that reduced caloric intake indefinitely. Maintaining a low drug-assisted body weight may require consuming less than the recommended 2,000-calorie daily intake to meet nutritional needs.

Although some people might be able to cycle on and off these medications successfully, we don't know if that will be possible for most people. Can a person stay on these drugs for life? Will they? Can someone sustain sufficient weight loss after they have gone off the drugs to make having gone on them worthwhile? These are important questions that must be considered when determining if anti-obesity medication is the right choice for any individual.

15

. . . .

Managing Major Weight Loss

The fundamental reason for taking GLP-1 drugs is that they change our relationship with food. But what should that new relationship look like? Nowhere on the drugs' prescribing information do manufacturers disclose how many calories people can (or should) consume while on the drugs. That's a serious oversight. We have a powerful new tool for adjusting human biology, and it comes without a user's manual.

Any kind of weight loss requires well-considered dietary and behavioral changes. The rapid, significant changes that commonly occur for people taking GLP-1s make such considerations especially urgent, though, and they raise significant questions. What is it like living with the new anti-obesity drugs long term? Do people who take the drugs end up eating so little that they could create new medical issues, even while obesity-related conditions recede?

At a meeting of the American Diabetes Association focused on a discussion about optimizing the use of GLP-1s, I asked some of the experts presenting how many calories patients were consuming while they were rapidly shedding weight. "I think it depends on how quickly they're losing weight, but when it is very quick, we would suspect between 500 and 800 calories each day. It's very, very low. Because their appetite is suddenly gone, their calories are just dropping into the toilet," said Maureen Chomko, a registered dietitian and diabetes educator in Seattle. To be clear, 500 to 800 calories is generally considered a semistarvation diet. I would not be surprised if the number of calories users are consuming during the acute weight-loss stage while taking these drugs is a bit higher, closer to 1,000 calories a day. In any case, the number is quite low.

Dr. Robert Kushner of Northwestern's Feinberg School of Medicine, a clinical investigator for the GLP-1 trials, estimates that people who leveled off and were maintaining their weight during the clinical trials consumed between 1,200 and 1,600 calories a day. Other studies provide additional insights into dietary changes of people taking GLP-1 drugs. In a published article, GLP-1 manufacturers report that people taking the drug ate an average of 415 calories for lunch, compared with controls who ate 640 calories. A study by Seattle-based obesity medicine specialist Sandra Christensen reported a reduction in average energy intake ranging from 16% to 39% among people taking the anti-obesity drugs. In another study, by Dr. Martin Friedrichsen of Novo Nordisk, lunch caloric intake was reduced by 47.1%.

Those numbers indicate a drastic change in eating patterns and nutrition. In other contexts, we might consider such a sudden drop in calories indicative of an eating disorder. For instance, the reduced eating reported by Dr. Friedrichsen falls into the same range of caloric reduction as was seen in a study of people being treated for anorexia by Dr. Matteo Martini from the University of Turin, in Italy. These caloric intake levels also fall below the number of calories needed to meet nutritional needs, according to US national dietary guidelines, although the number of calories needed to maintain one's weight varies. Someone who goes from 350 to 290 pounds will have different caloric needs than someone who goes from 200 to 140 pounds, for example.

The Minnesota Starvation Experiment, carried out by the physiologist Dr. Ancel Keys during World War II, provides a useful reference point for the effects of extreme caloric reduction. In the experiment, conscientious objector volunteers spent three months eating a baseline diet of 3,200 calories a day, followed by a six-month "semistarvation" period during which they received 1,570 calories daily. Note that 1,570 calories was considered semistarvation for these men. The participants lost 25% of their body weight, and they also developed fatigue, decreased sexual interest, emotional distress, and a preoccupation with food.

At a conference held by UT Southwestern Medical Center's Nutrition and Obesity Research Center, an obesity medicine specialist in the audience asked for clinical guidance about a patient who had lost considerable weight on one of the GLP-1 drugs. "She came to me as a new patient. She had a

BMI of 36. Her BMI now is 19. She is feeling dizzy with low [blood] sugar. She is cold and clammy. At 19, I see all this malnutrition in her. I'm thinking, 'Oh my God, I've got to get this patient off the medicine.' But she's adamant she will not stop: 'I have such a strong sweet tooth; if you stop this, I will regain all my weight.' She's gone to the other end of the spectrum. I spent an hour with her. I finally stopped the medicine. She is coming back next week. Tell me, how do I deal with this?"

I listened closely to the response from Dr. Jaime Almandoz, an obesity expert at UT Southwestern Medical Center: "Your patient has had a good result from being treated with anti-obesity medications in that her weight has come down in a clinically meaningful way. The challenge is that she is in a zone that someone might consider borderline unhealthy. You speak to a challenge when people who have lived with obesity for many years find an effective treatment that has helped them feel more like themselves. We hear from patients that this has been game-changing for them, and when they hear this may be taken away from them by a healthcare provider, it can create an adversarial relationship. What I have done before is to approach this from a perspective of safety—not saying this is dangerous, but I am concerned that as patients start to drift down toward unhealthy BMI range, we begin to discuss at what point do we need to stop this? I don't mean stopping the medication, but shifting from active weight loss to weight maintenance. That can head off a lot of these difficult conversations." Dr. Almandoz went on to say, "With the medications, some patients will go on to develop what some call disordered eating patterns or behaviors, but what it is, in my opinion, is fear of weight recurrence."

Following up, I asked him, "These are highly powerful, very effective drugs, but aren't they also potentially very dangerous?"

"Absolutely," he responded. "The challenge is how we treat obesity effectively as a chronic and complex disease. We have agents that can potentially [help patients] lose as much weight as bariatric surgery. If someone is going down the road for bariatric surgery, there are specific guidelines about preoperative education and assessment and a curriculum of education. Currently, there are no guidelines for people who will start medications."

A State of Semistarvation

The lack of guidance about proper caloric intake brings me back to one of my core concerns about the GLP-1 drugs. The FDA approved these medications without understanding how they should be used long term in a healthy, sustainable way. Weight loss would bring tremendous health benefits to millions of people who struggle with obesity, but it comes with its own risks—especially when the weight loss happens rapidly, or when it leads to a sustained, ultra-low-calorie diet, as often seems to be the case with GLP-1s.

Dr. Almandoz's point about some people going on to develop disordered eating is very important. I followed up with Dr. Kim Dennis, an expert in eating disorders and head of SunCloud Health in Illinois. "This feels a lot like when OxyContin came out. The company said it was nonaddictive, it was improving people's functionality," she told me. That comparison may sound extreme, and she was not saying that GLP-1s are addictive, but she went on to explain her point. "We know people who are weight-reduced or weight-suppressed, meaning below their natural set point, which is different for every human; when you are in a state of weight suppression, reward sensitivity increases," she emphasized.

Food addiction is a genuine problem, but treating it with a drug that takes its users to near-semistarvation levels of eating should raise concerns, too. It's a question of openly evaluating risks and rewards. Yes, appetite can be reduced with GLP-1 drugs. Yes, stimulation of the aversive system can tamp down reward sensitivity. Yes, the weight-loss effects of the new drugs will reduce body fat, including visceral fat, with many attendant health benefits. But users of these drugs need to understand the risks that come with sudden, drastic reduction in caloric intake. GLP-1s have the potential to put people into a state of semistarvation. At minimum, doing that requires close medical monitoring.

Once people are in semistarvation mode, it is critical to be on the lookout for metabolic and other complications. There is a rare metabolic condition associated with starvation, called euglycemic ketoacidosis, that we are beginning to see associated with people who are taking GLP-1s. Euglycemic ketoacidosis can lead to a significant drop in pH levels of the blood; the resulting condition, metabolic acidosis, can be life-threatening. I found a 2024 case report of a forty-four-year-old diabetic woman who was on increasing doses of semaglutide and who experienced fatigue and nausea along with vomiting. Her doctors astutely made the diagnosis of euglycemic ketoacidosis, which they linked to her starvation state. In their published paper, they write, "If not recognized and treated, ketoacidosis may lead to arrhythmias, cardiovascular collapse, seizures, and coma, with increased likelihood of death."

I contacted one of the authors and asked if they were aware of other cases of euglycemic ketoacidosis with the use of GLP-1 drugs. "I suspect that we may not be looking for it, and a few cases may have been missed, considering the fast pace and high volume of patients hospitalists are challenged with daily," he responded. There is nothing on the label of the GLP-1 drugs warning about this unlikely but serious possible consequence.

The GLP-1 warning label does disclose the risk of pancreatitis. During the first year of use, there is a bump in pancreatic enzymes in asymptomatic patients. Patients need to be observed for persistent severe abdominal pain, which may or may not be accompanied by vomiting. There is also an increased risk of gallstones and inflammation of the gallbladder. Although weight loss itself can have these effects on the gallbladder, "there are possible direct effects of the GLP-1 drugs," Dr. Judith Korner said at a recent lecture at Columbia University Irving Medical Center. Another potential adverse event that has only recently been noted is the risk of nonarteritic anterior ischemic optic neuropathy, a cause of sudden blindness. Massachusetts Eye and Ear at Harvard Medical School reports a sevenfold increased risk for people on GLP-1s, based on a population study.

One disconcerting, though hardly deadly, side effect of any dramatic weight loss is a condition called telogen effluvium, better known as "hair loss." This condition is triggered by significant stress or a sudden change in the body. Telogen effluvium causes a higher percentage of hair follicles to enter the resting phase, leading to hair shedding. As one of my dermatologist colleagues explains, it's as if your body is saying it has more important things to do than grow hair. Once the stress is alleviated, hair growth usually resumes after two to three months. Telogen effluvium can unmask an underlying condition of androgenetic alopecia (commonly called "male pattern baldness" even though it can occur in women, too). Someone who has androgenetic alopecia but might not have noticed due to its gradual nature can get a rude awakening when the stress from rapid weight loss suddenly makes the condition apparent. A young person will likely regrow all their hair, but a sixty-five-year-old who loses weight rapidly might never regrow all their hair if they also have androgenetic alopecia.

Another inconvenient and potentially more significant side effect, one that I've experienced directly, is intense chills due to weight loss. I wrote to the GLP-1 companies and asked them what they knew about chills being associated with their drugs. Here is the response from Novo Nordisk: "At this time, Novo Nordisk has not conducted studies to evaluate this topic. In order to further research your inquiry, we conducted a computer-assisted literature search of the National Library of Medicine and other relevant medical databases. This search did not yield any relevant citations for Ozempic and cold sensation, as well as its mechanism."

Dr. Karolina Skibicka from Penn State is quite familiar with the association between GLP-1 drugs and chills, however. In a lecture, she reported three separate studies noting a significant decrease in body temperature for several hours after administering short-acting GLP-1 drugs to lab rats. She joked that her graduate students could quickly identify the animals treated with GLP-1s simply by touching their tails. I asked Dr. Skibicka about the clinical significance of these large temperature drops. "No one knows," she replied.

I asked Dr. Jennifer Gaudiani if chills could be an early clinical sign of malnourishment. "The very earliest signs are cold hands or a sense of feeling chilly," she said.

"I was chilly within three days of starting these drugs, but I was still overweight," I said.

"You can be malnourished and still be overweight," she told me. "It was an abrupt reduction in calorie intake. Your body was radically slowing its metabolism to try to save your life because you aren't eating enough."

As someone who has been responsible for the review and evaluation of prescription drugs and has studied the emergence of adverse events, I'm very aware that clinical trials cannot detect every adverse event caused by a new drug. Some effects emerge only years later, after long-term use. The effects of rapid weight loss and eating reduction alone provide plenty of reasons to be cautious. Weight loss is not something to be treated lightly. The most worrisome consequences of the GLP-1s may be the ones we don't know about yet.

Strength and Muscle Mass

When I began taking GLP-1 injections and losing weight rapidly, I knew I had to be losing some of my muscle mass in the process. This is a common experience among people who are taking the anti-obesity medications—a high-level side effect, in essence. Dr. Grant Tinsley, who studies body composition and sports nutrition at Texas Tech University, has shown that 40% of the weight lost in patients on once-a-week injections of semaglutide came from lean body mass. Approximately 29% of the lean-mass loss was muscle.

Weight loss from any method—be it bariatric surgery, GLP-1 drugs, or lifestyle interventions—leads to the loss of lean tissue in addition to fat. The problem is especially acute for older people. As individuals age, they normally lose up to 10% of their muscle mass per decade after their twenties and thirties, a process known as sarcopenia. The primary driver of age-correlated muscle loss is simple inactivity. Muscle loss is a major reason why older people become frailer and more prone to accidents and falls. Lack of exercise, specifically lack of weight-bearing activities such as resistance training, also contributes to osteoporosis, the loss of bone mineral density. Osteoporosis leads to brittle bones that fracture easily, which could potentially be catastrophic in the event of a serious fall or other accident.

Exercise is crucial for maintaining strength and for maximizing the health gains from a weight-loss, fat-reduction plan, especially one that includes the use of GLP-1s. Adding muscle mass increases the resting metabolic rate—muscle consumes approximately six calories per pound every day for maintenance, whereas fat requires about two calories per pound. Exercise also seems to be helpful for weight maintenance, including maintenance for people who go off the anti-obesity medications. A recent study out of Denmark found that patients who went off the drugs did significantly better than the control group at keeping weight off if they maintained a regimen of exercise.

Don't expect to lose significant weight through exercise alone, however; if you were to put on ten pounds of muscle, a significant increase, that would increase your daily caloric needs by only about sixty calories. The primary benefits of exercise are improved overall health, including reduced stress and inflammation, and increased metabolic flexibility, the ability to switch readily between burning fats and carbohydrates in response to the body's demands.

Even individuals who are committed to a weight-loss plan are likely to run into a time when they regain weight. Perhaps they decide to go off their GLP-1 medication, or they lose focus on their eating plan, or their life becomes more stressful. Regardless of the reason, exercise when people regain weight is just as important as, if not more important than, when they lose it. When people regain weight, they generally do not rebuild their muscle, resulting in unfavorable changes to their body composition. Their body fat percentage increases, even if they didn't regain all of the weight they lost. To lose weight safely and maintain weight loss, it's important to preserve and potentially build lean mass using a combination of strength training and cardiovascular exercise.

Many people get their exercise through daily activities such as walking. But that mild approach, though beneficial, is not sufficient for addressing the significant changes that happen when taking GLP-1 drugs. German fitness researchers Katharina Gross and Christian Brinkmann reviewed the recent studies and determined that walking 150 minutes a week did not prevent muscle loss during treatment with semaglutide. In contrast, resistance training, such as weightlifting, was effective in reducing muscle loss and maintaining a better fat-to-lean-mass ratio. The CDC, the American College of Sports Medicine, and many other health organizations recommend regular aerobic activity every week as necessary for cardiovascular health, as well as two sessions of total-body strength training.

There are drugs in development that seem to stimulate muscle growth and that may be helpful in maintaining lean body mass during treatment with GLP-1 drugs. One such drug, called bimagrumab, is currently being studied for general use, both alone and in combination with semaglutide, in obese and diabetic people. Until those studies are complete, strength training is the only option for people seeking to maintain or increase body muscle during weight loss.

Knowing the risks of weight loss without exercise, I consulted a widely used online source of medical studies data for physicians and health providers, where I found an evidence-based weight training article. It was co-authored by three physicians, two of whom were part of a company called Barbell Medicine. Not long after, I found myself in a gym in Los Angeles, attending a weekend Barbell Medicine seminar led by the company's founders, Dr. Jordan Feigenbaum and Dr. Austin Baraki. There were a few dozen of us, all there to learn the basics of barbell training.

I don't think I've ever felt more like a fish out of water. But I knew that building up my strength was an essential part of my journey against food addiction and toward a healthy body with less visceral fat. At the Barbell Medicine seminar, a coach named Tom Campitelli calmly showed my group the techniques of the squat, how to position the barbell, placement of the hands and feet, and more. I ended up persuading Tom to take me on as a client, but group training along with a basic gym membership works just fine.

Soon, dressed in sweatpants, I found myself in my cluttered basement, surrounded by shelving and storage boxes and doing squats with a barbell. I also learned how to use barbells to target specific muscle groups. These exercises use the large joints involved in the majority of daily activity: the hips, knees, shoulders, elbows, and to a lesser extent, the ankles and wrists. "We want to train the muscle groups that flex and extend these joints," Campitelli explained. "The muscles around the hips and knees compose a significant amount of the skeletal muscle mass in our bodies. By loading and moving these big joints through their respective ranges of motion, you can train the muscles that operate them to become stronger."

Many movements in strength training, particularly with barbells, can be grouped as follows: pushing with the arms, pulling with the arms, bending the knees, and bending at the waist (sometimes called hinging, as with a door hinge). Squats, bench presses, deadlifts, and rowing broadly address these movement patterns. I found the repeated, discrete choreography of the limited sets of movements I practiced both useful and comforting. In a typical sixty- to ninety-minute weight training session, only a few minutes are spent lifting the weights on the heaviest sets. Most of the time is spent warming up with lighter weights, loading the bar, and resting between sets. Yet that seemingly small number of repetitions is capable of providing the stimulus that prompts the body to build more muscle.

These exercises may seem daunting—they certainly were to me at first—but Campitelli says that strength training is less likely to cause serious injury than many popular sports. Contrary to popular belief, technique is not the most important factor for reducing your chances of getting hurt while lifting weights. You can lift "poorly" or "wrong" provided the weight is sufficiently light. Instead, using weights that are inappropriately heavy, either in a single session or chronically over longer training periods, is a bigger risk factor for injury. Whether the details of my movements were exactly correct was less important than the ritual of doing things in a particular way.

Someone who has been inactive for decades cannot be expected to start immediately lifting heavy weights, but any level of exercise is better than none. Inactivity is a major driver of sarcopenia and loss of function. Older people are often advised to go slowly with strength training, but the same processes that allow the body to get stronger at age twenty still work when people are sixty, or even eighty-five. There is plenty of data showing that older adults can and do respond positively to training. Older lifters increase their strength and muscle size by similar percentages to younger adults. Age does not reliably predict the magnitude of improvement.

If we are going to try to reverse some of the complications of obesity in older people, we need to make sure we do not put them at increased risk of muscle and bone loss. Clinicians are appropriately concerned about any skeletal muscle or bone loss in older people. Resistance training is the best solution.

16

· · · ·

The Path Toward Healthy Eating

We don't yet have detailed clinical information about what, or how much, people typically eat while using the new anti-obesity drugs. Despite that, we know quite a bit about how to eat a healthy diet when we are drastically reducing our caloric intake. Starting from there, we can build up detailed guidelines about how to eat whether on GLP-1s or not. We can put together the user's manual the pharmaceutical companies and nutrition communities have failed to provide.

People on GLP-1 drugs have distinctly different nutrition needs from people who are trying to lose weight without medication. GLP-1 users should be under the care of a dietitian or a nutritionist, in part because of the risks of ending up in a state of semistarvation. The huge upside of the drugs is that they can disrupt food addiction, setting people free from the burden of having their behavior dictated by their environment. Weight maintenance requires eating at a reduced caloric level for long periods, which in the past has almost always proved to be unsustainable. It is difficult to eat fewer calories because of the addictive nature of our food environment. That's why diets fail. For all their complexities, GLP-1 drugs are game changers. By reducing reward sensitivity and food noise, they make it possible to stop counting calories and make it easier to switch to a high-quality diet.

Staying at a reduced caloric intake for life, even in the face of the endless availability of ultraformulated foods, would be like chaining Odysseus to the mast to prevent him from succumbing to the lure of the Sirens. Addiction specialists call such intervention "binding." It is sustainable only if there is something quieting the addictive circuits. That is exactly what the GLP-1 medications do. They make it possible to exist on reduced caloric intake, without hunger, appetite, or preoccupation. They allow us to put together a new kind of eating strategy that goes beyond the initial weight loss to include a sustainable plan for long-term weight maintenance. And if that plan fails at times, as it almost surely will, the drugs can help guide us back onto it.

There is suggestive evidence in animals and humans that GLP-1s can tame the reward system. "We actually showed it clinically," said Dr. Sean Wharton, the lead investigator on a clinical trial for semaglutide. As part of the trial, the investigators studied responses to a questionnaire that measured craving, control of overeating, and desire for sweet and savory foods. "We studied it for two years and showed that there is a decrease in cravings and a decrease in wanting," Dr. Wharton reported. The authors found that semaglutide "improved participants' ability to control their eating and made it easier to resist food cravings than placebo."

Dr. Corby Martin at the Pennington Biomedical Research Center in Baton Rouge examined the impact of tirzepatide on energy intake and eating habits compared to a placebo. He and his colleagues randomly assigned 114 participants with obesity to receive either tirzepatide, liraglutide, or a placebo. They observed that tirzepatide significantly decreased all food cravings, including lack of control over overeating, the anticipation of positive reinforcement that may result from eating, and the intense desire to eat. In contrast to what usually happens when people go on diets, participants taking tirzepatide did not exhibit any signs that they were actively attempting to restrain their eating. The restraint people generally need to sustain a diet was unnecessary when they were on tirzepatide. Without desire or wanting, they had no need for that restraint.

"Tirzepatide significantly decreased appetite for palatable foods at three levels, including in the environment, on our plate, and in our mouths," said Dr. Martin. He also found that tirzepatide significantly decreased impulsivity, a characteristic that is associated with gambling, but also with compulsive eating and food addiction.

Because GLP-1 drugs are so effective at reducing appetite and thirst, the primary task is not restricting calories (which will be handled by the drug), but rather, ensuring adequate nutrition. This is especially true because people with obesity are at increased risk of certain forms of micronutrient deficiency. One high priority is making sure that GLP-1 users eat enough protein to reduce the risk of sarcopenia.

Dr. Harold Bays, chief science officer of the Obesity Medicine Association, emphasizes that people taking GLP-1s need to pay careful attention to proper hydration. They must also be careful simply to take in a sufficient amount of energy each day. It's not easy. People who are on the drugs want to lose weight, and they know they need to decrease their calories to do so. Some patients struggle to find the right balance between enjoying their reduced appetite and eating enough to stay healthy. As previously noted, these patients are at risk of developing eating disorders.

Anyone taking a GLP-1 medication for weight loss should prioritize eating nutrient-dense foods, and pay special attention to getting adequate protein (approximately 25 to 30 grams per meal), fiber (at least 25 grams per day for women and 30 grams per day for men), and water. Protein is vital for muscle synthesis, cell health and repair, metabolism, neurotransmitter signaling, and hormone formation. It also boosts metabolic calorie burn and promotes satiety, which is beneficial when consuming less food. Adequate protein intake also helps maintain lean muscle mass during significant weight loss. Dietary fiber, found in vegetables, fruits, legumes, and whole grains, is vital for satiety, rich in vitamins and minerals, and acts as a key prebiotic for the gut microbiome. Because the gut microbiome aids in maintaining a healthy weight, getting enough dietary fiber is crucial for healthy weight loss.

Caloric intake isn't the only factor controlling weight loss, but a calorie deficit is crucial for losing weight. Calorie recommendations vary based on age, gender, activity level, metabolism, and health conditions. Although there are many easily accessible tools to estimate your personal daily calorie needs, they can be quite inaccurate. The best and safest approach is to consult with a professional to determine your suitable daily calorie targets. Again, my big note of caution is to be on the lookout for malnutrition.

Adjusting therapy and monitoring progress are crucial for people on GLP-1 medications. As a general guide, users should follow up with their medical care providers monthly to quarterly in early stages of taking GLP-1s, and once or twice a year in the maintenance stage. It is also important to pick a doctor or caretaker who knows obesity medicine and is trained to work with nutritionists and dietitians. Common GLP-1 titration protocols, in which the doses in the injections are gradually increased over three months, are designed to help patients adapt to the drugs, but they can raise the risk of side effects as the dosage goes up.

If you decide to go on anti-obesity drugs, remember that every individual reacts differently. Just because a friend or family member had one experience does not mean yours will be the same. You should consult with your medical care providers to adjust your dosages based on your amount of weight loss, side effects, and overall tolerance. In general, patients are advised to take the lowest effective dose for weight loss.

The Role of Supplements

A physician recently told me about a patient who had contacted her about baffling symptoms. They included fatigue, a finger cut that wouldn't heal, mild joint pain, and spontaneous bruising that seemed to be getting worse. Tests showed no blood abnormalities. The patient was on a very-low-calorie diet and taking tirzepatide, prescribed by another doctor. The physician suspected the patient had scurvy, a severe vitamin C deficiency, and tests confirmed the hunch. This odd case highlights another section that belongs in the GLP-1 user's manual: How to Avoid Micronutrient Deficiency When Drastically Cutting Calories.

For centuries, scurvy was the scourge of sailors. Before modern refrigeration, they had no access to vitamin C–rich fruits and vegetables during long voyages. The condition is rare in the modern industrialized world. Many doctors have never encountered it in the flesh. In this case, it was linked to the patient's taking an anti-obesity medication. And scurvy is not the only micronutrient-related problem I've heard about in people taking the new anti-obesity drugs. Another physician told me about a patient, also taking a GLP-1 drug, with Wernicke-Korsakoff syndrome, a sudden, acute memory disorder caused by a lack of thiamine, or vitamin B_1.

Our bodies make only a few of the vitamins we need to stay well, and none of the minerals. We need to get essential micronutrients from our diet. It's not surprising, then, that severe caloric restriction leaves people vulnerable to micronutrient deficiencies. And yet, more than three years after the FDA approved GLP-1 medication for treating obesity, there is still no published research on how this class of drugs affects nutrient absorption or vitamin levels.

What we do know is that micronutrient deficiencies are common among people following low-calorie diets: More than half have been found to be deficient in vitamin D, 30 to 50% are iron-deficient, up to 30% are deficient in calcium, and 20 to 30% have low levels of magnesium.

Unfortunately, there is no reliable guidance on dietary supplementation for GLP-1 patients. The supplement industry has seized on this information vacuum by marketing products claiming to fill GLP-1 nutrient gaps. Whether these supplements are safe or efficacious is anyone's guess. In the United States, the industry operates with little government oversight. The absence of evidence-based recommendations and consumer protections is particularly troubling given that most candidates for GLP-1 therapy have micronutrient deficiencies before they even start the drugs. People with obesity are more likely to be nutrient deficient than the population at large.

Metabolic alterations, oxidative stress in fat tissue, and other biochemical changes that occur during major weight loss can increase the body's demand for micronutrients even further. So can interaction with other medications such as metformin, which is sometimes prescribed with GLP-1 drugs. German nutrition researcher Dr. Antje Damms-Machado and her colleagues studied thirty-two people who followed an 800-calorie-a-day liquid diet for three months and lost, on average, forty-three pounds. The participants were deficient in various vitamins and minerals before they began the regimen and showed no improvement from the diet, even though their meal-replacement formula was suffused with micronutrients at amounts often higher than recommended for the general population. In fact, even more people had low levels of vitamin C, zinc, lycopene, and calcium at the end of the diet.

Dr. Almandoz and colleagues offer general guidance to clinicians who prescribe weight-loss drugs: identify pre-existing nutrient deficits in patients, monitor their nutrient intake, and recommend supplementation with a complete multivitamin, plus calcium and vitamin D as needed. But even when patients receive advice like this, following it isn't simple. Vitamin and mineral supplements vary widely in quality and potency, and the FDA does little to test these products or to substantiate their safety.

Taking a multivitamin with additional calcium and vitamin D might be sufficient to compensate for the effects of caloric reduction, but an obesity medicine specialist will be able to provide more specific advice, including insights about other micronutrients, such as iron, magnesium, and zinc.

Why Nutrition Still Matters

The introduction of GLP-1 drugs is prompting doctors and patients alike to question whether the basic rules of weight loss have changed. In an era of such powerful anti-obesity medicines, is there still a role for traditional dieting strategies?

We know from decades of experience that diet and exercise regimens are ineffective at keeping weight off over the long term. Why not skip that step, go straight to the new drugs, and worry less about what we eat? Most patients want or need to achieve more than the 4 to 7% weight loss that diets typically provide, and they dread the prospect of restricting themselves forever to a limited palette of foods, knowing that weight regain is practically inevitable anyway. Meanwhile, the GLP-1 drugs can routinely provide weight loss in the range of 15 to 20%, seemingly even without major behavioral changes. Looking only at the numbers, it's tempting to turn to drugs as the first (and maybe only) line of defense against obesity.

But drugs alone cannot end food addiction. First and foremost, nutrition is an essential part of everyone's lifelong health journey. In addition, GLP-1s are unlikely to be a permanent solution. The evidence today suggests that most people who try the anti-obesity drugs will eventually stop taking them, for a variety of reasons. Once people go off the GLP-1 drugs, they must find a sustainable eating plan that supports both weight loss and weight maintenance.

A key benefit of the new anti-obesity medications is not that they replace dieting—or, to be more precise, "nutrition therapy"—but that they can enhance its effectiveness. The drugs can help people learn to eat more healthfully and, just as significant, to recognize when to stop eating. Medication can help people make healthier food choices. At different points, an individual might rely more on medication to lose weight; at other points, they might rely solely on diet to maintain weight. In other words, nutrition therapy can add to the long-term effectiveness of the drugs, and the drugs can ease the path to healthy nutrition therapy.

Still, the widespread embrace of GLP-1 drugs contains an important cautionary message: Traditional approaches to diet are not adequate for dealing with modern food addiction. We need to tailor nutrition therapy to help treat the addiction and reduced satiety brought on by ultraformulated foods. We need to reduce people's reward-responsiveness and increase their satiety. For a significant part of the population, we also need to reduce glycemic variability, the sharp swings in blood sugar and hyperinsulinemia that stress the body and can lead to cardiometabolic abnormalities.

Nutrition therapy is foundational to all weight management. In many ways, drugs are the easy part of a weight-loss strategy. Nutrition is more challenging, but it is crucial to address. You have to make hundreds of dietary decisions each day. You can decide to go on drugs or off drugs, but you need to eat for the rest of your life. The failure to get nutrition right over the last fifty years has plunged us into a public health crisis.

Food Is Not the Enemy

I want to be very clear on an essential point: Food itself is not the problem. Common diet plans often treat food as an enemy to be conquered. Many patients talk about GLP-1s as a cure for indulgence. Even the avolition and aversive effects of the drugs can reinforce that message, seeming to imply that the way to lose weight and gain health is to lose the pleasure of eating. The loss of pleasure is one of my serious concerns about GLP-1s, because it reduces one of life's greatest joys.

In its natural form—whether plant, meat, or dairy—food does not generally trigger the addictive circuits in a major way. The real problem is ultraformulated food, which is really a very complex type of drug. As with any drug, the rate of absorption correlates with the drug potency. Many natural foods resist the rapid absorption of their nutrients and extraction of their energy. That is why few people crave a whole potato, an entire slab of beef, or a stick of butter. They don't stimulate the reward system in the way that triggers an intense reward response. It's only when we process these foods and alter their structure that we run into problems with excessive and compulsive eating.

Modern ultraformulated foods are insidious; their chemical trickery is hidden at the microscopic or molecular level so that we cannot see what they are doing to us. By the same token, we cannot directly sense what makes other foods healthy. Food is more than what we can see, taste, and smell; it holds a hidden world beneath its surface. This invisible structure dictates not only the nutritive value of a food, but also how our body processes it. This means a calorie is not always a calorie, and the nutrition label printed on the back of food packages does not always tell the whole story.

The intricate microstructure of a food influences the way our bodies absorb its nutrients. Microstructure refers to the small-scale arrangement of proteins, fats, carbohydrates, water, and other elements. For instance, meat consists of protein fibers grouped into larger bundles, with fat and water interspersed throughout. Cheese is a network of proteins that hold fat droplets and water. Bread is a network of gluten proteins that capture air bubbles, resulting in light and fluffy texture. These microscopic arrangements provide food with their distinct characteristics and influence how these foods are broken down by the digestive system.

Simply consuming certain nutrients does not guarantee that the body will be able to absorb them. Even if two food products have the same calorie count and identical nutrition labels, different microstructures can change how our body reacts to these products.

Before our bodies can use proteins, carbohydrates, and fats, these components must first be cleaved into their basic components: amino acids, monosaccharides, and fatty acids. The process takes place throughout the digestive system, with specialized molecules called enzymes acting like tiny scissors, cutting larger nutrients into the smaller units that the body can absorb. Micronutrients—vitamins and minerals—do not need to be cut into smaller pieces, but they still must be in the right form for our body to use them. Typically, micronutrients must be water-soluble, or dissolvable, to be absorbed by the body. A food's small-scale structure can also help or hinder the absorption of micronutrients.

A classic example of the effects of food processing is the difference between eating whole wheat grains versus eating finely ground wheat flour. Both come from the same wheat, so it might seem that they should provide the same nutrients. In reality, the processing that converts a grain into flour alters the microstructure of the wheat. Grinding the grain into small particles breaks apart its cellular structures, releasing previously trapped starches that our body can now quickly digest. The processing that alters the microstructure of wheat is the reason why eating a slice of bread raises blood glucose levels much more than eating an equivalent weight of whole-grain wheat bulgur. Physical alteration of any food's natural microstructure greatly influences our eating behaviors.

It's especially important to be aware of foods that can sit on supermarket shelves for weeks or months on end. Transforming plants, animals, and dairy foods into long-lasting products often requires the addition of large amounts of salt or sugar, not only to enhance taste but also to act as a preservative. These preservatives prevent spoilage bacteria from growing, which reduces the risk of foodborne illness. Without such additions, the convenience of shelf-stable grocery items would not be possible. Yet, the food industry has gone well beyond essential stability to make food hyper-palatable, which is why ultraformulated foods are so problematic.

Plant-Based Foods

Many people are shifting toward diets mostly or entirely made up of plant-based foods. There are many good reasons to make that change, including environmental sustainability and animal welfare. Plant-based diets can also provide health benefits and support weight loss or weight maintenance. But as with pretty much every aspect of nutrition, the details are complicated.

Plants are living organisms with their own survival strategies. Over millions of years, they have evolved defense mechanisms to make themselves a less nutritious meal for hungry animals. But animals have evolved over millions of years as well, adapting to the ways that plants deliver nutrition when eaten. A key distinction between plants and animals is that plant cells have tough, rigid walls made of fibrous materials like cellulose, hemicellulose, and lignin. These cell walls form barriers that protect the proteins, fats, and carbohydrates within the plant cells. In legumes like lentils or chickpeas, the proteins are not immediately accessible to the human digestive enzymes because they are locked inside the plant's cellular matrix.

Due to these walled-off structures, plant proteins are typically harder for our bodies to digest than animal-based proteins. Plant cells also contain anti-nutritional factors that greatly hinder protein digestion. These factors naturally slow the pace at which whole plant foods can be absorbed. For instance, many plants are rich in phytic acid, which binds to proteins in the plant cell, making them less accessible for digestion. Tannins, commonly found in foods like legumes and grains, inhibit the activity of digestive enzymes. Plant-based foods contain protein, but the arrangement of these anti-nutritional factors reduces how much of that protein our body can readily use.

For ages (hundreds of thousands of years, apparently) humans have been developing ways to process plant foods, altering the microstructure and improving their digestibility. The first big breakthrough was fire. Roasting, boiling, and steaming plants can soften and even begin to break down the fibrous cell walls, making the plants' proteins more accessible during digestion; high temperatures can also destroy anti-nutritional factors like lectins and tannins. Soaking legumes, seeds, and grains can force the phytic acid to leach out of the cell and into the water, freeing the once-bound proteins. But these early forms of processing were quite limited in effect compared to modern techniques of extrusion and chemical alteration.

Similar to the entrapped plant proteins, fats are also locked away behind cell walls. When we eat whole nuts, the intact walls make it difficult for our digestive enzymes to break down the fat, slowing digestion and absorption. Slow digestion, in turn, promotes feelings of satiety and helps manage blood lipid levels. When nuts are ground, the cellular structure is ruptured, making the fats more readily available for quicker digestion and utilization. Grinding makes it easier for our body to absorb fat-soluble compounds such as vitamins A, D, E, and K, but it also produces a much faster rush of energy.

Plant-based foods are rich in starches, which are often housed within the cell walls alongside fiber. Due to their large and complex structures, some, but not all, plant carbohydrates are more challenging to digest than simple sugars. Starchy vegetables and legumes such as lentils and chickpeas are further packed into granules that must be broken down into smaller components before they can be absorbed. Resistant starches are hard to digest because of their molecular structure. Their slow digestion has certain benefits, such as promoting satiety, and can provide a feeling of fullness that can last for several hours. Additionally, the gradual release of glucose into the bloodstream helps prevent rapid spikes in blood sugar levels.

In contrast, when starch is cooked and gelatinized, the granules burst open and become more porous, allowing increased digestion. Or, building on the earlier example, when wheat is ground into flour and then baked, the human digestive system can get much more rapid access to the starches within the wheat grains.

Plant cell walls are also a source of dietary fiber, another obstacle to digestion that comes with compensating health benefits. Fibrous molecules (including cellulose, hemicellulose, and pectin) sustain beneficial bacteria in the gut. Soluble fibers, like those found in oats and legumes, increase the viscosity of the contents in the stomach, slowing gastric release and increasing our feelings of fullness. In processed foods, the fiber is often pulverized or stripped away. Processing has transformed our relationship with our food.

Animal-Based Foods

Foods derived from animals also possess unique microstructures. At its core, meat is made up of muscle fibers, long, cylindrical bundles of the proteins called actin and myosin. Surrounding these bundles is a network of collagen, connective tissue that provides support and structure. Fat can be found in two different places. Intramuscular fat, also known as marbling, is dispersed throughout the proteins that make up the muscle fibers. Subcutaneous fat sits outside the muscle fibers and connective tissue, acting as a layer of insulation. The intricate arrangement of proteins, fat, and connective tissue in meat contributes to its texture and flavor, and also plays a critical role in how the body uses its nutrients.

Animal proteins are generally more digestible than plant proteins, primarily due to the lack of fibrous cell walls that obstruct and slow digestion. Unlike plant proteins, animal proteins also contain all the essential amino acids that humans need for important bodily functions. ("Essential" in this case means that the human body cannot make these amino acids, so we must consume them.) With no cell wall in the way, the fat in animal-based foods is also generally absorbed more efficiently than the fat in plant-based foods. Animal fats can supply the body with a rich, easily accessed energy source.

Animal-based foods contain minimal carbohydrates, making them a crucial part of a low-carb diet. Meat also has a high bioavailability of essential minerals, including iron, zinc, and phosphorus. In animal tissue, these minerals are found right next to proteins, often bound to them, making them readily absorbed in the digestive tract. The iron in meat, which is bound to a protein called heme, will be immediately recognized in our intestines and absorbed, whereas the non-heme iron found in plants is more likely to pass through the body unused. Foods from animal sources also do not contain the anti-nutritional elements commonly found in plant-based options. Then again, red meat, poultry, and fish do not contain any dietary fiber, so animal-based diets do not contribute to gut health in the same way that fiber-rich, plant-based foods do.

Processed meats present a unique challenge to human health and food addiction. A study led by researchers at the Harvard T. H. Chan School of

Public Health examined different categories of ultraprocessed foods and singled out processed meats (such as frozen chicken nuggets) as the one most correlated with increased overall risk of mortality. A separate report, based on data from the Nurses' Health Study, found a 14% increase in dementia risk among people who ate two servings a week of processed meats. Another study out of the Harvard T. H. Chan School of Public Health examined ten categories of ultraprocessed foods, focusing on their impact on cardiovascular disease. Processed meat, poultry, and fish stood out as one of two categories clearly correlated with elevated risk. That finding aligns with a great deal of other research linking meat-rich diets with higher bloodstream levels of low-density lipoprotein, the "bad," heart-harming form of cholesterol. The evidence is clear: Processed meats damage human health, and should be avoided regardless of weight-loss approach or goals for this reason.

Dairy Foods

Milk is a complex food made up of many different components that affect how our bodies digest and absorb nutrients. Structurally, it's considered an emulsion—a collection of tiny fat droplets dispersed throughout a watery liquid. This liquid contains sugars, vitamins, minerals, and two main types of proteins, casein and whey. Casein molecules clump together to form larger structures called micelles. Whey proteins float freely in the liquid. When milk is processed into yogurt and cheese, its structure changes, transforming from liquid into semi-solid gel. The casein creates a protein network that holds everything together, which has a large number of pores that trap whey, water, and fat.

The casein and whey in milk react quite differently in our digestive system. Casein is relatively difficult for digestive enzymes to break down, so it releases energy gradually. Whey proteins are smaller and not clumped together, so our enzymes can cleave these proteins right away, providing rapid energy. When casein proteins form a gel, they become even more challenging to digest because our enzymes must navigate through the pores of the casein network. Delayed digestion is part of the reason dairy products like yogurt lead to longer feelings of satiety than does a glass of milk. Solid and semi-solid foods also generally linger longer in the stomach than liquids do, because they need more time to mix with gastric juices and enzymes before they can be released into the intestines.

The dispersed fat droplets in cow's milk are tiny (about 1/10,000th of an inch in diameter), which makes them easy for enzymes to break down. Consequently, dairy fats are more readily processed and absorbed than fats from plant sources. Milk does not contain any dietary fiber.

Dairy-based foods primarily contain carbohydrates in the form of lactose, also known as milk sugar. Unlike the long chain carbohydrates found in plant-based foods, lactose is a simple sugar that is easy to digest. In our intestines, an enzyme called lactase slices lactose into two simpler sugars, glucose and galactose, that our bodies can absorb directly. Note that some people are lactose intolerant (unable to digest lactose) because their bodies don't make lactase. This condition is often linked to ancestry. Populations with a long history of consuming cow's milk, such as white Europeans, typically have higher levels of lactase in their bodies. Additionally, it is common for lactase to start working more slowly as people age, which can lead to lactose intolerance later in life.

Mammals produce milk to provide essential nutrients for their young, so it makes sense that milk's minerals (most notably calcium, magnesium, and phosphorus) are easy for our bodies to take in. Lactose can enhance calcium absorption by creating a slightly acidic environment in the intestines when our gut bacteria convert it into lactic acid. This acidity helps dissolve the calcium so it can be absorbed by the bloodstream more efficiently. Casein proteins in milk assist with mineral absorption, too. They bind to calcium and phosphorus, keeping these minerals in a form that is easier for our digestive system to process and helping to transport the minerals through the gut and into the bloodstream.

Most dairy products are not particularly ultraprocessed. One thing to watch out for with dairy products is added sugar. A 10-ounce commercial yogurt drink can contain more calories than a can of soda. Also, be aware that butter and cheese are often incorporated into high-fat, energy-rich foods without the consumer realizing it.

An Individual Approach to Nutrition Therapy

What is the "right way to eat" for proper nutrition and for weight management? With or without anti-obesity drugs in the mix, an effective nutrition therapy plan needs to take into account the difficult food environment we all live in. The truth is that plant-based, animal-based, and dairy foods each offer distinct benefits. The key factor is eating the food in an unprocessed or minimally processed state. When the natural microstructure of foods is altered during processing, the nutritional effects are altered, too. Eating whole foods, and avoiding highly processed foods, must be a central tenet of any health-promoting nutritional therapy plan.

At a meeting of the Obesity Society, Dr. Holly Wyatt presented the case of an imaginary patient named Lucy S., a fifty-five-year-old who comes to her doctor's office for help in managing her weight. She is frustrated with her previous attempts at weight loss, even though she knows it's important to do so for her health. Her family and friends try to be supportive but their advice collectively amounts to, "Stop eating so much." Up until the age of thirty, Lucy maintained a weight of about 140 pounds and then started slowly gaining weight. She currently weighs 172 pounds and is 5 feet 3 inches tall and has a BMI of 30 to 31, putting her in the obese category. Her past medical history is significant for hypertension and depression. She has a family history of coronary artery disease; her brother had coronary bypass surgery two years ago.

"What would you do with diet for this patient? What's the most important dietary factor for weight loss?" Dr. Wyatt asked. "Raise your hand if you think it's the number of calories. What if it's the amount of fat in the diet?" A couple of hands went up. "What about the amount of carbohydrates?" Again, a few hands went up.

Dr. Wyatt stressed the difference between weight loss and weight maintenance phases. Weight loss takes place over a finite period, usually months, during which the patient is in a negative energy balance. Fat burning is necessary and a reduction in calories is required. Weight-loss maintenance, on the other hand, is forever, or certainly over a long period of time. During weight-loss maintenance, the patient is in energy balance, maintaining intake with expenditure. Metabolic flexibility is needed to match that intake with expenditure, which usually requires high levels of physical activity.

For patients like Lucy S., who need to start by losing weight, Dr. Wyatt had a simple message: The defining issue for weight loss is how to get into negative energy balance. "You have to eat fewer calories than you are burning to lose weight. Now, that's not to say the macronutrient composition isn't important," she continued. "Where fat and carbohydrates come in is how they may influence how many calories you eat. But it's a myth that you can eat 6,000 calories [daily] and you won't gain weight as long as there are no carbohydrates. If people lose weight on a low-carb diet, they are losing it because they are eating fewer calories than they are burning."

For every patient, the exact journey is going to be different, depending on how they live and what they want to do. There are multiple approaches to nutrition therapy, but the principles behind them are always the same: The scientific evidence supports the essential requirement for an energy deficit.

Here is the rub with all diets: In the face of the addictive brain circuits and a harsh obesogenic environment, they are not sustainable for most people in the long term. The problem is that weight loss from dietary interventions, historically viewed as the product of sheer determination and willpower, fights against the hunger that is generated from the brain's homeostatic system and the cue-induced wanting that characterizes the brain's reward circuits.

Diets don't make the brain's homeostatic and reward circuits that drive overeating go away. Diets don't deal with the increased appetite caused by the reward system's responsiveness to cues in the environment. Increased appetite limits the effectiveness of all dietary interventions, and increased reward responsiveness from the addictive circuits and a decrease in satiety signals persist long after weight loss. In addition, without new learning that lays down new circuits, the brain's reward circuits continue to pull us to ultraformulated foods and wreak havoc.

Nutrition therapy will remain a go-to strategy for many patients. Most of us have tried all the popular diets. We know that all diet books are too good to be true. It doesn't mean there is no role for nutrition therapy, however. We need to shift away from the old-school caloric-reduction gimmicks to achieving energy deficits by limiting addictive foods. We need to increase the foods that satiate, and do so on a foundation of a healthy diet. Limit consumption of ultraformulated foods. Increase whatever makes us feel full, including increasing fiber, fats, and protein. The details will look a little different for every individual depending on life circumstances, state of health, and personal preferences, and those details will also change over time.

I asked Dr. Frank Hu, head of the nutrition department at the Harvard T. H. Chan School of Public Health, for his general guidance on what constitutes the foundations of a healthy diet. He responded that there are multiple layers of dietary recommendations. He visualizes a personalized diet pyramid. At the base would be common principles of a healthy diet for everyone, including reducing ultraformulated foods and increasing fruits and vegetables. The next layer would be a little more individualized, perhaps low-carb, more protein, but focusing on healthy sources of protein and fat (such as olive oil, nuts, and fish) rather than saturated fat. And he recognizes that some people may prefer vegetarian or vegan diets.

I asked Dr. Hu if the method of restriction makes a difference in terms of the health benefits that can be achieved. "We don't know," he said. "Probably not much difference. The outcome is the level of BMI you're able to achieve and maintain. It can be done by daily caloric restriction or through time-restricted eating or other methods. But the goal is to achieve a lower BMI, within normal range of BMIs, through diet, exercise, and other lifestyle strategies, or nowadays, through GLP-1 agonists. We don't know if a lower BMI achieved through diet or lifestyle versus drugs has the same long-term outcome. That's going to be a very interesting research question."

"Separate out weight for the moment," I said to him. "For people living with obesity, if you don't change body weight, does eating healthy reduce cardiovascular risk?"

"The answer is very clear. Improving diet quality can have benefits on cardiometabolic risk independent of body weight," he replied. "Data from the largest dietary intervention trial on cardiac disease showed that after five years of diet intervention, cardiovascular disease was reduced by 30% despite very little change in weight among participants. Also, numerous observational epidemiological studies show diet quality is associated with lower risk of cardiovascular disease after adjustment for BMI."

It would be a terrible mistake to say that one should focus only on drugs for weight loss and maintenance. In the end, we need to change the food preferences that were set and reinforced in our brains for us by the food industry. We will need to make use of various tools—used holistically, in various combinations—to improve our health outcomes.

17

. . . .

The Role of Insulin Resistance

Long before GLP-1s were approved for use in treating obesity, they were developed and prescribed to treat diabetes. A common thread between diabetes and obesity is insulin, the hormone responsible for managing blood glucose and all body tissues, including muscle, fat, and liver. GLP-1 compounds help regulate insulin levels in the body, counteracting the modern diet—full of high-glycemic-index foods. When the body loses the ability to produce and use insulin properly, the result is a cascade of weight and health problems.

Insulin resistance occurs when certain tissues in the body become less responsive to insulin's function in aiding glucose absorption in skeletal muscles and fat cells. It is a significant metabolic dysfunction that involves a systemic miscommunication between insulin and other tissues in the body, including fat, muscle, and the liver. In muscle tissue, insulin resistance reduces the absorption of glucose from food. In fat cells, it strongly promotes fat storage. In the liver, it can trigger an overproduction of glucose, disrupting overall blood glucose balance.

Insulin signals the liver and muscles to store excess glucose in the form of glycogen, which functions as stored energy in the body. You tap into your glycogen reserves when you exercise, for example. But once glycogen stores are at capacity, additional glucose is converted into fats known as triglycerides and are transported to fat cells (adipocytes) for long-term storage. The liver and muscles serve as short-term reservoirs for glycogen, while fat cells offer almost unlimited capacity for storing triglycerides. This system allows the body to maintain a reliable supply of stored energy.

During periods of fasting, whether between meals, while sleeping, or through intentional fasting, insulin levels naturally decrease. The drop signals the body to draw upon its available energy, first tapping into glycogen reserves. As these reserves diminish, the body shifts to burning fat. When insulin levels are high, the body's ability to tap into fat stores for energy is reduced. Because insulin levels typically increase in response to rising blood glucose, a pattern emerges. Elevated glucose triggers more insulin, creating a reinforcing cycle in which high glucose and insulin levels persist, continually disrupting the body's ability to break down fat.

Under normal circumstances, insulin maintains blood glucose within a narrow range by promoting glucose uptake into cells for storage or energy use. In the case of insulin resistance, blood glucose levels rise. To compensate, the pancreas produces more insulin. Over time, this increased demand can overwhelm the pancreas, leading to persistent high blood glucose levels, or hyperglycemia. Hyperglycemia stimulates the liver to convert excess glucose into fat. Because the liver is crucial for managing glucose, this extra fat disrupts its function, further aggravating insulin resistance. Addressing both liver fat and insulin resistance is therefore a primary goal for diabetes management.

"It has become clear that the accumulation of fat in the liver is a direct cause of insulin resistance, setting the scene for the development of type 2 diabetes," says Dr. Roy Taylor, professor of medicine and metabolism at Newcastle University and a leading expert in diabetes research. His clinical studies show that a consistent reduction in calorie intake can eliminate excess fat within the liver. Insulin can operate effectively again, decreasing the liver's glucose release into the bloodstream, normalizing fasting blood glucose levels, and even fully resolving insulin resistance.

We know that insulin-resistant individuals should avoid carbohydrates. The conventional wisdom is that obesity leads to metabolic changes and insulin resistance. The mainstream medical view is that obesity comes first. Obesity results in increased adipose tissue mass. At some point, the fat mass can no longer handle the large number of fatty acids. Then the fatty acids spill over into the blood, leading to ectopic fat deposition in various organs, including muscle, which causes lipotoxicity (a harmful accumulation of fatty molecules in the body), inhibited insulin signaling, and the development of insulin resistance. Insulin resistance leads to elevated insulin levels and hyperinsulinemia.

I have long wondered whether it's the other way around and hyperinsulinemia causes insulin resistance. Insulin is produced and released by the pancreas in response to blood glucose levels. Secretion happens in pulses and is proportional to changes in glucose, other hormones such as GLP-1s, and nutrients, including proteins and fats. Secreted insulin enters the portal vein on its way to the liver. During this "first pass" through the liver, approximately two-thirds of the insulin is pulled out of the circulation and degraded by liver cells. The other third enters the general circulation, which acts on muscles and adipose tissue to promote glucose into cells and suppress glucose production in the liver. When the insulin circulates back to the liver a second time, insulin is further extracted from the circulation.

Dr. Jens Holst and his team in Copenhagen have shown that high carbohydrate consumption and excess energy intake can hinder the clearance of insulin by the liver, affecting the insulin concentration in the body. Dr. Holst and his team studied test subjects and found that short-term carbohydrate overfeeding leads to increased fasting blood insulin concentrations and reduced insulin clearance. Excess carbohydrate intake also promotes liver fat production, leading to increased triglycerides in the liver, which is associated with reduced insulin clearance. In turn, excess insulin secretion after eating a carb-rich meal can saturate the insulin receptors in the liver, further decreasing insulin clearance and leading to hyperinsulinemia. Conversely, a high-fat/low-carbohydrate intake increases insulin clearance.

Dr. Holst and his collaborators conclude that increases in energy and carbohydrate availability are important mediators in the development of systemic hyperinsulinemia. The bottom line is that a high-calorie, high-carbohydrate diet significantly decreases insulin clearance and increases fasting plasma insulin concentrations in the body. This effect is more pronounced with higher carbohydrate intake.

According to Dr. Holst, reduced blood insulin clearance is the initial culprit in the development of hyperinsulinemia. A team led by his colleague Dr. Annemarie Lundsgaard has gone on to demonstrate that diets with reduced carbohydrate and increased fat intake can improve whole-body glucose metabolism and reduce insulin resistance. These studies do not prove that consuming a lot of carbohydrates causes hyperinsulinemia. However, they do suggest a strong link between high carbohydrate intake and reduced insulin clearance, which contributes to higher insulin levels in the blood and reinforces the importance of reducing carbohydrates in the diet.

Hyperinsulinemia: Too Much Insulin

Hyperinsulinemia appears to be the key to metabolic disease. Hyperinsulinemia, insulin resistance, gain of visceral fat, and glucose metabolism are so intertwined that it has been difficult to determine what comes first. There are ways to tease them apart, however. Medical scientists sometimes look at certain genetic diseases as natural experiments that help unravel the mechanism underlying a disease or condition. Prader-Willi syndrome, a genetic disease of children who become ravenously hungry and have decreased satiety, may be very illuminating in this regard. Prader-Willi is a rare and distinctive syndrome, affecting about one person in twenty thousand worldwide, but I think the general mechanism leading to increased appetite can inform us about common obesity.

Individuals with Prader-Willi typically progress through several distinct nutritional phases during their lifetime. Before birth, babies show reduced movement and growth, leading to smaller birth size. After birth, infants start out with poor appetite and feeding difficulties, but their appetite improves and they gain weight typically. As children with Prader-Willi grow older, they start to gain weight rapidly, without an increase in appetite or food intake; then they show more interest in food but can still feel full, with rising insulin levels leading to more weight gain and increased fat mass.

Eventually, individuals with Prader-Willi transition into phase 3, which can span from childhood into adulthood. During this phase, they develop a ravenous appetite and engage in aggressive food-seeking behavior, struggling to feel full no matter how much they eat. This phase is characterized by high insulin levels, making the body resistant to these hormones and leading to constant hunger and severe obesity. "It's a remarkable syndrome in terms of going from virtually no appetite to this insatiable appetite," said Dr. Daniel Driscoll, a clinical geneticist at University of Florida who has studied Prader-Willi syndrome extensively.

The sequence leading to intense eating in Prader-Willi syndrome, Dr. Driscoll has demonstrated, begins in childhood, when insulin levels rise significantly, resulting in rapid weight gain without an increase in food intake. As insulin levels continue to rise, individuals develop their increased interest in food and gain fat mass. Finally, the transition to phase 3 involves the body becoming resistant to insulin. "They will eat food from the garbage, they'll steal food. Several individuals have had gastric necrosis and burst their stomachs from the insatiable appetite," said Dr. Driscoll.

Dr. Driscoll thinks, and I agree, that Prader-Willi syndrome can help us to understand the broader problem of obesity. Hyperinsulinemia is a probable trigger for the weight gain and massive overeating in individuals with the syndrome, Dr. Driscoll has concluded, with insulin acting both as an initiating factor and an ongoing driver of hyperphagia and weight gain. Elevated insulin signaling may be the driving force behind the transitions through the various nutritional phases. Dr. Driscoll says he can help young Prader-Willi patients control their eating using a combination of a low-carb/low-glycemic-level diet and drugs; early clinical trials show some success using diazoxide choline, a compound long used for emergency treatment of hypoglycemia. Both the dietary and drug interventions affect the onset and severity of obesity and hyperphagia in these children by controlling insulin levels.

While weight is important for improving overall health, improvements in insulin sensitivity may be as important. When I work on ways to reduce obesity, I am focused mostly on visceral fat. As we have seen, while all fat can cause health problems, visceral fat is unique in causing the inflammatory conditions that are associated with cardiometabolic disease. Treating metabolic disease that results from visceral fat may be more of a priority than treating weight. It is estimated that less than 10% of Americans are metabolically healthy. In addition, research suggests that metabolic damage begins very early in life. Children consume 67% of their calories from ultraformulated foods. It can even begin as early as the first days of life. Over the last several decades, according to an analysis by Dr. Dina DiMaggio of NYU Langone Medical Center, about half of all formulas contain corn syrup solids. Dr. Nancy Krebs at the University of Colorado showed that a measurement of insulin release called C-peptide quadruples in infants consuming such formulas with corn syrups.

Also, cancer is on the rise in young people, including breast, endometrial, and colorectal cancer. Deaths from cancer are two to three times higher in Black and Native Americans. I asked cancer biochemist Dr. Lewis Cantley at Harvard, who studies the drivers of cancers' growth, about the role of elevated insulin levels. "I'm pretty convinced that high serum insulin levels contribute to the growth of certain cancers," he said. He made the connection between elevated insulin and cancer because his laboratory discovered an enzyme called phosphatidylinositol 3-kinase, encoded by the PIK3CA gene. Mutations in that gene cause cancer and also lead to the enzyme becoming overly responsive to insulin. This heightened sensitivity significantly increases glucose uptake in cells with these mutations, which is essential for supporting cancer growth. Without the increase in insulin, Dr. Cantley says, the tumors would be held in check by other genes that suppress tumors. According to him, the strong correlation between obesity and cancer rates is probably due to the fact that people living with obesity have high serum insulin. While there are other hormones that can also activate the enzyme, none do it as effectively as insulin. It's critical that we sort out whether the rise in these cancers is being fueled by diet and insulin.

Both excess energy consumption and a high-carbohydrate diet drive hyperinsulinemia. Hyperinsulinemia is thought to drive the accumulation of visceral fat and the resulting inflammatory and metabolic damage associated with obesity. A recent study by UCLA's Chyue Wu shows the prevalence of hyperinsulinemia increased dramatically, from 28 to 41%, from 1999 to 2018. There is an epidemic of hyperinsulinemia that is unfolding.

Eating to Avoid Insulin Resistance

Hyperinsulinemia and insulin resistance often occur along with obesity and insufficient physical activity and are linked to health issues such as high blood pressure and elevated blood lipids. To detect insulin resistance, it's important to consider tests that reflect these connections. While specialized tests that measure insulin and glucose responses aren't easily accessible, simpler indicators such as waist circumference, blood triglycerides, and glucose levels are common measures.

An increased waist circumference typically signifies excess abdominal fat, a key indicator of insulin resistance. Abdominal fat, or visceral adiposity, releases free fatty acids and inflammatory markers that can disrupt glucose metabolism. Given that insulin is crucial for regulating fat metabolism, elevated triglyceride levels and other lipid abnormalities are commonly linked to insulin resistance. Fasting blood glucose levels offer a direct measure of how effectively the body manages glucose, with higher levels indicating the presence of insulin resistance.

A waistline over 40 inches in men and 35 inches in women, a fasting triglyceride level over 150 milligrams per deciliter (mg/dL), and a fasting glucose level over 100 mg/dL are signs of insulin resistance.

Dietary strategies for managing insulin resistance share similarities with strategies for managing type 2 diabetes, since both conditions involve impaired glucose metabolism. For insulin resistance, the emphasis is on foods that enhance insulin sensitivity and overall metabolic health. Managing type 2 diabetes involves stricter alignment of carbohydrate intake and blood glucose levels to coordinate with insulin or medication dosages. For insulin resistance and type 2 diabetes, weight loss is a primary goal. Dr. Katarzyna Gołąbek, dietetics expert at Wrocław Medical University in Poland, asserts that managing calories to reduce body mass should be the cornerstone of dietary recommendations, as reducing even a small percentage of body weight can improve insulin sensitivity.

The low-glycemic-index and moderate-carbohydrate diets endorsed by many of the nutrition and obesity experts also seem to be helpful in reducing insulin resistance along with reducing visceral fat. A study conducted by Dr. Valene Garr Barry at the University of Alabama at Birmingham demonstrated that, among middle-aged participants with insulin resistance, people who followed a low-carb, high-fat plan lost more visceral fat compared to those on a low-fat diet. Dr. Amy Goss, also at University of Alabama, has shown that a ketogenic diet in aging adults with obesity may improve body composition by reducing fat mass relative to lean muscle. Supporting these findings, a 2022 study involving two hundred participants living with obesity compared the effects of a low-carb ketogenic diet with a low-calorie, low-fat diet. The results showed that those on the low-carb diet had greater reductions in overall weight, fat mass, and visceral fat without negatively impacting cholesterol levels.

A study led by Dr. Hana Kahleova at the Physicians Committee for Responsible Medicine showed that a low-fat vegan diet also improved insulin sensitivity and led to weight loss in overweight adults. Dr. Christopher Gardner at the Stanford Prevention Research Center maintains that both low-calorie and low-carb diets can be effective if people can adhere to them over time. Ultimately, the most successful diet will be one that is easiest for an individual to maintain.

The Role of Fasting

Many people lose weight by altering not just what they eat, but *when* they eat. An especially effective timing strategy is intermittent fasting. It's another way to adjust your reward and satiety systems, reduce total caloric intake, and loosen the grip of food addiction. It's also a useful strategy for cutting carbohydrates and pushing back against insulin resistance by cutting overall caloric intake.

Intermittent fasting restricts eating to designated time periods. It has gained popularity because it offers a flexible and straightforward way to manage weight, and tends to appeal to those seeking an alternative to traditional calorie-restriction diets. It also fits well with the current trend in personalized nutrition, giving individuals the freedom to choose fasting periods that align with their preferences and daily routines. By alternating between periods of normal food intake and periods of very low or no food intake, intermittent fasting may help some people adhere to their eating plan by providing regular breaks from calorie restriction.

There is no consensus on the optimal duration, but some experts suggest a fasting window of at least fourteen hours. Most Americans consume food within a twelve-hour daily window. Typically, the fasting hours will coincide with sleep or occur when meals, like breakfast, are missed. To experience the benefits of intermittent fasting, the break from eating needs to extend beyond the standard twelve-hour time frame. Modified and intermittent fasting plans may allow between 50 and 500 calories on "fast" days. These calories are usually consumed as low-calorie liquids or supplements.

Dr. Lisa Chow at the University of Minnesota, who studies the treatment of insulin resistance and diabetes, has shown that many people eat for more than fifteen hours a day, with their only real break from eating occurring during sleep. "In short, people are eating all the time," she says. Her research links the length of a person's eating window to their body mass index, showing that a smaller eating window is associated with a lower BMI.

When eating is restricted to a set time window, many people consume fewer calories without consciously trying. This drop in calorie consumption helps create an energy deficit essential for weight loss. Additionally, intermittent fasting helps reinforce healthier eating patterns. Setting regular meal windows may encourage greater awareness of food choices and portion sizes, promoting habits that can support long-term weight management.

Several studies show that the caloric restriction that accompanies intermittent fasting is helpful in reducing insulin resistance.

Another potential benefit of intermittent fasting is improved metabolic flexibility. During fasting, the body transitions from relying primarily on glucose for energy to increasing fat oxidation, effectively utilizing stored fat. According to Dr. Courtney Peterson, a professor at the University of Alabama at Birmingham, this metabolic shift typically takes place after around fourteen to twenty-four hours of fasting, at which point a noticeable rise in fatty acid oxidation begins. The longer the fasting period, the more efficiently the body can mobilize fat reserves for energy.

As with every dieting and weight-loss strategy, I ask: How long does it last? The periodic and alternate-day fasting approach, which typically involves twenty-four hours of water-only intake repeated several times weekly or monthly, has been shown to be effective for short-term weight loss. However, it also tends to result in high hunger levels, complicating long-term adherence. There is conflicting evidence regarding its efficacy. For example, alternate-day modified fasting did not prove to be more effective for long-term weight loss than traditional dieting (continuous energy restriction), though it did show improvements in insulin sensitivity among people with insulin resistance. The high dropout rates suggest that maintaining this regimen long term can be difficult.

The good thing about intermittent fasting is that there are so many variations that people can adapt to their own preferences. I do not like to fast for prolonged periods, but I have little problem consuming a very low number of calories on some days.

The fasting mimicking diet, created by Dr. Valter Longo as an alternative to traditional fasting for cancer patients, shows signs of enduring efficacy. This diet mimics the effects of fasting while allowing limited food intake. The diet is low in calories, protein, and carbohydrates, with an emphasis on unsaturated fats. Typically, it's followed for three to five days and repeated no more than once a month. According to Dr. Peterson, "After doing three cycles spread over a period of three months of the fasting mimicking diet, participants did lose weight and keep that off in the long term."

Intermittent fasting is a behavioral adjustment as much as a dietary one, so people's personal responses have a big impact on their ability to maintain the program. Many fasters report positive experiences, and some individuals experience improvements in metabolic markers, such as enhanced insulin sensitivity and better blood glucose levels. For others, the real benefit is simplified meal planning, which makes it easier to prioritize healthier food choices.

Still, some dieters struggle to maintain longer fasts. Fasts of eighteen hours, for example, can interfere with social eating situations and other aspects of daily life. A serious difficulty for most people is hunger or intense cravings during fasting periods, which can lead to overeating or opting for less nutritious foods during timed meals and snacks. Intermittent fasting should be approached with caution during pregnancy or by people who are managing diabetes or hypoglycemia. It is also risky for people who have eating disorders, as Dr. Nicole Spartano of Boston University School of Medicine notes: "If someone has a tendency toward anorexia or binge eating, fasting could worsen those issues."

Overall, though, intermittent fasting is proving to be an effective component of a comprehensive weight management strategy. Adjusting the times you eat is a quintessential example of behavior change. The documented benefits of intermittent fasting demonstrate that, in addition to drugs and nutrition, behavior is an important factor in the journey toward achieving and maintaining a healthy weight.

18

. . . .

Eating to Support Health

Every five years, the US Department of Agriculture and the Department of Health and Human Services provide updated guidelines on what people should eat and drink to meet their nutrient needs, to promote health, and to prevent disease. But these guidelines are written for healthy people at a time when the number of people who fit that description is dwindling.

Nearly a thousand deaths a day are linked to diet-related disease in the United States alone, and about 90% of the annual $4.5 trillion healthcare spending is attributed to managing and treating chronic diseases and mental health conditions. We need dietary guidelines to address the needs of the majority of the population that is overweight, obese, and/or insulin resistant or prediabetic. And we need guidelines that are flexible enough to provide vital health benefits for people whether or not they are taking antiobesity drugs.

There is also a whole other emerging need: dietary rules for people who stop taking the GLP-1s, a new and fast-growing population. There is proof that people can sustain weight loss after stopping GLP-1 drugs. The key is to find another effective tool for after the medications are stopped.

Virta Health, a company that specializes in providing carbohydrate-restricted nutrition therapy for patients with type 2 diabetes, studied individuals who took either semaglutide or tirzepatide and later discontinued those medications. Company researchers showed that patients who stopped taking medication and went on a low-carbohydrate diet with nutrition counseling were able to maintain their weight after stopping the medication. Weight remained stable during the eighteen months that patients were followed after they stopped taking medication. Not only did the program involve a low-carbohydrate diet, but it also provided intensive behavioral coaching. That built-in accountability is in no small part the reason for the success.

The conventional wisdom is that low-carb diets are hard to sustain for the long term. I asked the study's principal investigator, Dr. Shaminie Athinarayanan, at Virta, about the number of patients dropping out of the study. "With the right support and guidance, this lifestyle intervention can be maintained over the long term," she said. "In our clinical trial, we observed remarkable retention rates. At two years, 74% of participants remained in the study. We extended the trial and 87% of those who stayed through the two-year mark opted to continue." When I asked if she thought a healthy low-carb diet could really work when a patient was off the drug, she responded, "Yes, absolutely. A healthy low-carb diet can be effective if it is highly personalized to suit individual needs and preferences."

Surprisingly, this is the only study that has explored dietary interventions for after the medication is stopped. Then again, maybe I shouldn't have been surprised, because it's not in the pharmaceutical industry's interest to come up with alternatives. But those studies will happen, and we will learn more about how to sustain weight loss after going off GLP-1 medications. If people need help resetting their weight, going back on medication for a period of time is certainly an option.

There is an important question about intermittent use that needs to be answered. In discussions with colleagues at the FDA, some wondered if there was a chance the GLP-1 medications would become less effective over time if one adopted an on-and-off strategy. With certain other drugs that affect the brain, there is a change in receptors that can lead to the drugs' diminished efficacy over time. There's no evidence of this at present with the GLP-1 drugs, but it's a question that needs to be investigated.

With all that in mind, I sought out experts in health and nutrition and asked for their views on improving our diets—not for some idealized, healthy population, but for a population that is increasingly burdened by toxic visceral fat and insulin resistance, and that is increasingly turning to pharmaceutical treatments for help.

A surprising trend I noted in their replies was consensus on a diet that is lower in rapidly digestible carbohydrates, especially processed carbs, and is generally lower in grains overall. In particular, nutrition experts are zeroing in on the hazards of carbs with a high-glycemic index, which is a measure of how a food affects blood sugar levels after being consumed. High-glycemic carbs break down rapidly and flood the body with glucose. It is those carbohydrates that are causing metabolic chaos and dragging down our health.

Carbohydrate Quantity and Quality

Until recently, doctors and scientists who advocated low-carb diets were viewed as on the fringe. They had separate meetings and had to form their own societies. The meetings had a cult-like feeling, with zeal sometimes mixed with a reluctance to fully understand the range of consequences of their approach. Despite that, it appears they were right about the deleterious role of processed carbohydrates on human health.

"Low-carbohydrate" typically means getting less than 10 to 20% of daily calories from carbohydrates. In contrast, general dietary guidelines recommend that 45 to 65% of daily calories come from carbohydrates. Low-carb diets also tend to increase the proportion of protein and fat intake, which promotes satiety, leading to prolonged feelings of fullness. In the context of weight management and appetite regulation, low-carbohydrate diets help stabilize blood glucose levels, which prevents the sharp fluctuations that can trigger hunger. Additionally, as the body shifts from using glucose to using ketones—produced from the breakdown of triglycerides—as an energy source, hunger is further suppressed.

Due to these metabolic changes and appetite reduction, low-carbohydrate diets often result in more rapid initial weight loss than other diets. This rapid weight reduction prompts questions about whether the lost weight is predominantly fat or water. For managing insulin resistance, the primary objective is to reduce liver fat.

But the focus solely on low-carb diets misses an important point, says Dr. Walter Willett, a professor at the Harvard T. H. Chan School of Public Health. "It's about the *quality* of carbohydrates. The carbs should be whole grain and high fiber. Avoid foods strongly associated with weight gain, like refined carbohydrates, potatoes, corn, and peas and instead consume whole grains, yogurt, fruits, and vegetables." According to him, the optimal diet for the insulin-resistant population has recommendations similar to the average population, focusing on reducing refined carbohydrates and high-glycemic foods.

Dr. Gardner is even more negative than Dr. Willett in his views toward carbohydrates. Dr. Gardner says the optimal diet for an insulin-resistant person is a plant-based Mediterranean diet with no added sugar and no refined grains. He suggests that 50 to 55% of calories come from fat and fewer calories from carbs. "Whenever you say 'low carb,' it's low carb *compared to what*? Compared to the dietary guidelines recommendation of 45 to 65% of calories from carbs? Yes, people should be eating less than that because most of that is wheat," he says.

Dr. Gardner reports that for the average American, 40% of calories come from refined grains and sugar. "If there's anything I'm willing to give up, it's grains, all grains. Even with durum wheat and whole-wheat bread, it's still processed, with the same glycemic index as white bread. Americans eat so much wheat, it's amazing—most of the US grains are bread, pizza crust, bagels, and such." He says he'd like to see the average American follow a high-fat Mediterranean diet with about 40% of calories from carbs. What he calls the "Mediterranean-Plus" diet has the additional restriction of avoiding added sugars and refined grains.

Dr. Gardner's research has focused on the potential health benefits of various food patterns and dietary components. In a recent trial, he randomized 609 adults who were living with overweight or obesity to either a healthy low-carb or a healthy low-fat diet. Its results showed similar weight loss and improvements in metabolic health markers with a low-fat diet and a low-carb diet. He says low-fat and low-carb diets can both work for weight loss; the choice is more about which route is easier to adhere to for a given individual.

Dr. Gardner's study aimed to determine whether improvements in diet quality or changes in macronutrient composition were associated with differential weight loss when someone was on either a low-carb or a low-fat diet. But the study also tracked individual differences in insulin production and certain genetic components that have been shown to alter an individual's response to dietary macronutrient composition. The researchers found that there was a difference between low-carb and low-fat diets for reducing visceral adipose tissue. "Low carb was better," he says.

At the University of California, Irvine, Dr. Matthew Landry is researching the optimal diets for preventing chronic disease. His current work focuses on the benefits of plant-based diets. "At the end of the day, I think both low-fat and low-carb diets end up with a lot of the same health outcomes," he said recently. "Taking a step back, I think the bigger thing that impacts health is a plant-based diet, removing meat. That has always been of bigger interest to me."

As an optimal diet, Dr. Landry recommends a moderate low-carbohydrate plant-based diet. "Going completely to the vegan side is ambitious for many individuals," he says. "I still think we can get some benefits at just a vegetarian diet, or even just this flexible mostly vegetarian but occasionally omnivorous diet. You can still do some dairy, some eggs. I might exclude whole grains for the insulin-resistant person."

Lower Carb Versus Ketogenic Diets

Within the obesity medicine field, there is a debate on whether to follow a more moderate low-carb eating pattern or a more restrictive, ketogenic pattern. "There are two camps. There's the camp that follows a low-carb ketogenic diet, and there is a camp that recommends a modified lower-carb, higher-protein diet based on what the patient can sustain," said Dr. Angela Golden, who runs an obesity management practice in Flagstaff, Arizona.

I spoke to one expert on ketogenic diets, Dr. Eric Westman, director of the Duke Keto Medicine Clinic in North Carolina, who defended the keto diet, arguing that the formula for weight loss can be boiled down to one direct, uncomplicated statement: If you can push your metabolism into ketosis by cutting carbohydrates instead of using glucose for fuel, you will start burning body fat. "Fat burning, or ketosis, happens naturally," Dr. Westman said. "After two or three days of fasting, everyone goes into nutritional ketosis. If you eat carbs, you'll burn the carbs before you can burn the fat off your body. To burn fat, just don't eat carbs."

What Dr. Westman doesn't deal with is that if you cut carbs but eat fat instead of those carbs, the body has to burn that additional fat, resulting in no net loss of fat. Even though he doesn't tell people on low-carb diets to restrict calories, they are restricting calories. Although the specifics of ketogenic diets can vary, most focus on significant decreases in carbohydrate consumption. A healthy ketogenic diet will also avoid ultraformulated and refined foods. Ketogenic diet plans generally allow balanced intake of saturated, monounsaturated, and polyunsaturated fats. Such diets are also associated with negative outcomes in some patients, including raising low-density lipoprotein ("bad") cholesterol (LDL-C) and causing fatigue and brain fog at some stages of the diet.

To achieve ketosis, you have to limit your carb intake to between 20 and 30 grams per day, maybe up to 50 grams for some people. Dr. Westman acknowledges that the advice "just don't eat carbs" will be difficult to follow for patients who suffer from cravings for sugar or bread, but he claims that high-protein, very-low-carb diets have the same effect on appetite as GLP-1 drugs. "In my practice, I don't use drugs. You can get the same result, the same reduction in appetite as GLP-1, if you just cut out carbs. The food noise goes away," he told me.

The big question I had for Dr. Westman was how sustainable the keto lifestyle is. My experience has been that people can stick with Atkins or similar diets for a time and lose weight, but sooner or later, they will revert to their old eating habits and gain it all back. He insists that a low-carb approach can be sustainable. "I've had people on very-low-carb diets for twenty years."

I asked Dr. Westman if he had a diet for people who want to get off GLP-1 drugs and sustain their weight. "The company wants you on them forever. The State of North Carolina stopped paying for the drugs because they are breaking the bank," he first said. Then he answered my question: "It's low-carb keto." But most doctors working in obesity medicine are a lot more flexible than Dr. Westman is in their views of a strict ketogenic diet.

What I am hearing in talking to the experts is a general convergence on a lower-carbohydrate (or moderately lower-carb), plant-predominant eating pattern. Interestingly, I note that some of the people who had advocated for a high-fat, hard keto diet have eased up on that recommendation because, for some people, such an eating plan is hard to sustain. It seems that everybody is meeting in the middle: lower carbs; healthy fats; lean, non-processed meat; lots of whole, non-starchy vegetables; and low-glycemic foods. And everyone agrees that ultraformulated, high-glycemic-index foods are the enemy of weight loss and good health.

Addressing Concerns About Low-Carb Eating Patterns

Cardiologists for decades were focused on reducing fat in the diet, especially saturated fat. Yet, in talking to three of the leading preventive cardiologists in the world, Dr. Peter Libby, Dr. Brian Ference, and Dr. Jorge Plutzky, I learned that none were overly concerned about patients choosing a low-carbohydrate diet that might increase their fat or saturated fat intake.

They want to see their patients who have increased visceral adiposity lose weight. "For most people, you don't worry too much about saturated fat in reasonable levels; it's not going to affect people that much. It won't change their metabolic parameters," Dr. Plutzky told me.

I asked Dr. Libby directly, "What do you think about patients who are trying to lose visceral fat who cut out rapidly digestible carbs but increase saturated fat?"

"The health benefits are going to be terrific," he said. "I am cool with that."

"If their LDL-C bumps to a point that I don't want, then we will have a shared decision-making about treating that," he said.

Reducing LDL-C, a type of blood lipid that circulates in the blood and is referred to as "bad cholesterol," has dramatically reduced the incidence of atherosclerotic cardiovascular disease and cardiovascular deaths. The more one can reduce LDL-C, the more one can reduce cardiovascular risk. I am a strong believer in getting LDL-C as low as reasonably achievable and for as long a period of time as possible. Reducing the incidence of smoking and making available effective lipid-lowering agents has dramatically changed the course of people dying from atherosclerotic cardiovascular disease.

Some individuals on a low-carbohydrate diet will have an increase in their LDL-C levels. Further testing, such as for particle number, which is the amount of ApoB (a protein molecule) carried on lipoproteins, may bring clarity to their cardiovascular risk. In any case, elevated LDL-C is easily treatable.

It is not the whole picture, however. In the face of increasing obesity and diabetes, the prevalent blood lipid picture that is emerging is one of high triglycerides. In addition to LDL, triglyceride-rich lipoproteins contribute to atherosclerotic heart disease. There is reason to believe that they, too, are a causal cardiovascular risk factor, Dr. Libby told me. "Triglyceride-rich lipoproteins promote inflammation much more than LDL." Refined carbohydrates stimulate production of those particles in the liver.

At the American Heart Association's 2024 annual scientific meeting in Chicago, I asked the experts on a panel that presented the Annual Lipid Update if they agreed that rapidly absorbable carbohydrates are a big part of the problem we are seeing with elevated triglycerides. From the organization that focused for decades on saturated fat, there was remarkable agreement that refined carbohydrates were a part of the problem.

Reduction in weight can dramatically change cardiovascular risk. Diet quality is important. Reducing both rapidly absorbable carbohydrates and switching to healthy fats will reduce cardiovascular risk. Still, as Dr. Libby pointed out to me, people focus too much on what they're eating rather than on how much.

Building on the Mediterranean Diet

Dr. Iris Shai, a professor of nutrition and epidemiology at Ben-Gurion University in Israel, conducted one of the most rigorous and important dietary clinical trials, designed to make direct comparisons between competing dietary approaches. She compared a modified Mediterranean diet to low-carb and low-fat diets on a group of 322 moderately obese test subjects and showed that a low-carb and Mediterranean diet outperformed the low-fat diet at two years. Participants lost weight more rapidly with the low-carb diet, but at twelve months, their results were not different from those on the Mediterranean diet. At six years, more people sustained their weight on the Mediterranean diet than those on the low-fat or low-carb diet.

A notable feature of the Mediterranean diet is its high intake of vegetables, legumes, fruits, whole grains, and nuts. The diet also includes moderate poultry and fish, while limiting red meat. People who follow this diet consume moderate amounts of dairy products like cheese and yogurt, low amounts of eggs, barely any sweets at all, and often a modest amount of wine with meals. In general, the Mediterranean diet is characterized by minimal consumption of saturated fats and sugar, which helps avoid high-calorie foods and highly palatable combinations of food that are high in fat and sugar.

In discussing her findings, Dr. Shai pointed out that for the Mediterranean diet, what you do *not* consume matters even more than what you do. "You are free of junk food, of trans fats, processed meats, sugars, and sodium, and you are consuming high amounts of vegetables, fruits, and all the good things that come from nature," she said.

Dr. Shai's comments hint at a valuable insight: The notion of a single "Mediterranean diet" is an illusion. Although people commonly talk about the "Mediterranean diet" as if it were a single thing, the Mediterranean is a vast region encompassing a wide variety of eating styles. Scholars such as Dr. Kate Gardner Burt at Lehman College have done a good job of debunking this generalization. Although there are many cultures and countries in the region that have similar elements in their diets, it is unclear whether the nutrient profile called the Mediterranean diet reflects the actual dietary pattern of any specific one of them. For example, pre-industrialization, the shepherds of Sardinia ate lard and cheese, and pork and lamb have long been staples of the Greek diet.

What we know today as the Mediterranean diet is an idealized version of what nutritional epidemiologists consider a healthful diet. The most notable healthy feature that characterizes the "Mediterranean" style of diet is its emphasis on whole foods and its lack of ultraformulated foods. That is the core healthy principle behind this style of eating.

The breadth of the Mediterranean diet is also its primary drawback. It provides an overall eating plan, but does not give guidance on specific portion sizes. Patients may find it ineffective because some people can be fooled into thinking that eating healthy food allows unlimited portions or allows eating more for extra nutrients, which can result in high calorie intake.

Dr. Ioannis Nikitidis, a medical doctor and registered dietitian in Crete, Greece, understands that the Mediterranean diet is limited as an anti-obesity plan because it doesn't necessarily address the issue of satiety or result in lower calories. "I don't think that the Mediterranean diet alone is the ideal approach to tackle obesity and to help a patient get the maximal results in his weight-loss attempt. Some elements of the Mediterranean diet must be combined with elements of other diets, i.e., keto, to get the best possible result for the patient," he says. "The feeling of satiety is of great importance when you try to help someone to lose weight. For me, satiety should be considered carefully."

The macronutrients of the Mediterranean diet are about 40% energy from fat, 20% from protein, and 40% from carbohydrates. "I don't think that this ratio of macronutrients is ideal for weight loss and satiety," Dr. Nikitidis adds. "I suggest a 25% fat, 35% protein, and 40% carbohydrate ratio. Increased protein means increased satiety. I don't go as high as the keto diet, but I get partly some of the keto diet benefits. My preferences when talking about protein sources are chicken, turkey, and low-fat dairy products to avoid an increase in the LDL cholesterol. And I suggest fish to ensure getting the beneficial omega-3 fatty acids. I understand that fish is easier to find in Greece than in other countries, but the cost is still high compared to meat."

Dr. Nikitidis recommends a modified Mediterranean diet with a high fiber content to address issues of satiety. "The number of vegetables, legumes, fruits, whole grains, and nuts that are consumed makes a good combination of fibers and complex carbs. They help you limit any constipation issues and feel better, and in addition, they hydrate you. Hydration is important because if you are dehydrated, the feeling of hunger is greater and comes quicker. Thus, high fiber intake combined with high water consumption is a great combo. In addition, the fruit-vegetables combination increases the intake of vitamins and minerals."

A Dietary Foundation

There is no such thing as a perfect nutrition plan. Given the diversity of individual biology and environment, how could there possibly be a single solution? But as we have seen, there are some foundational principles that can be broadly applied for better health. Nutritional plans that cut caloric intake, focus on whole foods, and reduce carbohydrate consumption while supplying enough nutrients and micronutrients to sustain the body, allow for weight loss. In order for such an eating program to be sustainable, it must also be consistent and satisfying.

GLP-1 medications don't change the fundamentals of healthy eating, but they do make it easier to change eating habits. Physicians who care for people with obesity celebrate that they can recommend that patients on medications focus on diet quality rather than on calories. With all our medical and technological advances, it is striking that we need to tell people to focus on diet quality. The food industry has been regrettably successful at separating calories from nutrition. I always thought phrases like "empty calories" and "junk food" applied to a side segment of our food supply. Unfortunately, those terms have come to represent an increasing portion of our food intake. The food industry has figured out how to, in the words of Dr. Lydia Alexander of Kaiser Permanente, decouple energy intake from nutrition.

On average, people with obesity make seven serious weight-loss attempts over their lifetimes, trying out multiple styles of diets. With so many options to choose from, I asked an obesity medicine colleague, Dr. Jennie Stanford, a nutrition expert physician, to extract a "foundational eating pattern" that can help guide sustainable weight management. The goal was to come up with principles of a healthy diet that are applicable whether someone is on medication or off medication. In general, such a pattern should emphasize a moderate intake of lean protein, be plant-predominant, focus on low-glycemic carbohydrates and minimally processed foods, include healthy fats, and avoid extreme caloric restriction.

This is the basic blueprint to guide eating for good health.

Moderate Intake of Lean Protein

Our bodies cannot function without protein, and if dietary protein intake is insufficient, our bodies will begin breaking down protein stores from muscles and organs. The building blocks of protein molecules are called amino acids. Amino acids are required to build and maintain muscles and soft tissue; they are also necessary for cell-to-cell signaling, DNA synthesis and replication, and the basic metabolic reactions in cells. Our bodies can make many types of amino acids, but there are nine amino acids that we can obtain only through diet.

Protein sources that contain all nine essential amino acids are called complete proteins, whereas protein sources without them all are referred to as incomplete proteins. Animal proteins tend to be complete. A few plant protein sources are also complete. Most plant protein sources are incomplete individually but can be combined to be complete in total.

Protein needs vary widely depending on age, sex, activity level, health status, and individual metabolic factors. The recommended daily allowance (RDA), set by the National Academies Food and Nutrition Board, is an established threshold that is meant to represent the amount of a particular nutrient that is adequate for body functions in healthy people. For decades, the amount of protein in the RDA was set at a suboptimal level, at a maximum of 0.8 grams per kilograms (g/kg) of body weight.

A substantial amount of evidence suggests a diet that has more protein than the current RDA helps optimize metabolism, regulate appetite, maintain a healthy weight, preserve lean body mass, promote healthy aging, encourage physical recovery, and support physical strength. Higher protein diets also promote satiety, increase calorie burn, and help maintain lean muscle mass. Evidence suggests that substituting more protein for refined grains also tends to reduce insulin resistance and other markers of poor metabolic health.

The current RDA defines protein needs according to body weight only. A better foundational principle is to estimate protein needs as part of the total caloric intake. The ideal percentage of total daily calorie intake from protein ranges between 25 and 40% for most people, depending on different situations. Protein provides four calories per gram, the same as carbohydrates. If protein makes up 30% of a daily intake of 1,600 calories, that equals 480 calories, or 120 grams of protein.

To easily calculate daily protein intake, aim for grams of protein to be at least 75% of your body weight in pounds. For example, if you weigh 160 pounds, consume at least 120 grams of protein per day. This recommendation might not be suitable for individuals with insulin resistance, those aiming for specific fitness goals, individuals recovering from illness or surgery, those taking medications for weight loss, or others with unique circumstances. Personalized nutrition plans are important for determining your specific requirements.

Bottom line: Protein should come from lean sources that contain a good portion of their calories in protein, with minimal healthy fats or other added ingredients. Good sources of lean protein include poultry breast or wing meat (like chicken or turkey), lean cuts of pork, bison, eggs, quinoa, legumes, fish, shellfish, and seafood.

Appropriate serving sizes of protein would be about six ounces of meat or fish (about the size of one's palm); two whole eggs or three to four egg whites; a half cup of quinoa or legumes; a half cup of Greek yogurt or cottage cheese; one cup of tofu; and one-quarter cup of nuts. Animal sources of lean protein should take up about one-quarter of the plate. Good sources of animal protein may also contain healthy fats, and good sources of plant-based protein will also contain low-glycemic carbohydrates.

Plant-Predominant Eating

Plant foods are some of the most anti-inflammatory options available in our modern food supply. Plants can be eaten in minimally processed form, which preserves their valuable nutrients and micronutrients, including vitamins, minerals, and antioxidants. Antioxidants suppress the formation of damaging, proinflammatory molecular fragments, called free radicals, that can increase the risk of many chronic diseases. Exceptional sources of antioxidants include berries, citrus fruits, green leafy vegetables, cruciferous vegetables, beans, sweet potatoes, and quinoa. Diets high in antioxidants have been shown to reduce the risk of cardiovascular disease, anemia, certain cancers, joint diseases, inflammatory diseases, and cognitive decline.

Most plant foods contain dietary fiber, an important element within a healthy diet. Fiber helps promote satiety, reduce calorie intake, maintain a healthy weight, control blood glucose, regulate bowel movements and digestion, and support a healthy gut microbiome. A diverse, balanced gut microbiome is important for human health in numerous ways, some of which are still being discovered. Dietary fiber is a prebiotic, meaning that it acts as food for the microscopic organisms living within the gut. Fiber is also a component of low-glycemic carbohydrates, which help control blood sugar. Many nutrition and obesity researchers now agree on the health benefits of a plant-predominant diet that does not contain ultraformulated foods.

Dr. Robert Kushner, the obesity medicine clinician at Northwestern University, uses "more plant-based, less red meat days, focusing on fruits, vegetables, and whole grains." What's the difference between vegetarian and plant-based diets? It's the absence of processed foods. For example, you wouldn't eat fried zucchini in the latter, although this would be fine in the former.

"Plant-based is still very scary for a lot of people," says Dr. Jennifer Ng, a New York City–based internist and obesity medicine specialist who is a proponent of plant-based eating. She thinks a plant-based diet with a small meat component (flexitarian) is generally more palatable to younger patients. According to Dr. Ng, studies show that plant-based diets are associated with weight loss and lower BMI, along with longer adherence to such diets, further reducing the risk of obesity. Randomized controlled trials indicate that plant-based diets can be more effective for weight loss than other diets, although some studies show similar efficacy across different diets. Plant-based diets aid weight loss through high fiber content and lower caloric density.

There is evidence that diets low in animal-based foods and higher in healthy plant foods are associated with a reduced risk of cardiovascular mortality and disease, and type 2 diabetes. These diets enhance insulin sensitivity in individuals who are overweight or obese. They lower LDL cholesterol levels, protect against gastrointestinal cancers, and reduce inflammatory markers.

Bottom line: The most healthful type of plant-based diet, called "plant-based whole-food eating," includes whole grains, fruits, vegetables, legumes, seeds, and nuts while avoiding unhealthy processed and refined plant-based foods.

Healthy Fats

In contrast to the low-fat-diet craze of prior decades, a foundational eating pattern includes healthy fats in the mix. The evidence of a relationship between saturated fat and cardiovascular disease is complex and hotly debated. However, there are fats that are clearly healthful and beneficial, and that fight chronic diseases. Unsaturated fats (polyunsaturated fats and monounsaturated fats), specifically omega-3 fatty acids and omega-6 fatty acids, are essential dietary components.

Omega-6 fatty acids are important for blood clotting, immune functions, muscle contraction, cell structure, and skin health. Omega-6s are found in plant foods like nuts and seeds, and in some animal products as well. There can be too much of a good thing, however. In recent years, the intake of omega-6 fatty acids in the typical Western diet has increased dramatically due to the seed oils that are prevalent in highly processed foods. Seed oils are cheap and can be used as sources of fat to improve food textures and extend shelf life, so many processed foods are made with them.

The problem is that seed oils (such as soybean oil, canola oil, corn oil, and safflower oil) are proinflammatory, and they contain an excess of omega-6 relative to omega-3 fatty acids. Before the prevalence of processed foods, people usually ate omega-6 to omega-3 fatty acids in ratios from 1:1 to 4:1. Currently, sources estimate that the ratio of omega-6 to omega-3 is 20:1 or higher, which leads to a proinflammatory diet.

A useful compensation is to increase intake of omega-3 fatty acids, which are important in cognitive functioning, reducing inflammation, improving joint health, aiding vision, promoting cardiovascular health, and decreasing the risk of many chronic diseases. Eicosapentaenoic acid (EPA) and docosahexaenoic acid (DHA) are two common omega-3 fatty acids. These can't be made by the body, so they must be obtained in the diet.

Bottom line: Good food sources of omega-3s include extra virgin olive oil, avocado oil, avocados, chia seeds, flax seeds, nuts, and fatty fish. How much omega-3 fatty acids are needed on a daily basis can vary based on a number of factors, but a general recommendation is at least 1.5 to 2 grams per day. For reference, four to six ounces of salmon contain about 3 grams of omega-3 fatty acids, and one tablespoon of chia seeds contains about 2.5 grams. Eating three servings of low-mercury fish per week or having a serving of chia seeds each day would help meet the omega-3 goal.

Extra virgin olive oil is another good way to get more omega-3s into your diet. It is a versatile cooking oil, available in a variety of flavor intensities, and it can be used to prepare a variety of foods. Avocado oil is another common healthy fat, rich in omega-3 fatty acids. It provides a strong flavor and is better suited for savory foods; it is also better than olive oil for cooking because it has a higher-temperature smoke point.

High-Fiber, Low-Glycemic Carbohydrates

Much of the confusion surrounding carbohydrates centers around definitions. "Complex carbohydrates" is a term that should have been retired a long time ago, because it includes both starches, which are digestible, and fiber, which is not. I think it's best to focus more clearly on the health risks from excess consumption of "rapidly digestible" or "rapidly absorbable" carbohydrates. Rapidly digestible carbohydrates include sugars and starches that are readily broken down into glucose, causing a rapid rise in blood sugar. Sugar and starch contribute to the highly palatable food combinations that drive our reward/addictive circuits.

Rapidly digestible carbohydrates contribute to metabolic disease, including visceral, liver, and epicardial (cardiac) adiposity. Under any eating pattern, starch and sugar need to be reduced as much as possible. High-carbohydrate diets act to increase visceral and liver adiposity and inflammation, especially in people who live with insulin resistance.

Dietary fiber is also a carbohydrate, but a very different kind. It is a nondigestible carbohydrate that plays a positive role in reducing gastrointestinal motility, feeding the gut microbiota, and helping to reduce inflammation. Soluble fiber contained in oats, legumes, fruits, and vegetables acts as a bulking agent that absorbs water and combines with bile acids and aids in reducing blood lipids. Insoluble fibers aid in gastrointestinal movement.

The federal Dietary Guidelines Advisory Committee uses the term "total grains," which include whole and refined grains, and has recently suggested the majority of the total grains that people eat be comprised of whole grains. But the term "whole grains" is complicated as well; it can include large amounts of starch as well as fiber and protein.

The case for whole grains is that they provide some nutrients and fiber beyond starch. For example, whole grains are naturally rich in B vitamins, especially folate, thiamine (B_1), riboflavin (B_2), and niacin (B_3). Most whole grains are rich in iron, magnesium, selenium, and zinc. The germ in whole grains contains essential fatty acids, such as omega-3s and omega-6s. Whole grains provide unique phytochemicals that are mostly lacking in refined grains, because these healthy compounds are concentrated in the bran and germ.

The case against whole grains is that they are a major source of starch, which contributes to visceral and liver fat in vulnerable people, and all of the essential nutrients they contain can also be found in other foods. The fiber in whole grains is primarily soluble fiber, which does have certain helpful mechanical properties for gastrointestinal motility. More useful soluble fibers could be obtained from fruits and vegetables.

One of the reasons the US Dietary Guidelines Advisory Committee has tiptoed around the issue of grains is that, back in the 1940s, the Food and Drug Administration decided, in the face of national nutrient deficiencies, to allow the fortification of refined grains with vitamins and minerals. The most recent of these efforts was the fortification of refined grains with folate to reduce the risk of neural tube defects during pregnancy. Ever since, the FDA has essentially used refined grains as the delivery system of choice to prevent folate deficiency and fetal neural tube defects.

At the meeting of the 2025 Dietary Guidelines Advisory Committee, members floated a proposal to reduce the recommended daily servings of total grains for everyone above the age of one. The chair of the committee declined to consider the idea, on the grounds that grains had been chosen as a carrier for vitamins and minerals needed to address common nutritional deficiencies. Dr. Deidre Tobias from the Harvard T. H. Chan School of Public Health objected that "refined grains should not be consumed just to get multivitamins." For now, the US dietary guidelines continue to promote a diet heavy in total and refined grains, even though such a diet is causing metabolic chaos in a large segment of the population.

A helpful way to evaluate the quality of a carbohydrate is to look at its glycemic index. Glycemic indices are broken into three groupings: low (less than 55), meaning the food has minimal impact on blood glucose; medium (56 to 69), meaning it has a moderate impact on blood glucose levels; and high (above 70), meaning it causes a significant rise in blood glucose. Glycemic load is a related concept, a calculation based on the total amount of carbohydrates in a portion of food combined with that food's glycemic index value.

To be considered a low-glycemic diet, the total daily glycemic index should be below 45. Evidence suggests that low-glycemic diets decrease insulin resistance and lower fasting insulin levels, so following a low-glycemic diet is important in an overall foundational eating pattern. In addition, some studies show that in patients who have BMIs in the overweight or obese ranges, a low-glycemic diet may promote weight loss. However, results are mixed. What we do know is that following a low-glycemic diet helps preserve optimal metabolic health, which helps not only maintain a healthy body weight but also reduces the risk of chronic conditions related to abnormal insulin and glucose metabolism.

Starchy vegetables contribute high amounts of starch but do provide some protein as well. Sweet potatoes contain more beta carotene and phytochemicals than white potatoes. "Potatoes consistently have glycemic index values above 70, sometimes in the 90s. Instant potatoes are even higher. It's possible that wild varieties of potatoes were lower in glycemic index," Australian nutritionist Dr. Jennie Brand-Miller told me. "I suspect that breeding was designed to find the biggest potatoes and inadvertently, this made them higher in glycemic index because the starch was more branched."

Legumes such as beans, peas, and lentils have moderate amounts of digestible carbohydrates. They are an excellent source of nonanimal protein, have healthy soluble fiber, and are good for sustainability.

Fruits can easily be divided into low- and high-glycemic categories. Low-glycemic fruits include berries, apples, pears, oranges, and kiwis; they provide phytochemicals such as vitamin C, which can be difficult to get from other sources, and minerals like magnesium, potassium, and zinc. "Generally, fruit is low to moderate in glycemic index. They are a mixture of glucose, fructose, and sucrose so the ratio of glucose to fructose is around 1:1, on average. Fructose has a glycemic index of only 20 because it is oxidized quickly. Fruits have acids and fiber that slow down digestion too," Dr. Brand-Miller says.

Focusing on low-glycemic carbohydrates helps moderate the release of insulin and control blood sugar. Low-glycemic carbohydrates include fiber, protein, phytonutrients, antioxidants, and other beneficial nutrients that slow the breakdown of carbohydrates, helping to blunt the rise in blood sugar and better promote sustained energy release. Following a low-glycemic diet preserves optimal metabolic health, which helps not only maintain a healthy body weight, but also reduces the risk of chronic conditions.

Everyone can benefit from focusing on the quality of carbohydrates we eat. Everyone can benefit from minimizing starch and sugar and starchy vegetables and maximizing low-glycemic-index fruits; using legumes to maximize our protein sources; and eating non-starchy vegetables that are high in fiber.

None of this guidance should obscure the fact that carbohydrates form much of the basis of our current food supply. Pizza, hamburger rolls, bread, pasta, and baked goods are hard to avoid. This is where the concept of harm reduction becomes very useful. Some of us will be able to limit our consumption of refined sugars and starches and high-glycemic fruits. For others, that is far from realistic. Perfection is not a requisite for managing weight and reducing visceral adiposity. The goal is to limit the harm as best we can. We all encounter tremendous numbers of foods that stimulate the addictive circuits. Any positive incremental change is beneficial.

19

• • • •

A New Way of Viewing
Behavioral Therapy

The fact that the new anti-obesity drugs have worked with such dramatic success underscores a long-overlooked truth about behavioral therapy as a treatment for overeating and weight loss. Though behavioral change has long been at the core of many weight-loss programs and forms of therapeutic treatment, it hasn't always been as effective as other methods because, by and large, it has not been designed to address the neurobiology of food addiction. That anti-obesity medications help people lose weight doesn't prove that gastrointestinal hormones are the *cause* of obesity. Similarly, painkillers may reduce pain and inflammation and yet still not address the cause of the problem. But the effectiveness of these drugs does show that biological interventions at the molecular level can influence the disease process.

Dr. Judson Brewer, a professor of behavior and social sciences at Brown University's Mindfulness Center, puts it more bluntly: Cognitive behavioral therapy treatments, he says, have not been shown to produce successful results. The low long-term success rates of cognitive behavioral therapies, he says, "may stem from the fact that attempts at top-down regulation over behaviors rooted in lower-level reward-based systems are unlikely to persist, as they do not actually modify reward valuation processes motivating these behaviors." What's needed are behavioral therapies, according to Dr. Brewer, "that influence addictive behaviors by altering the lower-level reinforcement learning mechanisms responsible for instilling these behaviors in the first place." In other words, change needs to happen at a level below thought. Behavioral therapy must address automatic behavior by shifting our perception of food as a reward, thereby affecting the underlying biology of addiction.

There are dozens of large-scale neural circuits in the brain involved in shaping the behavioral outcome of any choice we make that governs functions like reward, emotional memory, cognitive control, and urges; they involve learning, memory, habit, and motivation. Addiction is a complex interplay of all these brain functions, areas, and circuits. Together, these functions produce the clinical symptoms of impulsivity, craving, wanting, preoccupation, and seeking that define the disease. The complex nature of addiction means that successful treatment often requires a comprehensive and integrated set of therapeutic interventions. But, also, more particularly, it requires taking a page from the recovery playbook and viewing behavioral therapy through the lens of addiction, creating practices that address ultraformulated food as a habit-forming substance that changes our biology.

Addiction has long been viewed as a war between our dopamine-mediated reward pathways and the executive inhibitory control circuits of the prefrontal cortex of the brain. This theory can be traced all the way back to Plato's comparison, in *Phaedrus*, of the soul to a winged chariot pulled by two horses—one noble, representing our intellect and reason, the other ignoble, representing our base impulses and appetites. A better model for viewing addiction, however, is one that incorporates the notion that the most emotionally impactful stimulus in our environment at any given time is what will prevail in terms of our behavior. This stimulus, be it a slice of pizza or a tray of cookies, leads to an infinite regress of feedforward loops and neuronal firings across networks that capture our attention and ultimately create addictive behavior. (Salient stimuli can work in the other direction, too. That is, I might be ready to give in and buy that soft-serve ice cream cone I've been thinking about from the moment I saw the neighborhood truck, but when my grandchild breaks free from my hand and runs into the busy street, my attention shifts, because there is nothing else around me that will reach that level of emotional salience.) Ultimately, with addiction, unless we're able to change the salience, or draw, of the emotionally impactful stimulus that is ultraformulated food, treatment is bound to fail.

This is crucial because emotionally salient stimuli change how we feel. And how we feel—not just how we think or behave—drives addictive eating behavior. Emotions have a subjective experience, a physiological reaction, an expressive component, and a behavioral response.

That subjective experience gives rise to an affect, or a feeling state, and to autonomic arousal, a response that takes place when the autonomic nervous system is activated, causing physiological changes like increased heart rate and rapid breathing—essentially the "fight or flight" reaction. When this occurs, it can feel negative or discomforting, and we automatically seek to alter that feeling back to baseline.

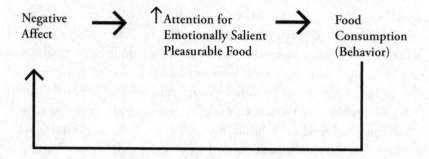

Throughout the day, we experience multiple internal, or interoceptive, stimuli—thirst, energy, glucose levels, hunger, sadness, stress, and boredom among them—and external stimuli—stressors or cues—that can change how we feel. These subjective feelings lead to nervous system activation and, eventually, actions or behaviors. If eating is the behavior—and if eating makes us feel either better or simply less bad—then this becomes reinforcing and addictive.

Stress particularly sustains food addiction. The stressor can be anything that challenges bodily homeostasis, anything that pushes the brain or body out of its ideal functioning state. It can be as simple as a significant spike or decline in blood glucose or as devastating as the loss of a loved one. We can conceptualize the brain as having two large neural networks, one for salience and another for the executive control system. Stressors change the allocation of resources to favor the salience network, focus attention, and direct behavior toward emotionally salient stimuli. In the face of such stress, automatic behaviors take over. This is the very definition of "stress eating." But remove that stressor, and we resume the day-to-day balance between executive control and emotional salience. So, how does successful long-term behavior change occur? Drs. Maren Michaelsen and Tobias Esch, of Witten/Herdecke University in Germany, searched scientific literature for what mechanisms enhance behavior change in addiction generally. They came up with three methods that may alter or shift our perspective on what is salient, thereby changing the perception of reward as well.

The first method employs substituting one reward for another. Drs. Michaelsen and Esch call this approach motivation. If we have experienced ultraformulated food as pleasurable in the past or hold a positive view of it, we will automatically move toward it—the goal here is to create a new behavior attached to a different stimulus until "motivation takes over," supplanting the addictive behavior.

The second method is called avoidance motivation. With this, we move away from an object or substance that has become negatively valanced, or associated. In doing so, we feel relief at avoiding an unfavorable outcome, which can become its own reward, or motivation. This is indeed what happened with smoking. Recall that, at the beginning of the twentieth century, the tobacco industry did everything it could to make smoking appear glamorous. It took another fifty years to undo that association, to change the perception so that people began to view the cigarette for what it really was, an addictive and deadly product.

The third method is called assertion motivation and involves achieving a state of homeostasis, or balance. Drs. Michaelsen and Esch argue that achieving a state of calm can be its own reward and help sustain behavior change. This state is linked, as the authors put it, to "the 'not-wanting' system and is associated with inaction, acceptance, or contentment." Achieving this state, in which the reward is a sense of inner peace, activating the parasympathetic autonomous nervous system and soothing brain chemicals, can hold more value than engaging in unwanted behaviors.

These methods all have in common a singular effort that behavioral therapy must strive to make to overcome addiction. To change addictive behavior, the behavior must be understood as driven by a powerful stimulus response. In the following sections, I explore a variety of behavioral therapies that aim to disrupt food addiction by shifting our perception and, ultimately, address our underlying neurobiological system.

Changing the Environment to Shift Behavior

One of the first physicians who studied how to modify eating behaviors was the psychiatrist Dr. Albert "Mickey" Stunkard, who spent most of his career at the University of Pennsylvania, where he founded the Center for Weight and Eating Disorders. As behaviorism—a school of thought that suggests that our behaviors and actions are shaped through conditioning and environmental stimuli—evolved throughout the 1960s and 1970s, Dr. Stunkard applied some of its principles to his theories about eating patterns, such as suggesting to patients that they keep food records. He was also one of the first to connect obesity to socioeconomic factors, and was a pioneer among medical professionals in advocating for the destigmatization of obesity.

Early in his career, Dr. Stunkard received a phone call from an insurance executive who was struggling with obesity. This man had recently had a heart attack and knew that he needed to lose weight. He'd seen Dr. Stunkard's research papers and wanted to know more about this "behavior modification" he'd written about. The insurance executive then created a self-help group called TOPS (Take Off Pounds Sensibly) that expanded to many chapters in the Philadelphia area. Dr. Stunkard was struck by the effective results many of these groups achieved. They were, indeed, better than those reported by medical studies—the average weight loss was just under fifteen pounds.

Dr. Stunkard began a study involving twenty-two TOPS chapters. He observed that there was a strong emphasis on self-discipline and a lot of competition among individuals to lose weight. Nobody could miss any meetings and there were weekly prizes given in recognition of people's weight loss achievements. Moreover, according to Dr. Stunkard, people were able to keep the weight off if they stayed in the program.

A few years before his death in 2014, I asked Dr. Stunkard: What is the most important thing someone can do to sustain weight loss? His answer was simple: reduce caloric intake, primarily fats and sweets. I asked him if he thought the people in the TOPS program had been successful because they were exceptionally disciplined, or if the program itself had been beneficial in changing their behavior.

"It must be just straight restraint," he replied. He again noted the rigid rules of TOPS. "If you drop out of this program, you're not allowed back in."

"It doesn't change the biology?" I asked.

"No," he answered without hesitation.

Instead, the change came from attaching more importance to the discipline and, perhaps, to the shared sense of accomplishment created by the group (not to mention the prizes) than to overeating.

This kind of social support group, which creates self-imposed barriers between oneself and an addictive substance, is a collective form of what is also known in the field as "self-binding." While Professor Thomas Schelling first used this term in the context of behavioral economics in the 1970s, the concept grew to encompass an alternative approach to abstinence, especially with alcohol abuse. Self-binding involves limiting exposure to the addictive substance, or the cues associated with it, to decrease use. We know from the opioid epidemic, for instance, that the wider availability of these drugs correlates with increased use. Self-binding can be a challenge in terms of entirely removing addictive substances, especially in the case of commercially available products such as alcohol and food.

There are other ways to view self-binding, however, which are somewhat more achievable in relation to food addiction. Dr. Anna Lembke of Stanford University School of Medicine divides self-binding into three categories. There is physical self-binding, which, as I mentioned, removes the substance and its cues from the environment—but, here, Dr. Lembke stretches this to include bariatric surgery, because this procedure makes overeating impossible; chronological self-binding, which limits the time during which a person is exposed to a substance, such as intermittent fasting; and categorical self-binding, which eliminates exposure to different forms of the substances, such as diets that restrict a certain type of food. The value of rules is that they can take the ambivalence out of decision-making. Ambivalence often presents the weakest link in our efforts to refrain from engaging with a substance because it allows for rumination and gives rise to craving.

And yet ambivalence about our desires is real and should be confronted. Not every part of us wants to change. Denying the ambivalence, says Dr. Andrew Tatarsky, founder and director of the Center for Optimal Living, only nurtures that part of ourselves that will ultimately sabotage our efforts. Rules in and of themselves may work for short periods of time, but unless there is meaning or consequences associated with those rules, their usefulness is limited. When we fast during a religious holiday, for instance, it is often only as the end approaches that urges increase. If deeply ingrained, a rule can decrease the reward value of a substance, but only if there is meaning attached to that rule.

Self-binding is also a form of harm reduction, which is an increasingly and hotly debated subject in addiction treatment. Rather than insisting on abstinence, harm reduction seeks, in the words of the late drug treatment pioneer Dan Bigg, "any positive change" that reduces the risk associated with the addictive substance. Harm reduction may be especially appropriate with food addiction given the wide availability and accessibility of ultraformulated foods.

Dr. Tatarsky believes that we need to shift from viewing substance abuse as a "limited disease model" that gives primacy to the medical issues toward one that understands the "multiple meaningful responses" in these complex behaviors, recognizing that there isn't just one way to treat addiction. We need to tailor treatments to meet people's unique motivations and relationships with these addictive substances.

There are also commonsense approaches to eating that foster the harm reduction ethos. At a recent meeting at Columbia University, Dr. Lisa Young gave a lecture on behavioral treatment, including cultivating healthy habits, portion control, and awareness and engaging in mindful eating. Dr. Young's research focuses on portion size. Over the last several decades, she says, it's the portion size of ultraformulated foods that has increased the most. She cited evidence that portion and package size influence food consumption. "People that were given large portions actually ate more," she explained. "And they found that by offering smaller portions across the whole diet, that could reduce daily energy intake by close to 30%."

She also said something after the lecture in a question-and-answer session that struck me. When asked how patients can balance mindful eating and obsessing about food, she replied, "It's why I'm not a fan of calorie counting, and I'm not a fan of weighing and measuring their food. You have to focus on the big picture. When you focus on mindfulness, you're focusing less on obsessing over the calories of what you're eating and focusing more on how you feel and tuning in. I think so many patients are disconnected from what they feel: Do I like what I'm eating? How do I feel? Am I hungry? Am I full? Can I stop? The food's not going away. And I think that doesn't create obsessional thinking. I think tracking the calories of everything they eat creates more of the obsession."

Many strong eating programs that use a form of harm reduction focus only on sugar abstinence. Bitten Jonsson, the Swedish internal medicine nurse who trained several of the obesity doctors I spoke to about food addiction, is one of the pioneers who runs programs to help people get off the offending substance. Another trailblazer is Dr. Vera Tarman, who started a website in 2008 called Addictions Unplugged, which helps educate the public about food addiction. There is also an international group called Food Addicts in Recovery Anonymous, as well as Overeaters Anonymous, the organization that goes back the longest, founded in 1960.

While I too am convinced that sweetness and sugar are at the heart of food's addictive properties, an alternative to abstinence, as these programs suggest, would be to practice what Dr. Lembke might include in her "categorical self-binding" by cutting back on their use. For example, one could cut out fat-sugar combinations or limit carbohydrate intake to 20, 30, or 50 grams daily.

Citing the work of the late Dr. Alan Marlatt, Dr. Tatarsky argues that harm reduction grows out of "compassionate pragmatism." Treating weight loss and management certainly could use a strong dose of that. There will never be one set of rules that applies to everyone because of the variations among individuals. Moreover, rules will need to change as we change our environments, treatments, and mindsets. While taking anti-obesity medications, for instance, the rule may be to "eat what you need" whereas, off drugs, this may shift to restricting carbohydrates if insulin resistant.

Applying the right level of pressure to allow oneself to follow the rules is also key. As harm reduction recognizes, rigidity can backfire, leading to disordered eating and other damaging outcomes. It is also critical to recognize, as Dr. Sean Wharton, medical director of the Wharton Medical Clinic in Toronto, says, that we all internalize biases, including about ourselves. When we are dealing with an addiction that is influenced by an array of physiological and hormonal influences, we need to jettison notions that using medication is a form of cheating. Being able to reduce caloric intake without being self-restrained to the point of obsession is an essential component of successful weight loss.

Craving

Battling cravings can be dispiriting for a variety of reasons. Sometimes it seems that everyone has one quick fix or another, but even the best tips, for example, "urge surfing," which simply means waiting for a time for the craving to pass—most cravings subside within a short time—seem to work only in the short term. In part this is because the human brain is designed to "lie" to us, as Dr. Omar Manejwala has written. "The ways that your cortex can rationalize acting in self-destructive ways is only limited by your own creativity. These erroneous beliefs are designed to protect your sense of self and the sense that you are in control."

When I spoke to Dr. Manejwala directly about resisting cravings, he didn't discount the power of thinking to "change the brain," but he suggested fixes that are ultimately meant to change habits or the environment. To start, he recommended doing a thorough assessment of one's circumstances, which he jokingly refers to as "an autopsy." Because cravings are so complex, you might have to dig deeper to understand them. "The challenge becomes understanding which of the contributing factors are driving your craving," he told me. "Is it a pattern? Is it a habit?" If you find yourself dealing with a late-night sugar craving, take a look at what you last ate to see if it could have been tweaked to avoid it. Perhaps you could have had more protein with dinner, or larger portions of vegetables throughout the day. "Do I have fewer cravings when I exercise more in the evenings versus in the mornings? Can I take a bath? Are there certain smells that can reduce this? Is it tied to my use of nicotine? Is it when I get into a fight with my spouse?" Only by determining the nature of the craving, Dr. Manejwala advises, can you figure out potential strategies for fighting it. Doing so successfully might require some experimentation, because no two people, and therefore no two cravings, are alike: While one person might feel that adding more fiber to her evening meal curtailed her desire for cookies later, another might find such a change does little or nothing. "Build logs, build patterns, analyze, and then test hypotheses," Dr. Manejwala says, a tedious prospect, perhaps, but a potentially rewarding one.

It's important to have tools to fight cravings as they occur, but even more crucial, Dr. Manejwala says, is preventing them in the first place. "Very little of dealing with cravings is what I have to *stop* doing. Most is what I need to *start* doing." If a craving usually occurs around a particular time, as with my own late-night eating, then "maybe you need to alter your life in some way so that you're not awake at that hour, or you're doing other things that are more immersive," he says. Even though you can't totally avoid food in life, you can manipulate your immediate environment to make cravings harder to fulfill. If you filled your fridge with solely healthy fare, then you'd have no choice but to eat those foods, after which your craving would likely subside because you'd be satiated.

There are also larger, more holistic changes that could prove beneficial.

Dr. Manejwala suggests engaging in fulfilling group activities, like religious services, exercise classes like running groups, or, even better, volunteering or giving back in a way that has a social component. Altruism and social connection can trigger the same reward pathways as intoxicants. "This is the reason why people in recovery really focus so much on doing positive, affirming activities," he says of those in twelve-step support groups. "They develop social relationships and friendships, and they emphasize altruism because of the hit or buzz that gives them." Many of these more significant lifestyle changes might appear to have nothing to do with cravings themselves, but because they help us feel better about ourselves overall, they can have significant ripple effects.

20

· · · ·

Tricks of the Mind

In addition to shifting our external circumstances by becoming more aware of the ways in which we perceive food psychologically, we can create changes that help subvert addiction.

Dr. Denise Ratcliffe, a cognitive behavioral therapist and the author of *Understanding and Managing Emotional Eating: A Psychological Skills Workbook*, helps people develop strategies to manage their emotions and thoughts about food. Her work draws on a blend of practices, including compassion-focused therapy and commitment therapy.

"It's a bit like a dartboard," she says when explaining the components of a person's emotional relationship to food. "The outer ring is the influences of society, the messages that people pick up about food, and the way things are marketed. On the next circle in, there's the family environment, the domestic environment where food is used in certain ways that form this individual's relationship with food."

Dr. Ratcliffe constructs a unique emotional eating map for each of her patients, exploring the individual ways each learned and developed a given emotional eating pattern, and then identifies exits from this automatic cycle. Each map serves as a representation of a dynamic journey, illustrating both the old routes and the new diversions.

"There is an important distinction between a destination and an endpoint," she elaborates. "A destination is usually a place that you navigate toward with a specific intent (for example, the short-term function of eating is to boost mood or distract from difficult feelings), whereas an endpoint is a place where you might unintentionally end up (the short-term function is quickly replaced by feelings of regret, shame, and frustration)." The intended destination might be temporary relief or distraction, while the unintended endpoint often involves negative consequences like regret, guilt, or distress over one's weight. This understanding is crucial, she believes, for recognizing the gap between short-term rewards and long-term impacts. These highlight the cyclical nature of emotional eating, where temporary relief is followed by enduring negative outcomes.

To counteract these patterns, Dr. Ratcliffe proposes creating alternative routes. Just as a pilot flying a plane may need to deviate by one degree over sixty miles to end up on a significantly different course, she leads clients to pursue small changes to arrive in a completely different place. This "rerouting" strategy includes identifying starting point triggers—such as a work problem or an argument—which create automatic reactions.

Instead of focusing on *what* a person is eating, the program identifies instead what happens just before someone engages in this behavior. Dr. Ratcliffe emphasizes the importance of recognizing the feelings that precede the urge to eat—a constellation of boredom, anger, stress, guilt, helplessness, and other emotions, typically.

She also believes that altering one's physical state can be a way to jolt someone out of automatic eating. Physical movement is a powerful tool to release tension and interrupt cycles of being emotionally overwhelmed. She draws a parallel to animals "shaking off" stress, suggesting that humans can benefit from similar practices, by dancing, swinging their arms, or simply moving to a different location. These movements serve as an effective outlet for pent-up emotions; they can also provide a sense of control and create a pause in distress. In addition, her approach emphasizes the role of sensory engagement in managing emotional eating, which can include listening to music or engaging in hands-on activities.

Long-term strategies focus on fostering emotional awareness and self-compassion. This involves examining critical self-talk and challenging negative beliefs. Both exacerbate emotional distress, making people feel ashamed and powerless, and perpetuate the cycle of emotional eating. By cultivating in her patients a kinder, more supportive internal voice, she is better able to help them begin to address the root causes of their emotional eating behaviors.

Experimentation is very important in this process. Individuals are encouraged to try different approaches and observe the outcomes, noting what works and what does not. Anticipating and managing setbacks is a crucial step as well. Dr. Ratcliffe acknowledges the tendency to revert to familiar patterns due to ingrained habits and the brain's established pathways. She stresses that these setbacks are natural and should not be viewed as failures.

Her work also aims to track emotional thinking patterns and an "emotional eating thought ladder"—the lower the rung, the more the thoughts and beliefs are out of our conscious awareness. She says automaticity, the ability to perform a task without conscious effort or thought, usually due to repetition, goes by many names but often is associated with psychological powerlessness.

The starting point for the emotional eating thought ladder is that people have intrusive thoughts about food, cravings, and wanting a specific type of food. "Usually that's the first layer of thinking," she says. "Above that is another layer of thought, which is the decision to act on that or not. It's the giving oneself permission to act on them, a way of rationalizing the decision to go ahead." She spends time with her patients differentiating between "wanting thoughts" and "decision thoughts."

From here, her clients work on recognizing, rerouting, and navigating emotional eating, building in pauses, "exits," and other responses to manage triggers. "To feel uncomfortable is an aversive experience, and so often people want to get rid of those feelings. One of the common things that I hear people talking about is that they use food as a way of suppressing challenging emotions, pushing them down. They're worried about what will happen if they allow those emotions to remain." Her advice is that people become more comfortable with being uncomfortable. "It's important to recognize that ups and downs are normal," she adds, "and we don't necessarily need to 'do' anything about difficult emotions."

For people with obesity, she says, there may also be negative feedback loops that are hard to sever or reroute. "People become distressed about their weight, so they may eat in unhelpful ways," she explains. "For other people, it's more than that. They may have depression or have had past experiences of abuse or trauma that they have learned to connect to food." The role of psychology in her work, she says, is to help "mop up some of the other pieces that get in the way of other interventions like surgery or medication."

This is just the kind of psychological support that people can use, either on its own or in conjunction with another tool, such as medication, to create enduring change. Indeed, Dr. Ratcliffe points out that, while anti-obesity drugs won't permanently change a person's emotional relationship with food, they *can* help when people's eating behaviors are driven by feeling that they have nowhere else to turn. "With the meds, they aren't feeling as distressed or trapped in a cycle," she explains. "They are feeling more hopeful."

Present Bias

One of the great mysteries in human behavior is why we so often decide to do something in the short term, knowing that it is not in our long-term interest. Why do we eat that piece of cake, knowing full well we will regret it later? Behavioral economist George Ainslie became interested in the topic as a medical student working in the Harvard Laboratory of Experimental Psychology. He focused on how choice varied in relation to time. This interest stuck with him even after he graduated medical school and began to work at the Veterans Administration in Pennsylvania, where he still works as a psychiatrist.

Dr. Ainslie's research in both humans and animals led him to see that we tend to overvalue a potential reward that is available immediately versus one available at some time in the future. However, the extent of this overvaluation diminishes depending on how far into the future a person must contemplate. For example, someone might prefer to receive $100 immediately over $200 one year from now, but if the choice is instead between $100 received in ten years and $200 received in eleven years, it becomes more likely that they will opt to wait for the larger sum, even though the interval between receiving the two rewards remains the same. When the possibility of an immediate reward is removed—and therefore also the reactive urge we might feel along with it—it becomes possible to weigh the two options on their own merits. And the perceived value of the reward diminishes the longer one must wait for it. This phenomenon of variability in the way a person values rewards over time is referred to as hyperbolic, or delay, discounting, and has been a major focus of Dr. Ainslie's work.

Dr. Ainslie's work with veterans affected by addiction led him to consider the problem of delay discounting in a new light. Specifically, he observed that a person with addiction is less able to inhibit urges, and therefore less able to logically decide between immediate versus future rewards. This impulsiveness is part of the wiring of addiction.

Effective long-term decision-making—what some call willpower—requires us to consider that today's actions can undermine tomorrow's goals. Dr. Ainslie described the compromises people make in considering immediate versus future rewards as "intertemporal bargaining"; it is the method by which a person makes a self-conscious decision by considering both external incentives and "shifting self-predictions," as Dr. Ainslie puts it. The neural circuitry of addiction makes it very difficult for people to improve self-destructive behaviors over the long term.

In addition, repeated failures to control impulses may turn into a negative feedback cycle. If a person cannot imagine future success, it becomes harder to act in accordance with their goals. At this point, they must find a different motivation. As Dr. Ainslie describes it, the person "needs to reestablish a relationship with her prospective future selves."

According to Dr. Ainslie, overcoming food addiction requires us to make the salience of the future cost or harm of our choices more resonant in the present. If I am obese at thirty-five and struggle with food addiction, for instance, my health at age seventy doesn't have as much concern for me, or salience, as the pleasure that food is going to give me in the moment. Somehow, I need to find a way to care more, at thirty-five, about my health at seventy. Someone who is seventy, on the other hand, may have an easier time being more motivated by their health because their mortality likely weighs more heavily on them; that person may view their future self with more emotion and, therefore, will be able to summon more resources. Recognizing earlier on in our lives how ultraformulated foods rob us of our future health—and what the food industry is doing to us—will help us make more rational decisions in the face of food addiction.

Overall, it's critical to identify what goal is most emotionally valuable to you and then try to tilt the balance of your behavior toward it.

The Importance of Sleep

When it comes to mental and physical health, sleep matters a lot. And as a population, few of us get enough of it. It is recommended that adults get at least seven hours of sleep a night. But more than a third of us don't reach that minimum. Three-quarters of Americans have at least one symptom of a sleep disorder, which can lead to sleep deficiencies. Doctors know that insufficient sleep is contributing to unhealthy body weight. But the relationship, clear as it is, is even more fraught than most realize.

"The less sleep you get, the higher your body mass index tends to be," says Dr. Lawrence Epstein, the assistant medical director of the sleep disorders service at Brigham and Women's Hospital in Boston and an assistant professor in medicine at Harvard Medical School. Sleep deprivation alters neurohormones and increases reward sensitivity. This leaves a person struggling to feel full even as they're eating more. And what are they eating? Mostly ultraformulated foods. Not to mention that because they're sleeping less, they're awake more, which means there are more opportunities to eat. Various studies have found that sleep deprivation leads to an increased intake of between 200 and 450 calories per day.

Even as a person is taking in more fuel in the form of food, they're using it up less. The sleep-deprived body burns fewer calories at rest, and is often too tired to exercise and will take the elevator rather than climb the stairs.

Food addiction, as we know, occurs when executive control is unable to sufficiently tamp down the desire to eat, and sleep deprivation diminishes executive control. A sleepy person, therefore, is powerless against cravings. Indeed, research suggests that sleepiness dampens regulatory activity in the brain while also amping up the brain's hedonistic response to addictive foods, creating a destructive combination.

Dr. Marie-Pierre St-Onge, an associate professor of nutritional medicine at Columbia University, cites a small study in 2013 in which researchers at Harvard Medical School's Social, Cognitive and Affective Neuroscience Lab imaged people's brains while showing them pictures of high- and low-calorie foods. They also asked them about their sleep habits and tendency to overeat. Those who reported more daytime sleepiness showed decreased activation in the ventromedial prefrontal cortex, an area of the brain involved in regulating emotions and behavior. Of that group, the women (though not the men) said it was hard for them to resist eating more than they'd intended. "Sleep problems may contribute directly to disordered eating via a reduction in executive function," write Drs. Lawrence J. Nolan and Allan Geliebter.

Dr. St-Onge's own fMRI research has produced complementary findings. She showed pictures of food and other objects to subjects who either had or had not gotten sufficient sleep that week. When sleep-deprived participants were shown pictures of food, especially unhealthy food, their addiction circuits were activated. Other imaging work has found that when tired people are shown pictures of food, there is an increase in activity in both the amygdala, the brain's emotional nexus, and the hypothalamus, which responds to hormonal signals to regulate food intake.

Tired people are getting hunger cues from both sides, the pleasure centers and the homeostatic ones. Conversely, Dr. St-Onge found that the participants in her study who had gotten adequate sleep showed increased activation in the brain's control centers: "Individuals who are well rested could make better decisions about their food intake and . . . food choices."

The negative effects don't apply only to those with chronic sleep deprivation. Just one night of insufficient sleep is enough to put your brain on autopilot, leaving you without the cognitive control to resist the pull of addictive ultraformulated foods. People with high sleep variability, who can't count on consistently getting a good night's rest, have been found to eat more, especially foods that are high in saturated fat. Men who have trouble falling asleep or staying asleep are hungrier and heavier. Dr. Virend K. Somers from the Department of Cardiovascular Medicine at the Mayo Clinic says that periods of restricted sleep don't just lead to weight gain, but also seem to change the way the brain and body process excess calories. In a small 2022 study, young, healthy, nonobese adults who slept four hours a night for two weeks ate more than 300 extra calories per day and put on about a pound or two. Not so surprising. Yet, when Dr. Somers analyzed their body composition with CT scans, he found that the weight gain was due largely to an 11% increase in visceral fat, the deep belly fat associated with cardiovascular and metabolic diseases and obesity.

The good news is that most of this is reversible. Improving sleep quality and quantity lowers daily caloric intake. If you can take the necessary steps to sleep better, it will be easier to lose weight or maintain your weight. That means going to bed and, more importantly, waking up at the same time every day. It means putting down your phone or closing your laptop to reduce the amount of light you're getting in the final hour or two before turning in. It might mean investing in a white noise generator or a CPAP (continuous positive airway pressure) machine for sleep apnea.

There's something that no amount of sleep hygiene can solve, however, and that is the magnetic draw of ultraformulated foods, which call to us at our most vulnerable time: before bed. Indeed, people consume most of their daily calories between 6 and 10 p.m. This may be wired into our circadian rhythm, says Dr. Frank Scheer, a neuroscientist in the Division of Sleep and Circadian Disorders at Brigham and Women's Hospital, who has studied the link between nighttime eating and obesity. Hunger naturally increases in the evening. Dr. Scheer speculates that this might be one of the body's ways of preparing for sleep—a nighttime circadian drive for calories ahead of a seven- or eight-hour fast. "You're fueling up, so to speak, beyond your homeostatic need, which is beneficial because you don't want hunger to interfere with sleep," he posits. But, then, the body does not typically crave broccoli and carrots at that hour.

To tease out how late eating affects the body and increases risk of obesity, Dr. Scheer and his collaborators designed an experiment that studied physiological responses and hunger levels (as reported by subjects) of people who ate most of their calories earlier in the day versus when their calorie intake shifted toward the end of the day. In the early eating condition, participants ate breakfast an hour after waking up, followed by lunch a little after noon, and an early-bird dinner at 5:20 p.m. In the late-eating condition, subjects skipped breakfast and ate lunch and dinner four hours later than the early eating group, eating a full meal around 9:30 p.m., two and a half hours before going to bed. Everyone ate the same meals and limited their daily activities to control their energy expenditure during waking hours. Yet there was a clear difference between those who did and did not eat at night. People in the late-eating group were hungrier during the day and showed a pronounced drop in the hormone leptin. What's more, they burned fewer calories while awake, a recipe for weight gain. The results add an important dimension to our understanding of behavioral patterns when it comes to weight: *When* you eat matters.

Ironically, obesity itself increases the risk of sleep deprivation. An obese body is in a state of chronic low-grade inflammation, which activates parts of the brain that cause wakefulness. Fat around the neck puts pressure on the upper airways while lying down, which leads to obstructive sleep apnea, an extremely common and underdiagnosed condition that interrupts normal breathing at night, leading to fragmented sleep. (Obstructive sleep apnea also increases the risk of a host of medical issues, including high blood pressure, heart disease, type 2 diabetes, stroke, and depression.) And according to CDC data, many of the US states with the greatest level of sleep deprivation also have high rates of obesity.

Call it chicken-or-egg or just a vicious circle, but what's inarguable is that sleep and weight are closely linked. If you aren't controlling your sleep, you limit your chances of controlling your weight.

Changing Mindset

The predominant view of authentic change is that it takes a thousand tiresome, plodding tweaks, that it's the result of time and introspection and effort, often a great deal of it. If change doesn't follow that predictable path, we're inclined to be wary of it. But what if personal transformation, achieved by virtue of our own perceptual shifts, *is* possible? What if change of this kind *is* eminently doable, even preferable? Two modern profiles upend some of our preconceived ideas of how some people change and may provide guidance for some of those hoping to remake themselves in less onerous ways.

By many accounts, Allen Carr was a fairly unremarkable man. Born in 1932 to working-class parents in London, he attended a local school on scholarship. After service in the Royal Air Force, he worked, unhappily, as an accountant. Like many of his peers, he smoked cigarettes, though what would become an enduring habit had an inauspicious beginning. "At some stage in their lives most smokers suffer from the illusion that they enjoy some cigarettes, but I didn't," Carr writes. "I always detested the taste and smell, but I thought that a cigarette helped me to relax."

Still, over the decades, Carr tried to quit many times, but the environment was not a conducive one for this. For one, at the time that Carr picked up the habit, smoking was widely accepted: By some estimates, around 80% of adult men and 40% of adult women smoked in the United Kingdom in 1950. People smoked in restaurants, on airplanes, and even in hospitals. And though some of the negative health impacts of cigarettes were known, the connection between tobacco and lung cancer wasn't yet widely publicized; different cigarette brands advertised their products alternately as "calming," "filtered," or "mild" to preempt any concerns over safety. With little external pressure to quit, it was difficult to find the wherewithal to battle the physiological addiction. Carr once vowed to his own father, who was dying from lung cancer, that he'd stop smoking—and then lit up almost immediately after the conversation. He described his failed attempts to stop as "sheer hell."

And yet, a mere two years later, Carr did quit. Even more astonishingly, he was able to do so permanently, and without suffering withdrawal symptoms. What had changed?

Reflecting on the experience, Carr described two epiphanies he had in close succession. The first was that cigarette dependence was simply nicotine addiction, nothing more. All the myriad explanations for why smoking was so captivating were actually just people trying to create a narrative that allowed them to avoid quitting. This realization helped denude cigarettes of some of their valence: Whereas he'd previously believed that smoking provided a variety of often paradoxical benefits—it was a welcome distraction but also a focus aid, a stimulant sometimes and a relaxant at others, a social lubricant but also an excuse to take time for yourself—Carr now saw that cigarettes did none of these things. Therefore, giving them up wasn't a true sacrifice, as they didn't truly provide any real benefit.

Second, and perhaps more important, he realized he'd been viewing a crucial part of the withdrawal process "from back to front." Rather than the cigarette providing relief from the craving, he saw that, in fact, the cigarette *created* the craving in the first place. After all, before anyone starts smoking, they never feel a desire for nicotine. Instead, like him, many smokers "force" the nicotine into their bodies as youths, to appear sophisticated, and then interpret the cravings that develop, as with most addictions, as a desire for the substance itself rather than as symptoms of withdrawal. (In reality, the withdrawal process is fairly mild and manageable; what generally stops smokers from enduring it is the *fear* that it will be painful.) The relief a smoker feels once they take a puff is just the way a nonsmoker feels all the time: free of craving. "The whole business of smoking is like forcing yourself to wear tight shoes just to get the pleasure of taking them off," Carr quipped.

Once he'd had these realizations, he stubbed out his last butt and announced to his incredulous wife that not only had he quit for good, but he wanted to "cure" the world of its smoking habit. Smokers didn't need to be beaten over the head with grim statistics or reminded of the deleterious health effects of tobacco; they already knew these things, and still it hadn't stopped them. What they needed to be taught was not how to cope with the desire to smoke but, rather, to cease desiring cigarettes in the first place.

Carr became a nonsmoking evangelist, hosting seminars and opening clinics worldwide. In 1985, he published his book *Allen Carr's Easy Way to Stop Smoking*; by some estimates, it has sold around twenty million copies since its initial publication. His major lessons—that the cigarette does nothing for you; that the nonsmoker is not deprived at all; that when you think you're getting pleasure from smoking, you're actually just staving off a minimal amount of discomfort that is itself *caused* by cigarettes; that quitting is, despite everything the media and health officials say, extremely simple—

sink into the brain over the course of reading. By the end of the book, his confidence is infectious. "I won't wish you luck," he writes at the book's conclusion, "[because] you won't need it."

In the end, it would take years of cooperation among lawyers, policymakers, and public health officials to finally chip away at the prevalence of smoking in many Western countries. But Carr's ideas about dependence and desire, as well as the delusion involved in both, influenced many people, including some who were dealing with a different addiction altogether.

One of those people was a middle-aged executive named Annie Grace. Although she spent her childhood in a one-room cabin in the mountains of Colorado, by her mid-thirties, Grace was a high-powered, jet-setting marketer for a multinational corporation. Her days were often spent traveling between international offices, with brief stops at airport lounges to shower; in the evenings, she could be found at dinner or drinks with colleagues. At times, it seemed her profession all but required she drink. A boss early in her career even told her the best deals were made at the bar, not in the boardroom, so she'd better show her face at every company happy hour. But almost a decade after she'd begun rising up the corporate ranks, her drinking was no longer confined to the bar. Instead, she found herself downing two bottles of wine on average a night and then waking up in a sweaty panic at 3:33 every morning. She soon fell into a spiral of self-recrimination and promises of repentance. Occasionally, she'd even drink in those early morning hours, just to quiet the recrimination.

Grace's eventual recovery (although she likely wouldn't use that word) came via similar logic to Carr's. She knew she'd become addicted to alcohol and berating herself for this problematic pattern wasn't working. She had to eliminate her desire for alcohol altogether, which involved a kind of deprogramming effort akin to the kind you might perform on a cult member. She bristled at aspects of the twelve-step model, such as that certain people are alcoholics and others are not: Surely if alcohol is an addictive, toxic substance, which we know for a fact it is, then the problem doesn't come from within the individuals themselves, their genetics or their spiritual makeup or anything else. Such explanations, she felt, lulled the "normal" drinker into a false sense of comfort and let the rapacious alcohol industry off the hook. She also didn't like the idea of making alcohol into a bogeyman that she'd forever be trying to outrun, the way some people in long-term sobriety seemed to be doing. Instead, she wanted to make it "small and irrelevant" in her life. And she did, via a system she recounts in her book *This Naked Mind: Control Alcohol, Find Freedom, Discover Happiness, and Change Your Life*. "I drink as much as I want, whenever I want," she confides in her book. "The truth is I no longer want to drink."

Like Carr, Grace shows the reader how numerous beliefs about alcohol that have seeped into our collective subconscious—that it's relaxing, for example, or that it's an important part of social bonding, or that it's just plain old fun—are just false. These ideas take hold through the media, our friends and family, and other cultural inputs. Over time, alcohol instigates subtle changes in our brains that make us want to drink more; through reward pathways, dopamine, or myriad other neurological processes, the cravings, as ever, self-perpetuate and grow in intensity. Grace describes how long it takes for alcohol to leave the body and concludes that so much of our seemingly harmless desire for a simple glass of wine is really just a reaction to our system entering a withdrawal phase. But the body, Grace says, is a miraculous healing organism, and if we can see through the "groupthink" that perpetuates our wrong ideas about alcohol—an effort, she writes, that is harder than giving up alcohol itself—then we too can have the "freedom" she has found.

Both Carr and Grace are often blunt about how noxious and repulsive cigarettes and alcohol are. Carr calls cigarettes "poison" and cites cancer risks repeatedly; Grace compares alcohol to motor oil. This approach clearly worked to extinguish their addictions. Both successfully changed in the long term, accomplishing this in a way that allowed them to bypass all the resentment, frustration, and physical upset that many prospective quitters have assumed would characterize their lives. Some addiction researchers have theorized that what finally compels a person to recover is realizing the extent of their losses as if on a "balance sheet," as psychologist Jim Orford put it; Grace and Carr were able to do this in an unprecedentedly condensed way that worked for them.

To date, no one has quite done for ultraformulated food what Carr did for smoking and Grace for alcohol. After all, there are virtually no downsides to quitting cigarettes or abstaining from alcohol, but inculcating disgust for food could foster an overly rigid attitude in an individual, which itself can have physical and mental health consequences that could be potentially as devastating as obesity. Also, as ultraformulated food has become an increasingly significant portion of the Western diet, with most people's nostalgia now tied to Cinnabon or Dunkin' Donuts, it becomes harder to ask people to recall a more innocent past of whole foods like fruits and vegetables.

What would such a project look like? Taking cues from Carr and Grace, it might invoke disgust as an aversive agent. We might have to pay witness to grotesque and sickening images of modern food processing: chicken nuggets made from "meat slurry," sodas containing phosphoric acid, a corrosive agent also found in fertilizers and polishes. We might have to be reminded of the ways in which formidable and wealthy Big Food has preyed on us, using methods similar to the ones used by the tobacco and alcohol industries; indeed, it might be necessary to encourage consumers to feel rage at being manipulated in this way. We may have to focus on what psychiatrist, neuroscientist, and author Dr. Judson Brewer called the "pleasure plateau," the point at which consuming something like cookies or ice cream ceases to be enjoyable and starts to feel mechanical, even sickening, and explain how the urge to continue eating past that point is one that has been *created* by the sugar, salt, and fat, ingredients that fail to truly satiate.

But more than harping on the negative, this endeavor would have to remind people of the possibility that one can live just as happily, and with as much satisfaction, while eating a healthy diet, and that there may even be *more* happiness and satisfaction to be drawn from an existence liberated from food addiction. Flavor can be found in so many ways that you don't have to envision a future of deprivation. No animal body craves maltodextrin or butylated hydroxyltoluene; no child reaches out for guar gum. The period of aversion will pass, and then the food one used to obsess over will become like vapor. There is joy in biting into a crisp new apple or a succulent piece of fish. There is satisfaction in creating and consuming a meal replete with vegetables and healthy grains and protein and noticing how strong and energetic and alive your body feels afterward. There is satisfaction in feeling independent of corporations and entities that rely on us to buy their ultraformulated products. These ideas can be absorbed without resorting to discussions about weight. These things are true for everyone, everywhere.

Now, too, of course there is the possibility of using anti-obesity drugs to grease the wheels of such a transformation by automatically shutting off our attraction to food, and therefore our addiction, too. In this sense, anti-obesity medications can lay the groundwork for the perceptual shift both Carr and Grace preached was necessary for quitting an addictive substance. It is also possible that this perceptual shift—that ultraformulated foods are not necessarily more enjoyable than whole foods, that they have been designed to hold us in their thrall, that Big Food hasn't considered our health or wellbeing in creating them—can be maintained, beyond the drugs. Ultimately, the anti-obesity drugs are not in control of our mindsets; they make physiological changes that create the ability for us to do so on our own.

21

. . . .

Continuing the Journey

There is no single path to losing weight and regaining health. Everyone begins in a different place and follows a different route. And numerous patient trials, along with a vast body of clinical experience, affirm that unpleasant truth: Sooner or later, almost every weight-loss plan fails. Even GLP-1 medications have a high dropout rate. About half of the patients who try the drugs discontinue them within the first year, mostly because of side effects, costs, or availability. People will need to combine strategies, rotate them, and adjust them to their specific and ever-changing needs.

To clarify what we are all up against, I looked into one of the most-cited weight-loss clinical trials, DiRECT (Diabetes Remission Clinical Trial). Investigators studied three diets: a low-carbohydrate diet with no calorie restrictions, a Mediterranean diet that restricted daily intake to 1,500 calories for women, and a low-fat diet with the same calorie goals. Low-carb produced the best results at six months, but the people on it regained some, though certainly not all, of their weight at two years. Participants on the low-fat diet lost the least amount of weight overall, with their results peaking at six months. By the two-year mark, they had regained some (but, again, not all) of their original weight. (See graph on next page.)

When the same researchers followed up on the participants at six years, all of the dieters had regained additional weight beyond where they were at two years. People on the low-fat diet regained the most, returning nearly to their pre-diet weight. Participants on the low-carb diet regained about half

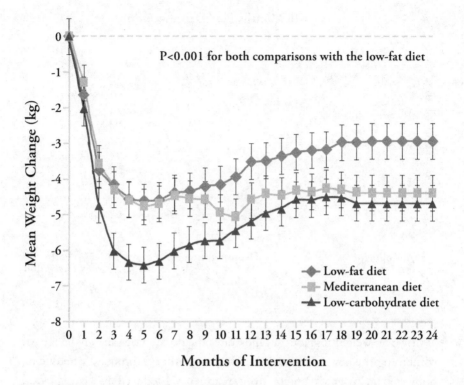

of their maximum lost weight. Those on the Mediterranean diet fared the best, but still rebounded from where they were after one to two years.

The new GLP-1 drugs can't fix the whole problem, but they do seem to promise a better, more effective way to navigate the weight-loss journey—if they can be taken in a sustainable way, combined strategically with dietary and behavioral adaptations. So far, there is no evidence of weight regain while people are taking GLP-1 medications, although we do not know the safety and efficacy of the drugs over a lifetime. We also do not know whether the drugs will maintain their efficacy if people use them intermittently. However, significant benefits may linger even after people stop taking the drugs.

As part of Virta Health's study of nutrition therapies, researchers monitored the weight of patients who took GLP-1 medications and then discontinued treatment. Those who were on carbohydrate-restricted nutrition therapy managed to hold steady or, more surprising, even to continue losing weight. Perhaps the drugs had helped them adjust their eating patterns.

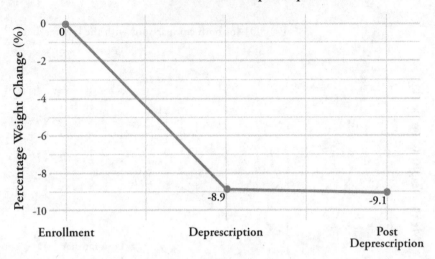

>18 Months Post Deprescription

My own weight-loss journey illustrates the possibilities and challenges of combining the new GLP-1 medications with other techniques for reducing body weight. After starting on drug treatments, I reduced my fasting blood glucose by twenty points, which took me out of the prediabetic range. My blood pressure normalized. My body fat dropped from 33 to 14%. My waist circumference decreased by twelve inches. My android-to-gynoid ratio (a measure of body fat distribution) decreased below one, indicating that I had lost a significant amount of visceral fat. In total, I lost 65 pounds.

I was on a GLP-1 drug for seven months before I decided I didn't want to stay on it indefinitely. I have been off the drug for considerably longer than that. At one point, when my weight fluctuated up, I took up the injections again. At other times, I've preferred to stick with nutrition therapy and behavioral changes. I've managed to keep my weight fairly stable ever since, with a much healthier level of visceral fat than before.

I am just a single example, a case study of one. There are many reasons for wanting to lose weight. No matter what the motivation, if weight loss results in a durable reduction of visceral adiposity and improves health outcomes, that is a net positive. GLP-1 drugs should be widely available, so long as they are prescribed in ways that lead to health benefits. Until now, treating excess weight, more specifically visceral adiposity, has been impossible for extended periods. This is because the addictive circuits in our brains are at work, along with gastrointestinal hormonal signals that perpetuate a dysregulated metabolic state. The GLP-1s help tame those circuits, opening up possibilities we didn't have before.

My blood glucose is highly sensitive to rapidly absorbable carbohydrates. I am strongly drawn to the feelings of satiety produced by fat and protein. When I go off drugs, I need to eat a reduced-carb diet or I will regain weight. At the same time, I need to be careful about shedding muscle along with visceral body fat.

I used GLP-1 drugs to reset my appetite so I could be in an energy deficit state. I used a diet to control my hyperinsulinemia so I could reduce my visceral adiposity. I do not view this as cheating or taking the easy way out. I improved my health, for now. What happens next month or next year is a whole other story. My journey, like everyone's, requires an ongoing effort.

Part IV

. . . . . .

THE ROAD AHEAD

22

• • • •

A New Landscape

Anti-obesity drugs have changed the landscape of weight loss. I have seen major drug discoveries transform other diseases. When I became commissioner of the Food and Drug Administration in 1990, there was one drug for HIV, and it did not work very well. By the time I left in 1997, there were many more drugs, and they had much greater efficacy. That advance happened because of the hard work of many researchers and drug developers, including people within the pharmaceutical industry. They did not cure AIDS, but they made it treatable. As with treatment for acute lymphoblastic leukemia (the most common cancer in children), we learned that combination treatment was important for durable efficacy in managing the symptoms of AIDS. Targeting a disease through multiple mechanisms can improve outcomes and reduce negative side effects.

We have reached a similar turning point with regard to obesity and visceral adiposity. We need to treat them through multiple mechanisms because there are multiple biological systems at play. Our brain has salience-detecting, reward-seeking circuits that result in addictive physiology. The aversive circuits that can protect us from poisonous substances can slow down gastric motility and temper addictive behavior. Rapidly absorbable carbohydrates and starches will raise glucose and affect insulin levels and increase the amount of toxic fat in our bodies. We live in an environment filled with ultraformulated foods that trigger continued eating. Food companies have a strong financial incentive to keep things that way.

What should an effective weight-loss journey look like in the age of

GLP-1s? Now that we have the tools to break food addiction, why not make them the default option for everyone who needs them? I've thought about these questions a lot.

Some physicians have publicly stated that diet and exercise alone are not enough to treat obesity and visceral adiposity, and that only medication and surgery are effective treatments. They are wrong. Diet and exercise are still the foundation of improved metabolic health. Medications are not the be-all and end-all solutions. They are tools that allow people to control appetite so that diet and lifestyle interventions can be effective.

These GLP-1 drugs are complicated and potentially dangerous. In some cases, they seem to steer users away from a state of addiction and into a state of near starvation. There is great variability of response. In some users, the drugs may lessen the joy of eating. We know that the drugs alone are not sufficient; they must be complemented with nutritional support and adequate strength training—especially for older people like me, who are susceptible to muscle loss and sarcopenic obesity.

Also, GLP-1s do not address the deeper problem of an industry pushing a supply of addictive, energy-dense foods. I don't want to see our society locked into a cycle in which one industry gets people hooked on addictive foods while another industry sells them the drugs to save them from that addiction. That's no solution.

The temptation of the simple fix is only going to get stronger. Many newer anti-obesity medications now in development are expected to reach the market in the next five years. They should be able to provide treatment for patients who need to lose up to 25% of their body weight. We all want one simple answer. This is *the* diet. This is *the* drug. But that is not how the biology of complex diseases works.

No one behavior will ensure continued weight loss. Different treatments at various points can mitigate treatment resistance over time and limit side effects from any one treatment. Weight-loss expert John Foreyt is fond of telling the story of one of his patients who lost weight and then ate the same meal every day for the rest of her life. The reason it stands out as a story is because it is so unusual, if not outright bizarre. Most of us cannot obsess over our behavior that way, and most of us would not want to even if we could. We are not going to come up with the one diet we are going to follow forever. Human beings don't behave that way.

Nevertheless, I am more optimistic than I have been in a long time that we as a society can make progress against obesity and food addiction. We can exert a strong pharmaceutical influence over our weight to an extent that has never before been possible. Now that we have these highly effective drugs, we can—if we make wise choices, and if we are fortunate enough to have access to quality healthcare—prevent and treat the health consequences of obesity and visceral adiposity.

No part of this process will be straightforward, so we are going to need help along the way. Pharmaceutical companies must be more transparent about the adverse gastrointestinal events associated with these drugs, including gastroparesis. They need to further study these drugs to help the public understand how to safely stop taking them, as well as comprehend the dangers of rapid weight loss. The FDA should mandate these studies and research on whether they can be used intermittently. Both the manufacturers and the FDA must also take steps to prevent the occurrence of malnutrition.

I am deeply troubled that the FDA approved GLP-1s for long-term chronic use without requiring the pharmaceutical companies to conduct enough studies. The pharmaceutical industry argues that these drugs have been around for decades, but not at such large doses and not for the treatment of obesity. Some people may be able to handle the drugs for life, but we just don't know. Right now we have only about five years of data at the current doses. I have not yet seen the FDA asking the hard questions. I don't see the medical community asking the hard questions either, in large part because there's so much money at stake. When I go to medical conferences, I note that nearly every physician speaker, it seems, has received some type of financial compensation from the industry. How can you trust a caretaker whose income depends on not offending the companies that make the drugs?

The FDA has a duty to ensure the safety of compounded pharmaceutical drugs and test what is being imported from China and elsewhere. The agency also needs to take action against medical devices that are promoted for weight loss and whose efficacy is questionable. The physician community must recognize that spending less than a minute reviewing a patient's medical record is not a sufficient assessment for determining treatment with GLP-1s. The surgical community needs to reassess the safety and efficacy of sleeve gastrectomies with high revision rates, likely restrict their use, and make their limitations clear to patients. Surgery will likely be relegated to those for whom medication is not effective. We need to use medications not only to treat obesity and visceral adiposity, but also to prevent severe obesity and decrease the need for surgical procedures.

The plastic surgery community and their colleagues in the med spa industry need to see weight loss for its health benefits and not as a way to attract patients for other cosmetic procedures.

Everybody in every industry that treats obesity should be working together on this issue to ensure the health and safety of patients.

Time for a Food Revolution

Using all the tools available to us, we can make improvements in our health that seemed out of reach even a few years ago. And yet, as good as the results can be, personal improvements do not address the underlying problem. We can tamp down the effects of the addictive circuits, but we're just masking the source of the addiction.

Our national body is ill. Our health has been hijacked during the last century by ultraformulated foods. The public is increasingly concerned about the rise in obesity, type 2 diabetes, heart disease, and other conditions. Americans have the lowest average lifespan among the world's twenty most developed nations, and that lifespan took a hit during the COVID-19 pandemic. I witnessed as obesity accounted for approximately two-thirds of hospitalizations from severe COVID-19 cases. There are about 678,000 deaths annually from food-related illness, with nutrition-related chronic disease costing about $16 trillion.

Food addiction and poor metabolic health begin as pediatric diseases, and a better awareness of these problems should begin in childhood as well. One in five children live with obesity. Increased weight causes type 2 diabetes, seen previously only in adults, to develop in children. Excess adiposity causes fatty liver disease, previously reserved for old men and people who drank alcohol excessively, in about 5 to 10% of children. Fatty liver disease has become as common as asthma.

Addictive behaviors are set during childhood. Starting in grade school, education about healthy eating, how the body and mind work, the importance of an active lifestyle, cooking skills, and emotional regulation may assist with prevention. Age-appropriate education that explains in simple terms how certain substances can trick the brain into wanting more and result in addiction can also be helpful.

Over the past few decades, a growing number of people in this country and around the world have joined the health populism movement. They have supported organic farming, farmers markets, whole foods, and plant-based diets. But the movement has remained stuck on the periphery of the national mainstream.

If we truly want to make America healthy, we are going to have to take on ultraformulated foods. No one likes what these foods are doing to our bodies. They are an assault on our health and, ultimately, our freedom and autonomy. We need to commit to ensuring every child reaches age eighteen at a healthy weight and in good metabolic health. We need a real food revolution.

23

. . . .

You Couldn't Have Designed
a Better Weapon

The food industry has profoundly altered our relationship with the things we eat, a relationship that is as old as our species. Consider the blueberry. Over millions of years, plants have evolved fruits to be consumed by animals, and animals evolved digestive systems to consume those fruits, resulting in a fundamental compatibility. A blueberry is a rich source of vitamins and antioxidants. Its microstructure is also well matched with the human digestive system: Packed with fiber, a blueberry releases its sugars slowly after being eaten, allowing the body to process them at a manageable rate.

Pick up a blueberry muffin at a café along with your morning coffee, though, and you get something else entirely. Now the blueberry has been cooked and sweetened. It has been combined with sugar, starch, bleached wheat flour, seed oils, and intense flavorings. The natural matrix of the fruit, not to mention the grains in the flour, has been completely altered. When a bite of that muffin hits the digestive system, it almost immediately releases a spike of glucose, contributing to metabolic chaos in a significant part of the population.

We used to think that food processing was good for us, and for a very long time we were right. Early forms of food processing were vital to our survival. Cooking enabled us to eat roots, stems, leaves, and other parts of many plants that would otherwise have been unpalatable to us. Simple forms of preservation, like salting and sun drying, provided a reliable food supply even during lean times. In the 1880s, pasteurization and canning made food safer, cheaper, and more widely available. Today, however, food processing poses a danger to human health.

Ultraprocessed, hyperpalatable foods present a constant challenge to people who are trying to limit their caloric intake, reduce visceral fat, and avoid insulin resistance. These foods are engineered to overcome all attempts to limit intake. They directly contribute to some of the most pressing health issues we face today: obesity, diabetes, and cardiovascular disease. They deliver intense flavors and pleasurable eating experiences that often combine fat and sugar; fat and salt; fat, sugar, and salt; or carbohydrates and salt in ways that are not typically found in nature. Extreme processing techniques dramatically alter the original microstructure and ingredients of these foods, adding to their addictive qualities and encouraging overconsumption, even by people who rationally know not to indulge.

Processing can alter the microstructure and nutritional qualities of meats as well. The natural microstructure of whole beef contains muscle fibers that surround the distributed fats, which slow digestion and lead to a sustained release of nutrients. In contrast, the muscle fibers are broken down and the fats are set free in finely ground, processed meats. The saturated and processed fats in hot dogs can therefore be more rapidly digested. Hot dogs also contain fillers such as sodium, preservatives, and even sugars. Those ingredients prioritize reward-system-activating flavor and shelf life over nutritional value.

You could not have designed a better weapon to blow up the human body.

Hyperpalatability and High Energy Density

Hyperpalatability is the outward face of food addiction: People might find it hard to resist a well-engineered cheeseburger with a large side of French fries, but at least they are aware (or superficially aware) of the foods they are eating. Energy density is an equally important aspect of food addiction, but it is inherently less obvious, because it is concealed within the density of calories as measured per gram or per fluid ounce.

Many familiar foods undergo transformations during processing that dramatically intensify their energy density compared to their natural sources. Professor Adam Drewnowski from the University of Washington has demonstrated that ultraprocessed foods have higher energy density and lower nutrient density compared to less processed foods. The removal of water makes the food shelf stable and cheaper to transport, but it is also a way to increase the food's energy density, along with the use of fat and sugar combinations. It's no surprise that these industrial formulations are cheaper than fresh food. For example, tomato sauce can be found in nearly every pantry. It is a go-to ingredient for quick pasta dinners on busy weeknights. Common, inexpensive supermarket tomato sauces are made from tomato paste, along with water, inexpensive fats like soybean or canola oil, and a considerable amount of added sugar. The processing begins with the tomato paste, which is created by cooking and straining tomatoes and then evaporating their water, resulting in a concentrated product that is lighter and easier to transport than whole tomatoes. The sugar added to the sauce gives a taste that appeals to consumers, especially children.

Other more expensive tomato sauces are categorized as "premium" and "super premium" and contain slightly different ingredients. Premium sauces typically contain less sugar and more whole tomato chunks, along with healthier fats like olive oil, but they often include dried herbs and vegetables that may not offer the same nutritional benefits as fresh ingredients. Super premium sauces aim to appeal to health-conscious consumers, featuring fresh herbs and vegetables and generally avoiding the use of tomato paste. Regardless of style, the processing methods and the added oils in pasta sauces result in a much higher energy density compared to fresh tomatoes.

Processed foods often serve as delivery devices for more sugars, fats, various flavors, and additives, compounding their negative health impacts. Bread is perhaps the ultimate example. Commercial breads are already often packed with sugars, fats, and highly processed flour. Then a slice of bread becomes a palette for butter, mayonnaise, jam, and countless spreads. The combinations—of sugar, fat, salt, and carbs—melt in the mouth and efficiently activate the reward system.

Increased Eating Rate

When food is processed, it often loses elements that help regulate eating behaviors, leading to quicker consumption and increased calorie intake. Foods that are engineered to be softer require less chewing, which leads to a faster pace of eating. A study by researchers in the Netherlands and Singapore showed that softer textures can increase energy intake because they allow for quicker consumption without attaining the level of satiety signaling that accompanies a harder food that must be thoroughly chewed. In essence, many processed foods are designed to encourage a "quick chew, swallow, repeat" cycle. Think about how long it takes to eat a cut of beef, with its firm texture and muscle-streaked microstructure, compared to a hot dog, chicken nuggets, or slices of deli lunch meat. Extensive chewing and longer oral processing lead to a greater sense of fullness. In contrast, rapid eating delivers calories without the corresponding signals of satiety.

The form of a food—solid, semi-solid, or liquid—influences consumption rates. Research indicates that liquid foods can be ingested at up to 600 grams per minute, whereas solid foods are typically consumed at rates between 10 and 120 grams per minute. Liquids can be consumed more rapidly than solids because they don't require chewing or mechanical movement in the mouth. As a result, liquids provoke weaker satiety response compared to solid foods containing the same number of calories.

The physical sensations of eating affect consumption rates as well. Many processed carbohydrates are designed to melt in the mouth, creating a pleasurable experience. Starch forms soft, cohesive wads in the mouth that minimize the amount of time spent chewing and that facilitate easy swallowing. Puffed snack foods have a high surface area filled with tiny air pockets. In the mouth, saliva quickly seeps into these small pores, causing the structure to break down rapidly and, again, encouraging rapid consumption before satiety signals kick in. The seamless transition from crunch to melt, a key feature of many processed foods, is crucial in promoting overeating.

High Glycemic Index

Processing can significantly alter the glycemic load of carbohydrates, transforming natural plant foods into energy-rich, highly digestible forms. Many processed foods now resemble predigested starches combined with sugars and fats, creating sources of quick calories that lead to spikes in blood sugar and overabsorption of sugar in the body. Insulin resistance and hyperinsulinemia are directly related to those spikes. Perversely, the foods we eat train us to like the feel of those spikes.

The food industry has turned wheat into a particularly effective weapon of metabolic chaos and addiction. The natural wheat kernel consists of the bran (which is rich in fiber), the germ (which contains essential nutrients), and the endosperm (primarily composed of starch). When eaten together, these three parts create a balanced source of nutrients. When wheat is refined into white flour, though, the bran and germ are stripped away, leaving only the starchy endosperm. High-speed rollers transform grains into fine flour, breaking down their natural microstructure. This flour can be further processed through extrusion, in which starch granules are subjected to high heat and moisture. Extrusion causes the starches to gelatinize and swell. The end result can be digested and absorbed much more rapidly than the original wheat kernel, causing a faster rise in blood glucose levels.

Supermarket breads also typically include components like wheat gluten, sugars, and emulsifiers used to enhance texture, extend shelf life, and create uniformity in each loaf. Even ostensibly healthy "whole wheat" breads generally have lost much of the wheat grain's natural fiber and nutritional benefits, leaving behind a product that contributes to a high glycemic load. In general, the more a food's natural structure is broken down, the faster its sugars are absorbed by the body. Foods like instant oatmeal, rice crackers, bagels, and croissants have high glycemic indices.

The processing of fresh fruits into shelf-stable food products often results in immense changes in glycemic load there as well. Fresh cranberries, which are known for their tartness and high nutritional value, are processed into dried "Craisins" that are infused with large amounts of sugar to make them more palatable. The process involves soaking the cranberries in multiple sugar baths. Cranberries, which start with only around 4% natural sugar, end up containing as much as 65% sugar by the end of the process. The hyperpalatability that comes with all that sugar only increases the likelihood that someone will eat enough Craisins to get a significant glycemic jolt.

How to Defuse a Food Bomb

By stripping foods of their natural structure and enhancing them with sugars and refined starches, the food industry has put us all in a very peculiar place. The foods that look, smell, and taste most appealing are sometimes the same ones that drive glucose spikes, cause weight gain, and lead to the buildup of visceral fat. They are leading us as a society toward insulin resistance and a rising prevalence of type 2 diabetes, along with associated cardiovascular and gastrointestinal disorders. Modern food turns out to be an extremely effective weapon against our biology.

Test subjects absorb significantly more calories when consuming a diet of highly processed foods than they do when following an unprocessed diet. It's easy to see why. Grapes are about as sweet as a natural food gets, and a bowl of grapes contains about 67 calories per 100 grams. In contrast, processed snacks like cheese crackers and chocolate chip cookies pack 489 calories and 451 calories per 100 grams, respectively.

Regulatory bodies like the FDA set guidelines for food safety, but there are no regulations protecting the public from hyperpalatability, sky-high energy density, and processing techniques that trick the body by stimulating the reward systems while largely bypassing the systems designed to activate satiety and to stop us from overeating. Nobody is truly in charge of protecting the public in the United States from the metabolic impacts of ultraformulated foods.

Some countries, particularly in Latin America, have taken steps to regulate ultraformulated foods by implementing public health campaigns. Chile's attempts to limit the presence of these foods in schools and health facilities demonstrate that change is possible, but also highlight the complexity of the battle against an industry with deep pockets and strong political influence. The global scale and influence of transnational food companies make these efforts difficult to enforce. These companies invest heavily in marketing and lobbying, making it challenging to introduce meaningful regulations that could curb the production and consumption of ultraformulated foods.

Yet, there is hope for those looking to reconnect with real, whole foods. Farmers markets and local food movements are becoming increasingly popular, offering consumers the opportunity to eat foods that are fresher, less processed, and free from the preservatives and other additives required for long-distance shipping. One of the most popular courses in medicine is culinary medicine, in which health professionals come together to teach people to cook rather than relying on ultraformulated foods. By focusing on minimally processed foods, people can enjoy the natural process of eating—chewing, savoring, and experiencing true satiety—without the artificial enhancements found in processed products. The challenge lies in creating environments that support these healthier choices, making whole foods not just available, but desirable alternatives to their ultraprocessed counterparts.

Monitoring the Spikes

There is another, more personal way to push back against food addiction and the food industry that enables it. You can't fight that entire industry yourself, but you can equip yourself so that you know what food is doing to you. Then you can at least be more focused and strategic in shaping your response.

For about $50, you can now directly observe how the foods you eat affect your body, in real time. The data come from a small sensor called a continuous glucose monitor, typically placed on the skin on the back of your arm, which measures your blood glucose levels. The monitor records in precise detail the spikes in blood glucose that occur after a meal. Every time you eat a mouthful of food, you can see within minutes how it's affecting blood glucose.

Traditionally, continuous glucose monitoring was used almost exclusively by diabetics who needed to know their blood glucose levels so they could adjust their sugar intake to manage their hyperglycemia. But it is beginning to gain widespread popularity for those interested in healthy eating and weight loss. Dr. Grazia Aleppo, an endocrinologist at Northwestern University, believes that many people could benefit from using one. She notes that the number of people with insulin resistance and prediabetes is rising rapidly, especially in the United States. If people had better information about their blood sugar levels, she argues, they might be more inclined to improve their diet, and would have a clearer picture of just how harmful modern food addiction can be.

"If you start eating cereal, bagels, sugar, and soda, your blood sugar will go up over 140 mg/dL. The problem is, it's not one time. One time doesn't matter," Dr. Aleppo says. "It's the cumulative effects, the constant spikes over thirty years that matter."

I ask Dr. Aleppo who should care about their glucose spiking.

"Everybody," she responds.

"But don't we all spike when we eat foods that elevate blood glucose?" I inquire.

Dr. Aleppo points to data showing that the amount of time our bodies spend with our blood glucose above 140 mg/dL is associated with increased cardiometabolic risk. The goal is to limit the time between 70 and 140 mg/dL, especially in people with prediabetes, which includes many people living with overweight or obesity. An estimated 97.6 million people in the United States have prediabetes.

High levels of glucose in the bloodstream can damage the endothelial cells that line the blood vessels, which sets off a cascade of harmful effects. "Endothelial cells are very sensitive to changes in blood glucose levels due to constant exposure to glucose fluctuations; these in turn may increase cardiovascular risk by increasing inflammation and, eventually, contribute to arterial stiffness," Dr. Aleppo explains. Fortunately, that sensitivity also means that modest changes in food choices and eating patterns can meaningfully lessen the impacts. With a continuous glucose monitor, anyone can see the effects of little victories against food addiction. "Continuous monitoring can show early changes in postprandial hyperglycemia. Small differences in the glucose average may change prognosis long term," Dr. Aleppo says.

Medical researchers have long recognized that persistent hyperglycemia poses a serious and steadily increasing risk to health. Only recently have they come to realize that strong intermittent spikes in blood glucose levels also cause damage. The numbers that appear on a continuous glucose monitor become more meaningful when connected to the actual biochemical effects they represent. Once people can make that connection and directly witness the link between food and glucose spikes, they may want to change what they are eating.

Dr. Aleppo narrates the consequences of a glucose spike. "When blood sugar levels are high, the endothelial cells cannot limit glucose exposure," she says. Those cells become stressed and release a molecule called DAMP (damage-associated molecular patterns), setting off a cascade of destructive effects. DAMP molecules trigger the production of free radicals—reactive oxygen-bearing molecules—that accelerate aging and cellular breakdown. DAMP can also trigger overproduction of blood platelets, leading to clotting, and can lead to changes that disrupt cells in the bone marrow, where red blood cells are made.

Continuous glucose monitors can help make people aware of the biological troubles brewing within them. The devices might also help spark a bigger, society-wide change.

Addictive foods are not labeled or regulated in large part because their ingredients fall under a scientific standard known as "generally recognized as safe." Common substances are to be classified that way if there is a general recognition that there is a reasonable certainty of no harm. Data from continuous glucose monitors worn by a large number of people who are vulnerable to cardiometabolic disease could provide the crucial information to indicate that certain ingredients, ingredient combinations, and processing techniques do in fact cause harm.

Evidence that raises questions about the safety of a food or category of foods could be enough to challenge their "generally recognized as safe" certification. Data from continuous glucose monitors could help the public fight back, at least a little, against the companies that make food into an addictive delivery system for hazardous glucose spikes.

24
. . . .

The Food Industry Has Us
in Its Sights

Thirty years ago, when I needed to understand the advertising machine behind the tobacco industry's decades of lies and obfuscation about the dangers of smoking, I went to Richard Pollay, a professor of marketing and behavior at the University of British Columbia Sauder School of Business, who was and is the foremost expert on cigarette advertising. Professor Pollay consulted in early litigation against the tobacco companies for suppressing scientific evidence of the dangers of smoking and pushing consumers to buy an addictive and deadly product. He interpreted the industry's internal marketing research as well as planning documents and published dozens of studies that unraveled the twisted, ingenious nature of their advertising methods.

I recently called Professor Pollay and we met again. This time, we sat on opposite ends of a Zoom meeting, gazing into the face of another shrewd, powerful, and persuasive force: Tony the Tiger.

Professor Pollay was showing me a 1978 print ad for Kellogg's Sugar Frosted Flakes, in which a boy sits at the breakfast table, gleefully digging into a bowl of cereal. At the top of the page, a slogan announces, "No breakfast is nutritious until somebody eats it."

It's a clever piece of deception. Deeper into the ad copy, there is a host of carefully crafted claims, misleading but meticulously accurate. One claim: "When you're Kellogg's, it's pretty easy to put good nutrition into a cereal.

After all, we've been doing it for a long time." Yes, Professor Pollay says, the company does put in micronutrients—but only after first removing that nutrition through a refinement process that takes the grains and other ingredients from which Frosted Flakes are derived and stripping those foods of their inherent value. Another claim: "A one-ounce serving of Kellogg's Sugar Frosted Flakes cereal contains 25% of the US Daily Recommended Allowance of 7 essential vitamins. Plus 10% of the US RDA of vitamin D and iron." Professor Pollay scoffs: "If this is one out of three meals you're eating and you're only getting 10% of the recommended daily allowance, it's not all that rich a source of nutrition."

Kellogg's even winks at the addictive elements in its breakfast cereal. After boasting that Sugar Frosted Flakes is loaded with essential elements, the company's ad confides, "But that's not why kids like them. It's that sparkle of sugar frosting we add that gets the cereal out of the bowl and into the youngster." In other words: all that refined sugar, which doesn't seem as virtuous as the vitamins. Well, it's virtuous, too, because without it, you'd never get those vitamins into your kids. In this vision, sugar has nothing to do with obesity or glucose spikes, it's merely a tool for encouraging nutritious eating.

"A lot of the advertising isn't trying to convince you that this is the best thing," Professor Pollay tells me. "It's trying to de-stigmatize the product." Kellogg's sugar defense didn't deceive the public for long, but the company kept adapting. In 1983, the word "sugar" was dropped from the cereal's official name. By the start of the twenty-first century, the advertising for Frosted Flakes had morphed again, making the cereal seem practically like a performance-enhancing drug. Frosted Flakes became the "Official Cereal of Major League Baseball" and a NASCAR sponsor. In a print ad co-branded with the 2002 Olympic Games, there are just two words: "Get Supercharged!" Tony the Tiger is recognizable only by the blurry streak of his orange tail disappearing between slalom poles on a ski course. Another ad from that year features the same two-word slogan near a tiger-striped basketball hoop mounted eight stories high.

"The implications are that this product is associated with healthfulness and athleticism. Leaping tall buildings with a single bound," Professor Pollay says. There's almost no text, which is typical of the image-led advertising style that dominates what people see today. Marketers realized that people weren't taking in all the information they printed; it was a waste of space. And, conveniently, when your ad says virtually nothing, that protects against claims of false advertising.

During my call with Professor Pollay, I was struck by the parallels between the strategies used in food marketing and those used in cigarette
marketing. Both types of ads were designed to imply healthfulness in ways
that were at once effective in the marketplace and defensible in the courts.
Professor Pollay notes one important difference: By the 1960s, cigarette
companies could not have any credible claim to the healthfulness of their
products, whereas the reasonable assumption was, and still is, that food
should be good for you.

In reality, mega-corporations are making and marketing highly chemical, engineered edible products that can do serious damage to our biology.
Then the company's challenge is to convince people that their products are
healthful without alerting them to all the ways that corporate food engineers have sapped the goodness from the original food. The processed food
industry currently spends $14 billion a year in the United States pushing
products that contribute to overeating and weight gain. To make sure those
ad campaigns hit, companies race to stay ahead of the zeitgeist. They hire
market research firms to divine what the public likes and dislikes, craves
and fears, and whether ads are hitting their marks.

The food industry then plies the public with apparent antidotes to the
concern du jour. Companies slap "fat free" labels on products that would
never inherently contain fat in the first place. They throw around "gluten
free" labels, too, knowing full well that the labels frequently appear on
products that would never contain gluten, a protein found in some grains
such as wheat and barley. (Never mind that most humans tolerate gluten
perfectly well.) There is no shortage of other examples of this kind of misleading labeling: all natural, real fruit, GMO-free, no artificial colors. It all
serves to distract from the problematic aspects of a product. The labels are
psychological tricks to make unhealthy food seem healthy.

I acknowledge that serious, well-intentioned studies in nutrition science
helped enable these food-industry deceptions. Researchers broke food down
into its components and analyzed it as a collection of chemicals. Along the
way, we gave companies the ability to sell those components without having
to maintain the essential, original, functional structure of food.

One of Professor Pollay's criticisms therefore hits me particularly
hard. "Even the display of nutrition data on the sides of processed food
packaging—while it was meant to be informative to consumers—is kind
of a virtue signaling. It says, 'Oh, we have these elements and we're not
supplying 100% of every one, but look at all the things we *are* supplying,'"

he says. "I think the information panels that were mandated suggested that these foods had virtue."

When I was FDA commissioner, I had instituted those nutrition labels.

"We sort of missed this consequence," I admit. We made the sellers of processed foods print facts about the vitamins, minerals, and proteins in their products. We made them call out trans fats and added sugars. But nowhere did we require companies to reveal how the composition of these foods affects our bodies. We continued to allow companies to describe food in terms of unfamiliar, technical, confusing ingredient names in the ingredient panel. Still, nothing relieves the companies of their responsibility to ensure that their products provide a reasonable certainty of no harm.

"It takes me back to the tobacco case," Professor Pollay says. "You can expect that the regulators are playing checkers while the industry is playing chess."

When food companies decided to promote "zero calorie" diet soda, "lower sugar" juice, "light" mayonnaise, and "natural" protein and granola bars, they could point right to the ingredient label. There it is in black and white: zero calories, zero trans fat, healthy-looking names of nuts and grains. And food companies have many more places to duck from responsibility for the health consequences of what they sell.

Food Label 2.0

Many of the largest food companies seem to have forgotten that they are in the business of making food that their customers rely on to thrive. Instead, this industry is slowly killing its customers, and its executives have to know this, yet they have done little to improve the safety of their products. Government has also failed to act. Unfortunately, there is little political reality for major new regulations restricting the sale of ultraformulated foods or forcing manufacturers to change the way they are made. Still, there is a way that we can help the public: by giving them a much more complete and useful understanding of the foods they are eating.

At the most basic level, consumers don't know what is in their food and how it affects them biologically. That kind of information is essential for human health. Making available details about processing and its effects on insulin release and blood sugar is the least the industry could do, and yet it does not. Current food labeling lacks full transparency, and often it is outright misleading. I am here to make the case for a radically new and improved approach, one that keeps the current nutrition facts panel but provides additional information about the product.

The US Food and Drug Administration, founded to protect the safety of our food, has failed to keep pace with an industry that has replaced much of what was once food with cheap, ultraformulated products that go well beyond what can be made in the home kitchen. The FDA, starved of needed funding by a Congress that is heavily swayed by industry lobbyists, no longer ensures the safety of our food or the adequacy of our food labeling. I want my former agency to take action so consumers can make healthier food choices and so companies have strong incentives to design foods that help sustain public health while still meeting consumer demands for taste, cost, and convenience.

The additional labeling would emphasize transparency about food ingredients and their processing. It should make it easier for shoppers to know what types of ingredients and nutrients are in the food packages they buy, and why they are in there. In addition to revamping food labels, we must reconsider the Dietary Guidelines for Americans, which is still designed for metabolically healthy individuals, even though today they represent less than 20% of the population. We need guidelines for the 80% of Americans who are insulin resistant or are having trouble maintaining a healthy weight.

As part of the additional labeling, we need a label on the front of food packages that enables consumers to quickly know whether the main ingredients in the food they are buying are ones they can thrive on. An approach I favor is one that lists the top three ingredients in packaged food. I also favor putting warning labels on harmful foods, a technique that has been shown to be effective at reducing consumption of ultraformulated foods in other countries.

The FDA is aware of the problems, but its current approach is far too timid. The agency has been testing and recently proposed a new design for front-of-package labeling that would include a mild food warning notice. Although this design was favored by some consumers and food companies, similar designs have been shown in studies to be ineffective and confusing. The FDA's proposed version of the label lists key nutrients (saturated fat, sodium, and added sugars) and puts a High, Medium, or Low next to each. Listing multiple nutrients and matching them with quantitative descriptors seems like a great way to cause a mental traffic jam. One need only to imagine being at an intersection and seeing a traffic light that is red, yellow, and green at the same time to realize how confusing such a system could be. Also troubling, companies can clean their labels by replacing these nutrients through ultraprocessing.

To provide transparency, we also need a full product dossier to match the complexity of today's highly processed foods. I envision a label that lists all of the ingredients, their function, and their potential impact on our health. Such a label will require more space than is available on most packages—but that's fine, as many people now carry a smartphone. To create the additional labeling, we will need a database of all the ingredients and nutrients in the foods sold at any given store, along with phone apps that will enable consumers to scan a code on the package and get a list of information, written in clear language, customized to their specific concerns and health needs.

The FDA would need to set standards for the master food database to ensure that all of the crucial information is available, accurate, and up-to-date. The agency should list the questions companies must answer about the products they sell so consumers don't have to rely on company virtue signaling and marketing in choosing what to buy.

Not Just a Label—A Food Information System

Food companies might object to the extreme transparency I am proposing. I would say that they should have no choice. Consumers should know about the function and health impact of every ingredient in the packaged foods they buy. A truly transparent system needs to ask and answer the following questions:

- What is each ingredient in this product? Why is it there? Does it have an established health benefit or concern?
- Does the food contain pairs of fat and salt, fat and simple sugars, or carbohydrates and salt, translated into simple numerical values that indicate hyperpalatable foods?
- Is the product energy-dense?
- What is the product's effect on insulin and blood glucose?
- What are the processing steps for this product? How does processing change the food matrix, how food is digested and metabolized, and

how does that affect eating rate, satiety, and human health? Where was the food produced, from farm to the grocery shelf?

- Is this product sweet, measured on a scale of 1 to 5, where 1 is not sweet and 5 is very sweet? Does it include added sweeteners? Refined carbohydrates?

- Has this product or its combination of ingredients been shown in valid studies to be healthy or potentially harmful?

We also need to revise the ingredient panel on all packaged foods. The ingredient labels that currently appear on food packages allow companies to avoid listing some ingredients or to do so in a misleading manner. For example, the labels require that ingredients be listed in descending order of predominance by weight. This rule allows companies to use several sweeteners that, if grouped together, would be one of the top ingredients, but when listed separately, are buried deeper down the list. Food companies also frequently use names that most consumers don't recognize—for example, allulose, tagatose, thaumatin, and neotame, all of which are sweeteners.

The revised ingredient panel should group ingredients by type or function, so that sweeteners and possibly other ingredients would be listed together as needed to give consumers a better understanding of the nature of the food they are buying. The label should also require quantitative ingredient declarations, a rule that is required in numerous other countries. This rule requires that an ingredient be emphasized on the label through words or images if the ingredient is essential to characterize the food, or if the ingredient's quantity is important in distinguishing the product from similar foods.

In this way, consumers would quickly see the percentage of the product consisting of that key ingredient. And new rules should ensure the readability of the top-line printed ingredient list on food packages, setting graphic requirements such as type size and font, as we did for the Nutrition Facts label.

A new food information program—one that is integrated into a much more extensive public information system about food, processing, and health—could provide a huge boost to public health. It would help millions of people steer away from food addiction and improve their eating patterns, with or without the help of the new anti-obesity drugs. But labeling alone cannot address the enormous crisis created by the modern food industry.

The United States leads the world in science funding, and yet we chronically underinvest in nutrition research. I have long argued that this country needs a national institute of nutrition that would research fundamental issues such as food composition, eating patterns, human metabolism, and connections between diet and health. So far, however, there is no political movement to create such an institute. The National Institutes of Health spends most of its budget, currently hovering around $50 billion a year, investing in effective disease treatments at its institutes of cancer, diabetes, and heart disease, while largely ignoring nutrition, which is the cause of many of those illnesses. Less than 5% of the NIH budget goes to nutrition research.

Likewise, the FDA needs more nutrition resources to ensure that our food doesn't make us acutely or chronically ill. Some of that funding should be directed to the extensive new food information project I've outlined here, but there is so much more to be done. Aggressive federal food safety programs have succeeded in reducing acute food illness deaths in the United States to 1,400 per year. Meanwhile, chronic food illness kills more than that many people every day, but gets comparatively little attention. The FDA spends only $25 million out of a food budget of more than $1 billion on nutrition and chronic food illness. Inadequate funding is a key reason why we have made no progress in reducing chronic food illness deaths in more than fifty years.

The relatively low average lifespan of Americans and the rising incidence of chronic disease among our children should sound an urgent alarm. We faced a similar alarm in the 1980s when tobacco was the leading cause of preventable death in the United States and 25% of young people smoked. We acted and moved toward solving the problem. Scientists investigated and documented the risks. Legislators worked out solutions. Congress enacted laws to reduce youth smoking. Communities passed smoking bans. Today, our national youth smoking rate is less than 2%.

We can have similar success reducing chronic disease, starting, again, with our children. A new system of food labeling can be the first effective step in providing transparency, empowering consumers, and forcing food companies to accept that their primary mission is to provide the food we need to thrive.

25

. . . .

The Gold Rush of
Weight-Loss Drugs

When I watch the frenzied excitement around the GLP-1 weight-loss medications, I'm sometimes reminded of the old California Gold Rush, with its potential to change lives. For patients, the GLP-1s offer by far the most promising treatments yet found for breaking food addiction, affording millions of people a more achievable path to weight loss.

For pharmaceutical companies, the drugs have been a tremendous financial windfall. The market for weight management has ballooned to $90 billion in the United States and $275 billion worldwide. The combined revenues from Eli Lilly, which makes tirzepatide, and Novo Nordisk, which makes semaglutide, from their weight-loss drugs is projected to climb to between $80 and $150 billion a year within a decade in the United States alone. These extraordinary numbers have set other major pharmaceutical companies scrambling to develop their own GLP-1 drugs or combination drugs.

But I keep thinking about another aspect of the Gold Rush: It was a time of chaos and confusion, when lots of people were swindled, fell for false claims, or pinned their hopes on rumors in the absence of reliable information. I want to hold the food industry responsible for its actions, but I want to hold the medical and pharmaceutical industries to a higher standard as well.

If used properly, the GLP-1 medications show promise for treating obesity, but the intense marketing of the drugs, amplified by celebrity endorsements, media hype, and word-of-mouth messages, is already leading to misuse. Companies are producing copycat versions of the drugs and off-brand versions that put unsuspecting patients at risk of harm. Federal and state regulatory authorities appear overwhelmed, like a handful of security guards trying to stop a mob of thousands. And keep in mind that the makers of the drugs are still unsure of the exact mechanisms that cause the weight loss. Much more study is required simply to understand the biochemical and physiological workings of the GLP-1 drugs.

As the demand for the new GLP-1 drugs went viral, Novo Nordisk and Eli Lilly ran out of them, prompting the FDA to officially declare shortages of the semaglutide drugs Ozempic and Wegovy in August 2022. Four months later, the FDA added the tirzepatide drugs Mounjaro and Zepbound to their medication shortage list. Compounding pharmacies— companies that combine, mix, or alter ingredients to create a customized drug—jumped in to address the shortage with their own versions of semaglutide and tirzepatide injections, taking advantage of a regulatory opening created by the shortage designation. These alternate providers significantly undercut the standard cost, which is around $1,000 a month for the sanctioned drugs, and potentially pose unnecessary risks for patients.

In October 2024, the FDA removed the Eli Lilly drugs from the shortage list, and Lilly filed lawsuits against the compounding pharmacies producing versions of Mounjaro and Zepbound. Meanwhile, the compounders sued the FDA to retain the shortage designation. Patients are caught in the middle, faced with a confusing array of options, many of them potentially dangerous. For now, neither government nor private companies have the authority or inclination to mitigate the risks.

OppGen Marketing has put together *The Ultimate Weight Loss Marketing Playbook* to guide white-label clinics on ways to feed the vast demand for weight-loss drugs. (The practice of white-labeling allows companies to put their brand names on products or services provided by others.) OppGen notes that physical weight-loss clinics were economically battered by the COVID-19 pandemic, but sales of weight-loss supplements were a rich source of compensating revenue. Another company, MD Integrations, offers to help online companies set up a white-label practice within days. As a test, one of my researchers contacted FuturHealth, an online white-label weight-loss company boasting two hundred thousand patients. After informing them that his only goal was to lose weight as quickly as possible, and answering just a few questions about his general health, he was approved for branded or compounded weight-loss drugs and guaranteed a 15% weight loss.

White-label clinics prescribing alternatives to FDA-approved weight-loss drugs often partner with compounding pharmacies. Unlike standard pharmaceutical companies, compounding pharmacies have less stringent safety requirements. Patients sometimes pay the price for the looser oversight. In 2012, contaminated spinal injection products from a compounding pharmacy sickened 798 individuals with meningitis and resulted in the deaths of more than one hundred people. The CDC, in collaboration with state and local health departments and the FDA, tracked the contaminated steroid injections back to the New England Compounding Center in Framingham, Massachusetts. The owner of the firm was sentenced to prison for his role in the affair.

Consider the difference between the GLP-1 drugs made by Novo Nordisk and Eli Lilly and the compounded versions now flooding the market. FDA approval is required by law only for prescribed drugs. Pharmaceutical companies seeking approval must demonstrate safety and effectiveness initially through animal studies, and eventually conduct human clinical trials where the results are peer reviewed by independent scientists. The process must be transparent, and subjects of clinical trials must be fully informed of the risks before providing consent. Further, manufacturing plants producing prescription drugs are subject to inspection, and ingredients can be verified through chemical testing.

In contrast, many compounded versions of prescription drugs can be sold only if there is a shortage of the FDA-approved products. Once that happens, though, the compounded versions do not require clinical trials to prove they are safe and actually work. Their precise ingredients are rarely verified.

The situation is worse for pharmaceutical products or components produced in foreign countries, where many drugs sold in the United States are made. The FDA's overseas inspection program traditionally has been underfunded, forcing the agency to conduct inspections (either on site or upon entry at US borders) mainly in the small number of cases where there are grounds for suspicion. The United States' line of defense against contaminated products from offshore companies is so porous that the auditing arm of Congress, the Government Accountability Office, placed the FDA's foreign inspection program on its list of "high-risk" federal programs, finding it inadequate to protect public health safety. Government analysts have noted that the FDA's foreign inspections are severely limited because they "have generally been preannounced" and "may rely on the establishment being inspected to provide translation services."

As a result, potentially millions of patients are receiving weight-loss drugs without knowing their actual ingredients or the source of their manufacture, and without the assurance that the drugs they are taking were made in facilities that were inspected prior to their shipment. Poison control centers across the country are reporting illnesses related to knock-off GLP-1 drugs. The American Medical Association (AMA) documented a 1,500% increase in poison incidents related to weight-loss drugs. The AMA also found in August 2024 that approximately half of the online pharmacies selling GLP-1 compounded versions were operating illegally. The National Association of Boards of Pharmacy, representing state agencies, separately reports that at least 35,000 online compounding pharmacies are acting illegally.

In early 2024, the FDA confirmed that it had received "adverse event reports" about compounded versions of semaglutide and cautioned that "patients should not use a compounded drug if an approved drug is available. Patients and healthcare professionals should understand that the agency does not review compounded versions of these drugs for safety, effectiveness, or quality." The agency further warned, "Patients should only obtain drugs containing semaglutide with a prescription from a licensed healthcare provider."

My former agency seems caught in a quandary between tightly regulating the newly approved drugs and loosening the supply by allowing copycat versions of them. Meanwhile, compounded weight-loss drugs remain prevalent and easy to obtain.

Telemedicine dominates the field of obesity medicine, which further complicates efforts to take strong action against compounded and illegal versions of GLP-1s. For patients, telemedicine can have many upsides. It improves access to healthcare in large regions of the country, eases the ability to practice proactive patient care, and reduces unnecessary costs. But it is largely unregulated, lacks sufficient laws to protect patients, and has minimal if any hands-on oversight by federal, state, and local agencies. This is a dangerous environment in which to launch large-scale medical outreach operations to tens of millions of patients with obesity.

The medical director of one large online weight-loss clinic privately related to me that his screeners often spend just a minute assessing forms online before prescribing new GLP-1 drugs. Some states do not allow telemedicine for weight loss, so companies created "medical spas" to provide weight-loss services for patients. Such spas sometimes operate unsafely, use mainly compounded drugs, and do not conduct comprehensive patient evaluations before selling GLP-1 knockoffs.

Meanwhile, compounded, off-label, and outright fake versions of GLP-1s have become a global problem. The World Health Organization reports that it has observed an "increased demand for these medicines as well as reports on falsification," adding that "to protect themselves from falsified medicines and their harmful effects, patients who are using these products can take actions such as buying medicines with prescriptions from licensed physicians and avoid buying medicines from unfamiliar or unverified sources, such as those that may be found online." In issuing a warning, the WHO noted that falsified drugs had been detected in Brazil and the United Kingdom in addition to the United States. In Australia, the government was so concerned about the dangers of compounded weight-loss drugs that it totally banned their use in 2024.

Americans should not accept a system so full of loopholes that patients with obesity are routinely sold unsafe or ineffective drugs and supplements. The FDA, despite its legal limitations, could do more than issue warnings and alerts to a handful of the many white-label sites and compounding pharmacies. It should add resources and regulatory reforms that provide more than lip service to the problem. The FDA should also reform its process for declaring drug shortages to ensure it is not wantonly used to allow the proliferation of compounding pharmacies to replace the approved therapies. Such a change would not require additional funding or new legislative authority.

"There's an urgent need for better post-marketing surveillance, to look at questions around safety. We have a complete blind spot for compounded medications. We desperately need to know what's happening there," said Dr. Kristina Henderson Lewis at a symposium on long-term use of anti-obesity medication in 2024.

We need new weight-loss drugs like the GLP-1s, but not at the expense of patient safety. In the nineteenth-century Gold Rush, people accepted danger and uncertainty because they were taking risks knowingly, hoping for a great reward. In that regard, the current gold rush is completely different.

Too often, people do not know where their weight-loss medications are coming from, who produced them, who inspected them, or even what is in them. And the reward they are chasing is not a self-indulgent dream of great wealth, but the basic human values of living a healthy life, unbound by food addiction.

There has never been a greater need for solutions to obesity, and there has never been a greater need for careful oversight of those solutions. At a time when we should go forward safely and proceed with caution, we are doing neither. White-label companies and compounding pharmacies will continue to compete for larger shares of the GLP-1 market, and obesity patients will remain at their mercy.

26

· · · ·

Economics and Equity

We all understand the stigma and discrimination against people with obesity. It has been part of the culture for many decades. People with obesity are viewed differently from others in employment, healthcare, and social relationships. Society sets thinness as an ideal. People with obesity don't meet that ideal and are discriminated against. And even if they are treated as if they have a disease or an addiction, we don't support them accordingly.

Before the signing of the Affordable Care Act in 2010, what insurance covered was governed strictly by contract. An employer and the insurance company would enter into a contract that set out the conditions the insurer would cover. Section 1557 of the Affordable Care Act changed that by preventing insurers from discriminating in those contracts based on race, color, national origin, sex, age, or disability. The purpose of Section 1557 was to eliminate discrimination in how insurance carriers designed their benefit packages. The law prohibits designing a benefit that targets people with a disability. Today, many insurers cover prescription drugs for conditions such as heart disease and cancer, but have an exclusion in their policy that states they will not pay to cover therapies to treat obesity.

Other sections of the Affordable Care Act reinforce the fact that the purpose of Section 1557 was to prohibit insurers from denying coverage to a group of people with a condition for which other insureds are entitled to receive coverage. The exclusions to cover highly effective medications for obesity, in my opinion, fall within the prohibition of Section 1557 because they target people with obesity, which is a disease, impairment, and disability, and excludes effective medications from coverage.

The insurance companies argue that obesity is not a disability. Informally, we all know that is not true. Certain state and federal courts have agreed, ruling that obesity is always a disability. These courts have held that, in those individuals living with obesity, the condition impairs life activities sufficient to meet the definition of a disability. Under federal law, if a medical professional diagnoses a condition, that condition is an "impairment," and if the condition results in a substantial impact on a daily activity, it is a "disability."

Behind the argument over these legal disputes regarding obesity coverage is the stereotype that obesity is the result of a lack of willpower and that people should be able to control their eating—in essence, that obesity is a personal failing, not a medical condition. We know this is not true, and we now know the reason. Obesity is the result of living in a society in which we are all surrounded by ultraformulated foods. Those foods have altered the reward circuitry of the brain and impaired satiating mechanisms, causing a dysregulated appetite that results in an energy balance at a higher-than-normal body fat mass associated with adverse health consequences and impairments.

The obstacle to recognizing this reality is that four federal courts of appeals have ruled that obesity is not a physiological condition or impairment. They have bought into the arguments of the insurance companies that obesity is not itself enough of an impairment and that there needs to be a secondary underlying condition. They are wrong medically, and they are wrong on the law. We know that obesity is the central and causative element of diabetes and cardiometabolic disease. It also triggers other serious obesity-related conditions such as sleep apnea, osteoarthritis, and certain forms of cancer. Another argument the insurance companies make is that they are not discriminating against people with obesity; they are discriminating only against weight-loss drugs. That is like saying the companies could deny coverage for people with cancer because they would not be discriminating against the cancer patients, only against chemotherapy.

I have tried to understand what is going on with these judges in these US courts of appeals. They may have grown up at a time before we understood that obesity is a disease. They may be resistant to recognizing the true medical nature of obesity because of the enormous costs associated with anti-obesity medications and they are concerned that paying for them would overwhelm healthcare budgets. The law often depends on a judge's understanding of science, or on a judge's feelings about budgets and spending. But, the law should prevent discrimination. We can no longer discriminate against people living with obesity.

There are two immediate problems caused by the discrimination against protecting people living with obesity. Because insurance doesn't cover weight-loss medications, people who need them but can't afford them may resort to sources with questionable product safety. In addition, the use of these medications is not being administered under good clinical care. In a fair society, the care and monitoring of weight loss for people with obesity has to be viewed as an essential aspect of medical care that will be reimbursed by health insurance. To do otherwise is discrimination.

Cost-Effectiveness

Insurance companies can deny coverage for other reasons. They can say that a medication is not cost-effective. In some ways, this is their most powerful argument, because it sidesteps legal questions about discrimination and even moral arguments about fairness. In this view, if the cost of the drugs is greater than the value of the health benefits they provide, it is simply not the job of the insurance company to cover them. The companies can now frame it purely as a matter of practical economics.

That has always been a dubious argument. The marked cardiovascular benefits associated with the new GLP-1 anti-obesity medications mean that it may also be an obsolete argument, especially as the costs of these medications come down. The insurance companies have put exclusions into their policies specifically denying coverage for weight-loss drugs because they know that they will lose if they have to litigate that these medications are not medically necessary. The legal standard for whether something is "medically effective" is whether it is effective and whether it is a less costly alternative. These new anti-obesity medications are undoubtedly effective. Given the enormous healthcare expenses associated with obesity, treatment is also a bargain in the long run. The trouble is, insurance companies don't typically prioritize the long-term payoff from preventive care. If they did, patients would ultimately benefit and overall healthcare costs would be lower.

The best economic argument the insurance companies can make is that the weight-loss drugs are not really cost-effective after all, because patients will eventually gain the weight back. Either they will stop taking the drugs, or the drugs will lose their ability to control body weight. If the companies are right, that will be a serious blow to the millions of people who have pinned their hopes on the new GLP-1 drugs. The new anti-obesity drugs are not a cure-all, and for most people, I expect, they will not be the solitary answer, but it is already clear to me that these drugs improve our ability to tackle food addiction and its nasty side effects.

The pressing question for patients and companies alike is how well the GLP-1s will work over many years and decades. If researchers can put together strong evidence of significant long-term cost-saving health benefits, that will torpedo one of the insurance companies' most powerful rationales for denying coverage. Put simply: The best argument for equity is efficacy.

For some insight, I checked in with Dr. David Arterburn, a health services researcher at Kaiser Permanente who has spent his career exploring the complexities of treating obesity. His work focuses on balancing the promise of anti-obesity medications with the realities of how they are used in the real world. His interest in obesity began during his medical residency, at the height of the controversy over fen-phen, the diet drug combination that was ultimately pulled from the market due to safety concerns. Seeing firsthand how difficult it was to manage obesity, Dr. Arterburn transitioned from direct clinical care into research on the safety and effectiveness of anti-obesity treatments.

Over the years, his focus has shifted from bariatric surgery to anti-obesity drugs, and now specifically to understanding the cost-effectiveness of the new GLP-1 drugs like semaglutide and tirzepatide. These drugs have shown impressive potential for helping people lose significant amounts of weight, but he wanted to know whether healthcare systems can afford them, and if they will prove sustainable, affordable, and accessible in the real world, where patients have to deal with the thorny issues of cost, access, and long-term adherence.

Insurance coverage will depend heavily on the cost-effectiveness of these medications, which involves weighing both the immediate costs of the drugs and the long-term savings they might generate by reducing obesity-related complications such as type 2 diabetes, heart disease, and stroke. For now, the upfront costs of GLP-1 medications are significant. Even with price pressure from compounding and increased production by Eli Lilly and Novo Nordisk, dosages of the drugs, often exceeding $1,000 per month, could save the healthcare system substantial money if the drugs help people achieve lasting weight loss and avoid costly chronic conditions. But that's a big "if." Even in integrated healthcare systems like Kaiser Permanente, spending on GLP-1 medications has skyrocketed as more patients seek access to them.

Dr. Arterburn told me that the price of these medications is a huge concern for doctors and hospitals in addition to insurance companies. "It's almost untenable for healthcare systems to afford to pay for the number of people who would like to be treated," he told me. Healthcare payers are faced with increasingly difficult decisions about how to allocate resources effectively, ensuring that those who need these treatments the most can access them without overwhelming the system financially. They, too, need to know whether the long-term savings generated by these medications will be enough to justify their upfront costs.

If weight loss achieved using GLP-1 drugs leads to fewer hospitalizations, fewer cases of type 2 diabetes, and lower rates of heart disease, then the initial investment could pay off in the long run. But that kind of return on investment may take years—or even decades—to materialize. "Cost savings from these medications aren't coming soon," Dr. Arterburn said. Moreover, real-world use of these medications often doesn't match the results seen in clinical trials. In carefully controlled studies, patients remain on the medications for extended periods, and the weight-loss results are impressive. But when patients are just living their normal lives, they frequently stop taking the drugs long before they've achieved meaningful, lasting weight loss.

"More than 90% of patients stop taking anti-obesity medications within a year, with many discontinuing after just six months," Dr. Arterburn said. Early discontinuation significantly undermines the potential long-term benefits of these medications. When patients stop taking the drugs, they often regain the weight they lost—sometimes at an even faster rate than they lost it. "The slope of weight regain is often steeper than the slope of weight loss, and that's a real concern," he told me. As noted, this phenomenon, known as weight cycling, has its own set of negative health consequences, including increased risks for cardiovascular disease and metabolic disorders.

In many ways, the issue of adherence lies at the heart of the debate over the cost-effectiveness of anti-obesity medications, and so ultimately over the whole issue of equitable access. The impressive weight-loss numbers that GLP-1 drugs can produce don't mean much if patients discontinue the medication too early. For these medications to be considered cost-effective, they need to help patients achieve and maintain long-term weight loss over a large portion of a lifetime. But achieving long-term adherence to these medications is no small feat, especially given the financial barriers and potential side effects patients face.

Dr. Arterburn's research highlights the need for support systems that can help patients stick with their treatment plans. This could include counseling, education, and financial assistance programs aimed at reducing barriers to adherence.

Given the high cost of anti-obesity medications, Dr. Arterburn advocates for step therapy models, which provide a structured approach to managing costs while ensuring that patients have access to effective treatments. That approach might not satisfy patients who have heard about GLP-1s and want to get instant access to these drugs. Under the step therapy model, doctors would first direct their patients to less expensive interventions—such as diet, exercise, and counseling—before prescribing more costly medications like GLP-1 receptor agonists. If the initial treatments fail to produce meaningful results, then the more expensive options can be introduced. The problem with this approach is that the less expensive options have only a fraction of the efficacy of the new drugs.

By prioritizing less expensive treatments as the first line of defense, Dr. Arterburn explains, healthcare providers can reserve the more costly medications for patients who are at the greatest risk of developing severe obesity-related complications. The argument is that this approach helps ensure that resources are used efficiently and that patients receive the most appropriate care based on their individual needs. Dr. Arterburn acknowledges that step care models have their limitations, though. Not all patients respond well to lifestyle interventions or to lower-cost medications. The step care model also, by definition, places obstacles in patients' path to accessing more effective weight-loss treatments like GLP-1s. Considering the breadth of the food addiction problem, such obstacles go directly against the goal of equitable treatment.

Ultimately, the price of the new anti-obesity medications needs to come down. Cheaper drugs, more than anything else, will shift the cost-benefit relationship and put pressure on insurance companies to provide broader, fairer coverage. Dr. Arterburn is optimistic that the cost of these medications will decrease. He noted that there is already some movement in that direction, and not just from the lightly regulated compounders. "As more generic versions of GLP-1 medications come to market, we should see prices drop," he says.

The Fight for Equity

Insurance companies are not likely to provide expanded coverage without a fight. That is already happening. Cigna Health and Life Insurance was hit with a class-action suit over its failure to cover the cost of anti-obesity drugs. Lawyers for the patients argue that obesity is a disability, and so falls under the Affordable Care Act's anti-discrimination law. The company has argued vigorously that it is unreasonable to classify all obese people as disabled, claiming that 40% of the population would then fall into that category. Plaintiffs in a number of cases against the insurance companies counter by citing the authority of the American Medical Association. In a 2013 policy ruling, the AMA recognized obesity as a "disease state with multiple pathophysiological aspects requiring a range of interventions."

The fight for equity is making some slow progress. According to a survey by the International Foundation of Employee Benefit Plans, 34% of policies covered GLP-1 drugs in 2024, up from 26% a year earlier. Until there is a significant drop in prices for semaglutide and tirzepatide, though, it's hard to imagine insurance companies giving in. Even at a modestly reduced price, the budget impact of treating the whole population of US adults with obesity would be enormous.

One area where progress is being made is in reimbursement under Medicare Part D for use of these drugs in obesity. Currently, the Medicare statute prohibits payment for drugs for weight loss. The Centers for Medicare and Medicaid Services (CMS) in the Department of Health and Human Services has proposed reimbursing for GLP-1 drugs for the treatment of obesity by distinguishing the treatment of obesity from weight loss. The proposed rule must become final before reimbursement, which could take several years.

For now, the cost of these drugs makes them inaccessible to many people who could benefit from them. I don't think we've ever seen a similar situation in which there was such a moral and financial quandary between high cost and high benefits. Treatment for hepatitis C was probably the closest event, but that was a short-duration treatment for a much smaller population. In the fight against discrimination, as in the fight against obesity, we are in uncharted territory.

Epilogue

THE FOOD MOVEMENT IS HERE

What happened in Sardinia starting in the 1950s has been repeated over and over across much of the world, with the same tragic outcome each time. As food scarcity has been replaced with abundance, that abundance has come at a great cost. New techniques drastically increased agricultural productivity, new manufacturing techniques delivered a cornucopia of convenient snacks and prepared and packaged meals, but what we got was not an abundance of actual *food*.

Instead, we got a near-boundless supply of ultraformulated food products with built-in macronutrient imbalances of fat, sugar, and salt combinations. Those products have made it socially acceptable to eat or snack at any time. They assault us with rapidly absorbable carbohydrates, decreased protein, and destroyed food structure, setting off addictive eating patterns and metabolic chaos. These ultraformulated foods are toxic to our brains and bodies. The resulting health crisis is especially severe in the United States, where we have the highest levels of obesity among all large developed nations.

In our current environment, it is difficult to escape the pull of food addiction, overcome our built-in reward response, and find our way back to good health. Difficult, but not impossible. The development of GLP-1 anti-obesity medications provides an opening: a chance not just to help a lot of people lose toxic body fat, but also an opportunity to rethink our entire modern food industry.

We can now effectively treat obesity, even if we are only masking the root cause. It may seem absurd to have one industry make us sick only to have another industry develop drugs to treat that sickness, but that is where we are right now. We can start by making the best possible use of the GLP-1 medications. The food industry should be held accountable for the medical costs to rid ourselves of the damage their products have caused. At the same time, we must improve the quality of our diet. That element is nonnegotiable.

Great challenges await those of us who want to see real change happen, from the food manufacturers, who stand to lose profits, and other formidable forces. Climate change, including floods and droughts; infectious diseases that affect food-producing animals; plant blights; and geopolitical upheavals all threaten our ability to produce quality food. I've seen first-hand the effects of avian flu on poultry and dairy farms. I've seen how those industries, even now, resist needed public health interventions to stop the spread of the virus. And I've seen how easy it is for politicians to give them cover.

In contrast, I've also seen how families will take measures to protect their loved ones, how restaurateurs will work to provide healthy food, and how doctors are learning to provide compassionate care to people who struggle with their weight.

I wrote this book in part to give individuals clear and concrete guidance on how to free themselves from addiction to ultraformulated foods. I also view this book as a call to collective action. People across the political spectrum have had it with the food industry and what it has done to our health. The food movement is here. A healthier society is possible.

Acknowledgments

"It's David. I want to write a book, this time, about the mysteries of weight and to investigate how we can dramatically change weight and keep it off. I want to give readers the information they need to go about changing their bodies and health. There will be the usual years of research and thinking and traveling and, of course, hundreds of pages of citations and endnotes." Thank you to those who did not delete that email or block my calls.

Nell Casey and Corey Powell listened, read patiently, took my halting speech and endless sentences and helped turn them into readable prose. I am indebted to them for their skill and insight.

Without Tanya Boroff, I would have been buried in hundreds of drafts of this book and my family would have deserted me. Thank you for your masterful coordination and picking up the pieces. Your dedication and professionalism made this book happen.

Julie Will is the senior vice president and editor in chief, nonfiction, at Flatiron, but she has also been my champion for many years and I continue to benefit from her mind, talent, and friendship.

My agent of long standing is Kathy Robbins. Thank you, Kathy, for supporting and championing my enthusiasms. At the Robbins Office, thanks to Janet Oshiro, Grace Garrahan, and Alexandra Sugarman.

Enormous thanks to three people who have, once again, unfailingly demonstrated their belief in my work with generous financial support—Dagmar Dolby and Lynda and Stewart Resnick.

There are hundreds of interviews and correspondence referenced in the endnotes. No one person understands all aspects of this complex public health problem. My goal was to make the best thinking accessible to the reader. I am also indebted to the following writers, editors, thinkers, and sounding boards who put their minds and pens to my questions and thoughts: Alexandra Kazaks, Kelsey Osgood, Abbey Thiel, Tom Campitelli, Jerry Mande, Marc Smolonsky, Grace Flaherty, Jim Webster, Jennie Stanford, Caitlin Dow, Jelena Markovic, Ioannis Nikitidis, Stephanie M. Mull, Denise Ratcliffe, Kate Sherwood, Beverly Gearreald, Haile Frank, Ivo Pirisi, Andrew Schiff, and Yael Summerfield. Their expertise is unmatched.

I also benefited enormously from the writing skills of Sheila Himmel, Laura Reiley, Richie Chevat, Fran Smith, Amanda Schupak, Willow Gabriel, and Savannah Logan.

Without the talents of Jenna Dolan and Chris Jerome for copyediting, Kelsey Kudak for fact-checking, and Katharine Boggess for help checking quotations, I would be laboring still.

Thank you to Roanne Goldfein. There is no more supportive and patient friend and editor.

As always, I appreciate Elizabeth Dupuis for providing me with access to the library at the University of California, Berkeley. Kelly Close and her team helped provide valuable information.

I believe all of us can attest to the importance of proofreaders. Thank you to Richard Alwyn Fisher, Eliza Childs, Chris Jerome, Bob Land, Sheila Oakley, and Nina Questal.

I am grateful to Sedonia Thomas for transcription, Ava Lawla for video management, and Imran Hossain, Anže Ban Virant, Christina Gaugler, and Meighan Cavanaugh for graphics.

I hope that readers appreciate the endnotes that support the science and lead you to the sources and inspiration for my thinking. What I call the Endnotes Team has been of stout heart and brave in wrangling, organizing, and checking and rechecking. With gratitude to: Richard Alwyn Fisher, Beverly Gearreald, Willow Gabriel, Steph Hendren, Natalie Logue, Cynthia Yaudes, Dawn Bakken, Marissa Sariol-Clough, Alana Del Sordi, Katharine Boggess, Bob Land, Emily Loftis, and Jacqueline Cellini. Indexing is an art. Thank you to Lisa Rivero.

At my academic home, the University of California, San Francisco, I appreciate the help and support of Dean Talmadge King, Christopher Anderson, Raphael Hirsch, Miranda Chiu, Eve Claussen, and Lili Evans.

We all understand the importance of our IT/computer gurus who work night and day to keep us up and running. Mine are Ernie Franic and John Michaelsen.

My thanks to the team at Flatiron: publisher Megan Lynch, director of publicity and marketing Marlena Bittner, assistant editor Sydney Jeon, assistant managing editor Morgan Mitchell, associate editor Hallie Schaeffer, production editor Christopher O'Connell, proofreaders Donald Kennison and Sara Thwaite, and designer Kelly Gatesman.

I appreciate Susanna Lea Associates for handling the foreign rights. Thank you to Susanna, Stephen Morrison, and Mark Kessler.

My thinking owes a great deal to the organizations whose conferences and meetings were a source of information and a robust exchange of ideas. My thanks to the Obesity Medicine Association, the Obesity Society, the Society for the Study of Ingestive Behavior, the European Congress on Obesity, the International Congress on Obesity, the European Association for the Study of Diabetes, the American Diabetes Association, the American Heart Association, the Endocrine Society, and the Harvard Blackburn, Columbia-Cornell, and Boston courses in Obesity Medicine.

The dysregulation of weight is a disease. Its impact on our health is dramatic. Please get good medical care. I know that is not always easy. Always ask questions.

I appreciate that Mollie Van Lieu took in good stride my interrupting so many dinners with my questions about nutrition, food, and the politics of fruits and vegetables.

My family sustains me, understands my absences (mental and otherwise), tolerates my sleep schedule, and brings me joy. My love to Paulette, Elise, Ben, Mike, Mollie, Lena, David, Rosie, Barbara, Suzanne, and Dee.

Notes

The sources below include Works Referenced, Interviews and Correspondence, and Notes. They will lead the reader to the sources referenced and relied on in the text.

Introduction

Sources
Works Referenced

Adams, R. C., J. Sedgmond, L. Maizey, C. D. Chambers, and N. S. Lawrence. "Food Addiction: Implications for the Diagnosis and Treatment of Overeating." In *Eating Disorders and Addictions: Clinical Perspectives and Treatment*. Ed. Ellie Morrison. American Medical Publishers, 2023.

Bonder, R., and C. Davis. "Associations Between Food Addiction and Substance-Use Disorders: A Critical Overview of Their Overlapping Patterns of Consumption." *Curr Addict Rep* 9, no. 4 (2022): 326–33.

Florio, L., D. L. S. Lassi, C. de Azevedo-Marques Perico, et al. "Food Addiction: A Comprehensive Review." *J Nerv Ment Dis* 210, no. 11 (November 1, 2022): 874–79. https://doi.org/10.1097/NMD.0000000000001555. https://www.ncbi.nlm.nih.gov/pubmed/36302082.

Gearhardt, Ashley. "Food Addiction: A New Substance Use Disorder?" Lecture presented at the Annual Meeting of the American Psychiatric Association, San Francisco, CA, May 20–24, 2023.

Gearhardt, Ashley N., Kelly D. Brownell, Mark S. Gold, and Marc N. Potenza. *Food and Addiction: A Comprehensive Handbook*. Second edition. Oxford Scholarship Online. Oxford University Press, 2024.

Guleken, Z., and T. Uzbay. "Neurobiological and Neuropharmacological Aspects of Food Addiction." *Neurosci Biobehav Rev* 139 (August 2022): 104760. https://doi.org/10.1016/j.neubiorev.2022.104760.

Hayashi, D., C. Edwards, J. A. Emond, et al. "What Is Food Noise? A Conceptual Model of Food Cue Reactivity." *Nutrients* 15, no. 22 (November 17, 2023). https://doi.org/10.3390/nu15224809. https://www.ncbi.nlm.nih.gov/pubmed/38004203.

Jurema Santos, G. C., M. S. de Sousa Fernandes, P. G. Carniel, A. da Silva Garcez, C. Gois Leandro, and R. Canuto. "Dietary Intake in Children and Adolescents with Food

Addiction: A Systematic Review." *Addict Behav Rep* 19 (June 2024): 100531. https://doi .org/10.1016/j.abrep.2024.100531.

Koob, George. "Hyperkatifeia and Negative Reinforcement as a Driving Force in Addiction-Like Overeating." Lecture presented at the Annual Meeting of the American Psychiatric Association, San Francisco, CA, May 20–24, 2023.

Kwak, Y. E., R. McMillan, and E. K. McDonald IV. "Trends in Overweight and Obesity Self-Awareness Among Adults with Overweight or Obesity in the United States, 1999 to 2016." *Ann Intern Med* 174, no. 5 (May 2021): 721–23. https://doi.org/10.7326/M20–3882. https://www.ncbi.nlm.nih.gov/pubmed/33253038.

Laque, A., G. E. Wagner, A. Matzeu, et al. "Linking Drug and Food Addiction via Compulsive Appetite." *Br J Pharmacol* 179, no. 11 (June 2022): 2589–609. https://doi.org/10 .1111/bph.15797. https://www.ncbi.nlm.nih.gov/pubmed/35023154.

Milano, W., F. Carizzone, V. De Biasio, et al. "Neurobiological Correlates Shared Between Obesity, Bed and Food Addiction." *Endocr Metab Immune Disord Drug Targets* 23, no. 3 (2023): 283–93. https://doi.org/10.2174/1871530322666220627125642.

Pickard, Hanna, and Serge H. Ahmed. *The Routledge Handbook of Philosophy and Science of Addiction*. Routledge Handbooks in Philosophy. Taylor and Francis Routledge, 2019.

Rubino, D., N. Abrahamsson, M. Davies, et al. "Effect of Continued Weekly Subcutaneous Semaglutide vs. Placebo on Weight Loss Maintenance in Adults with Overweight or Obesity: The Step 4 Randomized Clinical Trial." *JAMA* 325, no. 14 (April 13, 2021): 1414–25. https://doi.org/10.1001/jama.2021.3224.

Schiff, Sami. "What Have I Learned from Bariatric Patients About Their Mind and Behaviours?" Lecture presented at the Annual Meeting for the International Federation for the Surgery of Obesity and Medical Disorders, Naples, Italy, August 30, 2023.

Senol, E., and H. Mohammad. "Current Perspectives on Brain Circuits Involved in Food Addiction-like Behaviors." *J Neural Transm* (Vienna) 131, no. 5 (May 2024): 475–85. https:// doi.org/10.1007/s00702-023-02732–4.

Stice, E., and K. Burger. "Neural Vulnerability Factors for Obesity." *Clin Psychol Rev* 68 (March 2019): 38–53. https://doi.org/10.1016/j.cpr.2018.12.002; https://www.ncbi.nlm .nih.gov/pubmed/30587407.

Sun, W., and H. Kober. "Regulating Food Craving: From Mechanisms to Interventions." *Physiol Behav* 222 (August 1, 2020): 112878. https://doi.org/10.1016/j.physbeh.2020 .112878; https://www.ncbi.nlm.nih.gov/pubmed/32298667.

Wang, Gene-Jack. "The Role of Reward Dysfunction in Overeating of High-Calorie Foods and Obesity." Lecture presented at the Annual Meeting of the American Psychiatric Association, San Francisco, CA, May 20–24, 2023.

Young, L. "Turning Down the Food Noise: Blockbuster Weight-Loss Drugs Are Revealing Secrets in the Brain About Appetite and Satiety, as Well as Pleasure and Addiction." *Sci Am* 331, no. 1 (July 1, 2024): 36. https://doi.org/10.1038/scientificamerican072024 -oPr5Gvp2GiG52cVWgx0tT; https://www.ncbi.nlm.nih.gov/pubmed/39017507.

Interviews and Correspondence with the Author

Koob, George (February 2024; May 2024).

Notes

2   **ultraformulated:** I would like to acknowledge a conversation with Dr. Kevin Hall in which he used the term *ultraformulations*.

2   **"no free ride":** Author interview with Koob, February 2024.

3   **change can be dramatic:** I want to acknowledge Dr. Lee Kaplan and Dr. Randy Seeley, who have used different diagrams to illustrate weight settling points that have served as a basis for designing this illustration.

1: Environment Is Destiny

Sources
Works Referenced

Blomain, Erik Scott, Dara Anne Dirhan, Michael Anthony Valentino, Gilbert Won Kim, and Scott Arthur Waldman. "Mechanisms of Weight Regain Following Weight Loss." *ISRN Obesity* 2013, no. 210524 (2013). DOI: 10.1155/2013/210524.

Blue Zones. "Sardinia, Italy: Home to the World's Longest-Living Men." https://www.bluezones.com/explorations/sardinia-italy/.

Buffa, R., G. Floris, M. Lodde, M. Cotza, and E. Marini. "Nutritional Status in the Healthy Longeval Population from Sardinia (Italy)." *J Nutr Health Aging* 14, no. 2 (February 2010): 97–102. https://doi.org/10.1007/s12603-010-0018-9.

Callahan, Alice. "Why, Exactly, Are Ultraprocessed Foods So Hard to Resist? This Study Is Trying to Find Out." *New York Times*, July 30, 2024. https://www.nytimes.com/2024/07/30/well/eat/ultraprocessed-foods-diet-study.html.

Deiana, L., L. Ferrucci, G. M. Pes, et al. "AKEntAnnos: The Sardinia Study of Extreme Longevity." *Aging* (Milan) 11, no. 3 (1999): 142–49. https://pubmed.ncbi.nlm.nih.gov/10476308/.

Digital History. "Torches of Freedom Campaign." Omeka, n.d. https://omeka.uottawa.ca/jmccutcheon/exhibits/show/american-women-in-tobacco-adve/torches-of-freedom-campaign.

Editors of Encyclopaedia Britannica. "Cigarette." Encyclopedia Britannica, n.d. https://www.britannica.com/topic/cigarette.

Edwards, Phil. "What Everyone Gets Wrong About the History of Cigarettes." Vox, April 6, 2015. https://www.vox.com/2015/3/18/8243707/cigarette-rolling-machines.

Fazzino, Tera, and Kaitlyn Rohde. "Why It Can Be Hard to Stop Eating Even When You're Full: Some Foods May Be Designed That Way." Salon, December 8, 2019. https://www.salon.com/2019/12/08/why-it-can-be-hard-to-stop-eating-even-when-youre-full-some-foods-may-be-designed-that-way_partner/.

Gupta, Dr. Sanjay. "How Worried Should You Be About Ultraprocessed Foods?" CNN Audio, May 7, 2024. https://www.cnn.com/audio/podcasts/chasing-life/episodes/e33ed732–8efa-11ee-ae9c-efadc2b27ac3.pdf.

Hales, Craig M., Margaret D. Carroll, Cheryl D. Fryar, and Cynthia L. Ogden. "Prevalence of Obesity and Severe Obesity Among Adults: United States, 2017–2018." NCHS Data Brief No. 360, February 2020. https://www.cdc.gov/nchs/products/databriefs/db360.

Hall, Kevin D. "Energy Compensation, Metabolic Adaptation, and Physical Activity."

Lecture presented at the International Congress on Obesity (ICO), São Paulo, Brazil, June 26–29, 2024.

Hall, K. D., A. Ayuketah, R. Brychta, et al. "Ultra-processed Diets Cause Excess Calorie Intake and Weight Gain: An Inpatient Randomized Controlled Trial of Ad Libitum Food Intake." *Cell Metabolism* 30, no. 1 (July 2, 2019): 67–77.e3. https://doi.org/10.1016/j.cmet .2019.05.008.

Helzer, J. E., L. N. Robins, and D. H. Davis. "Antecedents of Narcotic Use and Addiction: A Study of 898 Vietnam Veterans." *Drug Alcohol Depend* 1, no. 3 (February 1976): 183–90. https://doi.org/10.1016/0376–8716(76)90028–4.

Holmes, Chris. "Celebrity Smokes: A Gallery of Star-Powered Ads." Gray Flannel Suit, August 20, 2013. https://www.grayflannelsuit.net/blog/celebrity-smokes-a-gallery-of -star-powered-cigarette-ads.

Kessler, D. A. *The End of Overeating: Taking Control of the Insatiable American Appetite.* Harmony/Rodale, 2010. https://books.google.com/books?id=QFR1M3Vwe1wC.

Kessler, D. A. *Fast Carbs, Slow Carbs: The Simple Truth About Food, Weight, and Disease.* HarperCollins, 2020. https://books.google.com/books?id=UBWoDwAAQBAJ.

Kessler, D. A. *A Question of Intent: A Great American Battle with a Deadly Industry.* PublicAffairs, 2002. https://books.google.com/books?id=FGx-tjk30dMC.

Kugel, Seth. "A Tour of Sardinia, Full of Discoveries." *New York Times*, May 27, 2015. https://www.nytimes.com/2015/05/27/travel/a-tour-of-sardinia-full-of-discoveries .html.

Loviselli, A., M. E. Ghiani, F. Veluzzi, I. S. Piras, et al. "Prevalence and Trend of Overweight and Obesity Among Sardinian Conscripts (Italy) of 1969 and 1998." *J Biosoc Sci* 42, no. 2 (2010): 201–11. DOI: 10.1017/S0021932009990411.

Lushniak, Boris D., Jonathan M. Samet, Terry F. Pechacek, Leslie A. Norman, and Peter A. Taylor. "2: Fifty Years of Change, 1964–2014." In *The Health Consequences of Smoking—50 Years of Progress: A Report of the Surgeon General.* Centers for Disease Control and Prevention, 2014. https://www.ncbi.nlm.nih.gov/books/NBK294310/.

McDonald's. "Sardinia." 2024. https://www.mcdonalds.it/ristorante/sardegna.

MMWR Weekly. "Cigarette Smoking Among Adults—United States, 1991." Centers for Disease Control and Prevention, April 2, 1993. https://www.cdc.gov/mmwr/preview /mmwrhtml/00020103.

Monteiro, C. A., G. Cannon, J. C. Moubarac, R. B. Levy, M. L. C. Louzada, and P. C. Jaime. "The UN Decade of Nutrition, the Nova Food Classification and the Trouble with Ultra-processing." *Public Health Nutr* 21, no. 1 (January 2018): 5–17. https://doi.org /10.1017/s1368980017000234.

National Cancer Institute. "Psychoactive substance." NCI Dictionary of Cancer Terms, n.d. https://www.cancer.gov/publications/dictionaries/cancer-terms/def/psychoactive -substance.

Pedersen, H., and M. Altman. "Horizons of Authenticity." In *Phenomenology, Existentialism, and Moral Psychology: Essays in Honor of Charles Guignon.* Ed. Hans Pedersen and Megan Altman, 165–78, 175. Springer Netherlands, 2014. https://books.google.com/books?id =MgVNBQAAQBAJ.

Pes, G. M., A. Errigo, and M. P. Dore. "Association Between Mild Overweight and Survival: A Study of an Exceptionally Long-Lived Population in the Sardinian Blue Zone." *J Clin Med* 13, no. 17 (September 9, 2024). https://doi.org/10.3390/jcm13175322.

Pes, G. M., M. Poulain, A. Errigo, and M. P. Dore. "Evolution of the Dietary Patterns

Across Nutrition Transition in the Sardinian Longevity Blue Zone and Association with Health Indicators in the Oldest Old." *Nutrients* 13, no. 5 (April 28, 2021). https://doi.org /10.3390/nu13051495.

Pes, G. M., F. Tolu, M. P. Dore, et al. "Male Longevity in Sardinia: A Review of Historical Sources Supporting a Causal Link with Dietary Factors." *Eur J Clin Nutr* 69, no. 4 (April 2015): 411–18. https://doi.org/10.1038/ejcn.2014.230.

Pes, G. M., F. Tolu, M. Poulain, et al. "Lifestyle and Nutrition Related to Male Longevity in Sardinia: An Ecological Study." *Nutr Metab Cardiovasc Dis* 23, no. 3 (March 2013): 212–19. https://doi.org/10.1016/j.numecd.2011.05.004.

Poulain, M., G. M. Pes, C. Grasland, et al. "Identification of a Geographic Area Characterized by Extreme Longevity in the Sardinia Island: The Akea Study." *Exp Gerontol* 39, no. 9 (September 2004): 1423–29. https://doi.org/10.1016/j.exger.2004.06.016.

Poulain, M., G. Pes, and L. Salaris. "A Population Where Men Live as Long as Women: Villagrande Strisaili, Sardinia." *J Aging Res* 2011 (2011): 153756. https://doi.org/10.4061 /2011/153756.

Roberts, Joyce. "Vietnam Veterans and Illicit Drug Use." Master of social work thesis, California State University, San Bernardino, 2017.

Robins, L. N. "The Natural History of Drug Abuse." *NIDA Res Monogr* 30 (March 1980): 215–24.

Robins, L. N. "Vietnam Veterans' Rapid Recovery from Heroin Addiction: A Fluke or Normal Expectation?" The Sixth Thomas James Okey Memorial Lecture. *Addiction* 88, no. 8 (August 1993): 1041–54. https://doi.org/10.1111/j.1360–0443.1993.tb02123.x.

Robins, L. N., D. H. Davis, and D. N. Nurco. "How Permanent Was Vietnam Drug Addiction?" *Am J Public Health* 64, no. 12 Suppl. (December 1974): 38–43. https://doi.org /10.2105/ajph.64.12_suppl.38.

Robins, L. N., J. E. Helzer, and D. H. Davis. "Narcotic Use in Southeast Asia and Afterward: An Interview Study of 898 Vietnam Returnees." *Arch Gen Psychiatry* 32, no. 8 (August 1975): 955–61. https://doi.org/10.1001/archpsyc.1975.01760260019001.

Robins, L. N., J. E. Helzer, M. Hesselbrock, and E. Wish. "Vietnam Veterans Three Years After Vietnam: How Our Study Changed Our View of Heroin." *Am J Addict* 19, no. 3 (May–June 2010): 203–11. https://doi.org/10.1111/j.1521–0391.2010.00046.x.

Robins, L. N., and S. Slobodyan. "Post-Vietnam Heroin Use and Injection by Returning US Veterans: Clues to Preventing Injection Today." *Addiction* 98, no. 8 (August 2003): 1053–60. https://doi.org/10.1046/j.1360–0443.2003.00436.x.

Savelle-Rocklin, N. *Beyond the Primal Addiction: Food, Sex, Gambling, Internet, Shopping, and Work.* Taylor and Francis, 2019. https://books.google.com/books?id=KOOLDwAAQBAJ.

Schalow, F. *Toward a Phenomenology of Addiction: Embodiment, Technology, Transcendence.* Springer International, 2018. https://books.google.com/books?id=w3TuugEACAAJ.

Schiff, S. "What Have I Learned from Bariatric Patients About Their Mind and Behaviours?" Lecture presented at the Annual Meeting of the International Federation for the Surgery of Obesity, Naples, Italy, August 30, 2023.

Shirk, Adrian. "The Real Marlboro Man." *The Atlantic*, February 17, 2015. https://www .theatlantic.com/business/archive/2015/02/the-real-marlboro-man/385447/.

Spiegel, Alix. "What Vietnam Taught Us About Breaking Bad Habits." NPR, January 2, 2012. https://www.npr.org/sections/health-shots/2012/01/02/144431794/what-vietnam -taught-us-about-breaking-bad-habits#:~:text=In%20May%20of%201971%20two were%20actively%20addicted%20to%20heroin.

Tessier, S., and M. Gerber. "Factors Determining the Nutrition Transition in Two Mediterranean Islands: Sardinia and Malta." *Public Health Nutr* 8, no. 8 (December 2005): 1286–92. https://doi.org/10.1079/phn2005747.

Truth Initiative. "Sex Sells: A Look at the Tobacco Industry's Use of Sexual Themes to Sell Products." Truth Initiative, August 21, 2018. https://truthinitiative.org/research -resources/tobacco-industry-marketing/sex-sells-look-tobacco-industrys-use-sexual -themes.

Wadden, T. A., R. H. Neiberg, R. R. Wing, et al. "Four-Year Weight Losses in the Look AHEAD Study: Factors Associated with Long-Term Success." *Obesity* (Silver Spring, MD) 19, no. 10 (2011): 1987–98. https://doi.org/10.1038/oby.2011.230.

Wang, Chaoyue, Marco Murgia, José Baptista, and Massimo Marcone. "Sardinian Dietary Analysis for Longevity: A Review of the Literature." *Journal of Ethnic Foods* 9 (September 2, 2022). https://doi.org/10.1186/s42779-022-00152-5.

Yale University Library. "Selling Smoke: Tobacco Advertising and Anti-Smoking Campaigns." https://onlineexhibits.library.yale.edu/s/sellingsmoke/page/celebrities.

Zinberg, N. E. *Drug, Set, and Setting: The Basis for Controlled Intoxicant Use.* Yale University Press, 1986. https://books.google.com/books?id=yYBna18Bd4cC.

Interviews and Correspondence with the Author

Di Chiara, Gaetano (May 2024).

Pirisi, Ivo (May 2024).

Notes

8   **one study found:** Loviselli, "Prevalence and Trend of Overweight and Obesity Among Sardinian Conscripts."

9   **one such trial:** Callahan, "Why, Exactly, Are Ultraprocessed Foods So Hard to Resist?"

9   **"formulations mostly of cheap industrial sources":** Monteiro et al., "The UN Decade of Nutrition, the Nova Food Classification, and the Trouble with Ultra-Processing."

9   **people being studied:** Gupta, "How Worried Should You Be About Ultraprocessed Foods?"

9   **"People can achieve":** Hall, "Energy Compensation, Metabolic Adaptation, and Physical Activity."

10   **primarily men smoked:** Editors of Encyclopaedia Britannica, "Cigarette."

10   **cigarettes made up:** Edwards, "What Everyone Gets Wrong About the History of Cigarettes."

10   **Manufacturers began putting pictures:** Truth Initiative, "Sex Sells."

10   **the cultural icon:** Shirk, "The Real Marlboro Man."

12   **"The immediate access":** Schalow, *Toward a Phenomenology of Addiction.*

12   **"allure of his/her addiction":** Schalow, *Toward a Phenomenology of Addiction.*

12   **by 2030, about half:** Blomain et al., "Mechanisms of Weight Regain Following Weight Loss."

12   **older age groups:** Hales et al., "Prevalence of Obesity and Severe Obesity Among Adults."

13 **an official visit:** Spiegel, "What Vietnam Taught Us About Breaking Bad Habits."

13 **very well-conducted study:** Robins et al., "Vietnam Veterans Three Years After Vietnam."

13 **An estimated 5%:** Spiegel, "What Vietnam Taught Us About Breaking Bad Habits."

13 **"This surprising rate of recovery":** Robins, "Vietnam Veterans' Rapid Recovery from Heroin Addiction: A Fluke or Normal Expectation?"

13 **"narcotic use and narcotic addiction were extremely common":** Robins, "Vietnam Veterans' Rapid Recovery from Heroin Addiction: A Fluke or Normal Expectation?"

13 **Some experts:** My colleague Gaetano Di Chiara believes it is more appropriate to use the word "dependence" than "addiction" when describing the rewarding effects of highly palatable foods. For him, there is a quantitative difference in the levels of dopamine between cocaine or amphetamines and, for example, sugar and fat combinations.

14 **substance is psychoactive:** National Cancer Institute, "Psychoactive Substance."

14 **300 to 400 fewer calories:** Wadden et al., "Four-Year Weight Losses in the Look AHEAD Study."

14 **heart of addiction:** I would like to acknowledge Dr. Lance Dodes's book *The Heart of Addiction*.

2: The Addictive Power of Food

Sources
Works Referenced

Alexander, B. *The Globalization of Addiction: A Study in Poverty of the Spirit.* Oxford University Press, 2010. https://books.google.com/books?id=BgkWDAAAQBAJ.

Alexander, B. *Pathways of Addiction: Opportunities in Drug Abuse Research.* National Academies Press, 1996. https://books.google.com/books?id=xFIkdvSPZm0C.

Arbour, Nathael L. "You Are Not Alone!" Liberté Alimentaire. https://libertealimentaire.com/.

Auriacombe, M., F. Serre, C. Denis, and M. Fatseas. In *The Routledge Handbook of Philosophy and Science of Addiction.* Ed. Hanna Pickard and Serge Ahmed. Routledge Handbooks in Philosophy. Taylor and Francis Routledge, 2019.

Avena, Nicole. *Hedonic Eating: How the Pleasure of Food Affects Our Brains and Behavior.* Oxford University Press, 2015.

Barrett, Lisa Feldman. *How Emotions Are Made: The Secret Life of the Brain.* Harper Paperbacks, 2017.

Baumeister, Roy F., and John Tierney. *Willpower: Rediscovering the Greatest Human Strength.* Penguin, 2012.

Beth Israel Deaconess Medical Center. "Profiles in Medicine: Bruce Bistrian, MD, PhD, MPH." Beth Israel Lahey Health. https://www.bidmc.org/-/media/files/beth-israel-org/research/research-by-department/medicine/clinical-nutrition/bidmc-dr-bistrian-profile-032522.pdf.

Bishop, F. Michler. *Managing Addictions: Cognitive, Emotive, and Behavioral Techniques.* Rowman & Littlefield, 2001.

Bordeaux, Patrick, and George F. Koob. *Escaping Addiction: Resetting the Brain for Success.* Rowman & Littlefield, 2023.

Brownell, Kelly D., and Mark S. Gold, eds. *Food and Addiction: A Comprehensive Handbook.* Oxford University Press, 2012.

Califf, Robert. "FDA Commissioner Robert Califf Testifies Before Senate HELP Committee on Combating Diabetes, Obesity." YouTube, December 5, 2024. https://www.youtube.com/watch?v=5upGvDdCZyM.

Cassidy, Ryan Michael, and Qingchun Tong. "Hunger and Satiety Gauge Reward Sensitivity." *Front Endocrinol* 8, no. 104 (2017). doi:10.3389/fendo.2017.00104.

Cleveland Clinic. "Blood Glucose (Sugar) Test." November 16, 2022. https://my.clevelandclinic.org/health/diagnostics/12363-blood-glucose-test.

Cottone, Pietro, Catherine F. Moore, Valentina Sabino, and George F. Koob. *Compulsive Eating Behavior and Food Addiction: Emerging Pathological Constructs.* Academic Press, 2019.

DiClemente, Carlo C. *Addiction and Change: How Addictions Develop and Addicted People Recover.* Guilford Press, 2006.

Dodes, Lance. *Breaking Addiction: A 7-Step Handbook for Ending Any Addiction.* Harper, 2011.

Donovan, Dennis M., and G. Alan Marlatt. *Assessment of Addictive Behaviors.* Guilford Press, 1988.

Drummond, D. Colin. *Addictive Behaviour: Cue Exposure Theory and Practice.* Wiley, 1995.

Farber, S. K. *Hungry for Ecstasy: Trauma, the Brain, and the Influence of the Sixties.* Jason Aronson, 2012. https://books.google.com/books?id=eHl0l3TJXn8C.

Fauconnier, Marie, et al. "Food Addiction Among Female Patients Seeking Treatment for an Eating Disorder: Prevalence and Associated Factors." *Nutrients* 12, no. 1897 (2020): 1–19. doi:10.3390/nu12061897.

Fisher, Carl Erik. *The Urge: Our History of Addiction.* Penguin, 2022.

Fong, Benjamin Y. *Quick Fixes: Drugs in America from Prohibition to the 21st Century Binge.* Verso Books, 2023.

Frijda, Nico H. *The Emotions.* Cambridge University Press, 1986.

Garland, Eric L. *Mindfulness-Oriented Recovery Enhancement for Addiction, Stress, and Pain.* NASW Press, 2013.

Gordon, Eliza L., et al. "What Is the Evidence for 'Food Addiction'? A Systematic Review." *Nutrients* 10, no. 477 (2018): 1–30. doi:10.3390/nu10040477.

Greenberg, Leslie S. *Changing Emotion with Emotion: A Practitioner's Guide.* American Psychological Association, 2021.

Hall, F. Scott, Jared W. Young, and Andre Der-Avakian. *Negative Affective States and Cognitive Impairments in Nicotine Dependence.* Academic Press, 2016.

Heather, Nick, Matt Field, Antony Moss, and Sally Satel, eds. *Evaluating the Brain Disease Model of Addiction.* Routledge, 2022.

Hill, Daniel. *Affect Regulation Theory: A Clinical Model.* National Geographic Books, 2015.

Hughes, Carly A., Amy L. Ahern, Harsha Kasetty, et al. "Changing the Narrative Around Obesity in the UK: A Survey of People with Obesity and Healthcare Professionals from the ACTION-IO Study." *BMJ Open* 11, no. 6 (2021): e045616. DOI: 10.1136/bmjopen-2020-045616.

Ifland, Joan, Marianne T. Marcus, and Harry G. Preuss. *Processed Food Addiction: Foundations, Assessment, and Recovery.* CRC Press, 2017.

Institute of Medicine, Committee on Opportunities in Drug Abuse Research. *Pathways of Addiction: Opportunities in Drug Abuse Research.* National Academy Press, 1996. https://books.google.com/books?id=xFIkdvSPZm0C&printsec=frontcover&source=gbs_ge_summary_r&cad=0#v=onepage&q&f=false.

Jonsson, Bitten, and Pia Nordström. *Sockerbomben: bli fri från ditt sockerberoende.* Forum, 2004.

Kanoski, Scott E., and Kerri N. Boutelle. "Food Cue Reactivity: Neurobiological and Behavioral Underpinnings." *Rev Endocr Metab Disord* 23, no. 4 (2022): 683–96. doi:10.1007/s11154-022-09724-x.

Kassel, Jon D. *Substance Abuse and Emotion.* American Psychological Association, 2010.

Kessler, David. *The End of Overeating: Taking Control of the Insatiable American Diet.* Rodale, 2010.

Khantzian, Edward, J. *Treating Addiction as a Human Process.* Jason Aronson, 1999.

Koob, G. F. "Anhedonia, Hyperkatifeia, and Negative Reinforcement in Substance Use Disorders." *Curr Top Behav Neurosci* 58 (2022): 147–65. https://doi.org/10.1007/7854_2021_288.

Koob, G. F. "The Dark Side of Emotion: The Addiction Perspective." *Eur J Pharmacol* 753 (April 15, 2015): 73–87. https://doi.org/10.1016/j.ejphar.2014.11.044.

Koob, George F., Michael A. Arends, and Michel Le Moal. *Drugs, Addiction, and the Brain.* Academic Press, 2014.

Koob, George F., and Michel Le Moal. *Neurobiology of Addiction.* Academic Press, 2006.

Koob, G. F., and M. Le Moal. "Review: Neurobiological Mechanisms for Opponent Motivational Processes in Addiction." *Philos Trans R Soc Lond B Biol Sci* 363, no. 1507 (October 12, 2008): 3113–23. https://doi.org/10.1098/rstb.2008.0094.

Koob, George F., Patricia Powell, and Aaron White. "Addiction as a Coping Response: Hyperkatifeia, Deaths of Despair, and COVID-19." *Am J Psychiat* 177, no. 11 (2020). https://doi.org/10.1176/appi.ajp.2020.20091375.

Loreto, B. B. L., Anne Orgler Sordi, Melina Nogueira de Castro, Felipe Ornell, et al. "Proposing an Integrative, Dynamic and Transdiagnostic Model for Addictions: Dysregulation Phenomena of the Three Main Modes of the Predostatic Mind." *Front Psych* 14 (2024): 1298002. doi: 10.3389/fpsyt.2023.1298002.

Lowe, R., and T. Ziemke. "The Feeling of Action Tendencies: On the Emotional Regulation of Goal-Directed Behavior." *Front Psychol* 2 (2011): 346. https://doi.org/10.3389/fpsyg.2011.00346.

Maier, John Thomas. *The Disabled Will: A Theory of Addiction.* Routledge, 2024.

Manejwala, O. *Craving: Why We Can't Seem to Get Enough.* Hazelden, 2013. https://books.google.com/books?id=_vGBGSOaqTIC.

Maté, Gabor. *The Myth of Normal: Trauma, Illness, and Healing in a Toxic Culture.* Penguin, 2022.

McLellan, A. T. "Pre-addiction: An Overlooked Part of the Substance Use Disorder Continuum." Lecture presented at the International Society of Addiction Medicine (ISAM), Istanbul, Turkey, September 5–8, 2024.

McLellan, A. T., G. F. Koob, and N. D. Volkow. "Preaddiction: A Missing Concept for Treating Substance Use Disorders." *JAMA Psychiatry* 79, no. 8 (August 1, 2022): 749–51. https://doi.org/10.1001/jamapsychiatry.2022.1652.

Meule, A. "Food Cravings in Food Addiction: Exploring a Potential Cut-Off Value of the Food Cravings Questionnaire—Trait-Reduced." *Eat Weight Disord* 23 (2018): 39–43. https://doi.org/10.1007/s40519-017-0452-3.

Meule, A. "Impulsivity and Overeating: A Closer Look at the Subscales of the Barratt Impulsiveness Scale." *Front Psychol* 4 (2013): 177. https://doi.org/10.3389/fpsyg.2013 .00177.

Miller, Robert. *The Feeling-State Theory and Protocols for Behavioral and Substance Addiction: A Breakthrough in the Treatment of Addictions, Compulsions, Obsessions, Codependence, and Anger.* CreateSpace Independent Publishing Platform, 2018.

National Cancer Institute. "Homeostasis." https://www.cancer.gov/publications /dictionaries/cancer-terms/def/homeostasis.

Park, Jaeyoon. *Addiction Becomes Normal: On the Late-Modern American Subject.* University of Chicago Press, 2024.

Pickard, Hanna, and Serge Ahmed, eds. *The Routledge Handbook of Philosophy and Science of Addiction.* Routledge, 2018.

Recio-Román, Almudena, et al. "Food Reward and Food Choice: An Inquiry Through the Liking and Wanting Model." *Nutrients* 12, no. 639 (2020): 1–41. doi:10.3390 /nu12030639.

Samson, Andrea C., David Sander, and Ueli Kramer. *Change in Emotion and Mental Health.* Academic Press, 2024.

Sander, David, and Lauri Nummenmaa. "Reward and Emotion: An Affective Neuroscience Approach." *Curr Opin Behav Sci* 39 (2021): 161–67. https://doi.org/10.1016/j.cobeha .2021.03.016.

Schalow, F. *Toward a Phenomenology of Addiction: Embodiment, Technology, Transcendence.* Springer International, 2018. https://books.google.com/books?id=w3TuugEACAAJ.

Siegel, Shepard. *The Ghost in the Addict.* MIT Press, 2024.

Solomon, Richard L. "The Opponent Processes in Acquired Motivation." In *The Physiological Mechanisms of Motivation.* Ed. Donald W. Pfaff. Springer New York, 1982.

Stapleton, Connie. *Weight Loss Surgery Does Not Treat Food Addiction.* CreateSpace Independent Publishing Platform, 2017.

Szalavitz, Maia. *Unbroken Brain: A Revolutionary New Way of Understanding Addiction.* Picador, 2017.

Tarman, Vera. *Food Junkies: Recovery from Food Addiction.* Dundurn, 2019.

Tatarsky, Andrew. "Demystifying Harm Reduction." Lecture presented at Treating the Addictions, Cambridge Health Systems, Boston, MA, March 2, 2024.

Unwin, Jen. *Fork in the Road: A Hopeful Guide to Food Freedom.* Independently Published, 2021.

Valls, Pablo Oriol, and Alessandro Esposito. "Signalling Dynamics, Cell Decisions, and Homeostatic Control in Health and Disease." *Curr Opin Cell Biol* 75 (2022): 102066. DOI: 10.1016/j.ceb.2022.01.011.

Volkow, Nora D., Gene-Jack Wang, Joanna S. Fowler, and Frank Telang. "Overlapping Neuronal Circuits in Addiction and Obesity: Evidence of Systems Pathology." *Philos Trans R Soc Lond B Biol Sci* 363, no. 1507 (2008): 3191–200. doi:10.1098/ rstb.2008.0107.

Washton, Arnold M. *Willpower Is Not Enough: Understanding and Overcoming Addiction and Compulsion.* HarperCollins, 1990.

Wells, Pete. "After 12 Years of Reviewing Restaurants, I'm Leaving the Table." *New York*

Times, July 16, 2024. https://www.nytimes.com/2024/07/16/dining/pete-wells-steps -down-food-critic.html.

West, Robert, and Jamie Brown. *Theory of Addiction*. Wiley, 2013.

Yale University Library. "Selling Smoke: Tobacco Advertising and Anti-Smoking Campaigns." https://onlineexhibits.library.yale.edu/s/sellingsmoke/page/celebrities.

Zorrilla, E. P., and G. F. Koob. "Impulsivity Derived from the Dark Side: Neurocircuits That Contribute to Negative Urgency." *Front Behav Neurosci* 13 (2019): 136. https://doi .org/10.3389/fnbeh.2019.00136.

Interviews and Correspondence with the Author

Cywes, Robert (April 2024).

Dennis, Kim (September 2024).

Kalayjian, Tro (May 2024).

Koob, George (February 2024; May 2024).

Leduc, Nathaël (April 2024).

McArthur, Erin (April 2024).

Palavecino, Sandra (April 2024).

Small, Dana (February 2024; March 2024; July 2024).

Wilcox, Claire (April 2024).

Zorrilla, Eric (January 2024; February 2024).

Notes

15   **"Both substances and behaviors"**: Auriacombe et al., *Diagnosis of Addictions*.

16   **"'hook' of addiction"**: Schalow, *Toward a Phenomenology of Addiction*.

16   **a pressing unease:** Pickard and Ahmed, *The Routledge Handbook of Philosophy and Science of Addiction*.

16   **defines cravings:** Manejwala, "Craving: Why We Can't Seem to Get Enough."

17   **"food addicted"**: Muele, "Food Cravings in Food Addiction."

17   **"action tendencies"**: Frijda, *The Emotions*.

17   **"opponent process"**: Solomon, "The Opponent Processes in Acquired Motivation."

18   **"downregulation . . . upregulation"**: Author interviews with Zorrilla, January and February 2024.

18   **biochemical processes:** Valls and Esposito, "Signalling Dynamics, Cell Decisions, and Homeostatic Control in Health and Disease."

18   **derived from the Greek:** Koob, Powell, and White, "Addiction as a Coping Response."

18   **"the dark side"**: Author interviews with Koob, 2024.

18   **main drivers:** Muele, "Impulsivity and Overeating."

19   **amount of sugar:** Cleveland Clinic, "Blood Glucose (Sugar) Test."

19   **used in obesity medicine:** Beth Israel Deaconess Medical Center, "Profiles in Medicine."

20   **state of balance:** National Cancer Institute, "Homeostasis."

20   **Part of Being Human:** Khantzian, *Treating Addiction as a Human Process*.

20 **"chocolate inebriate":** Cottone et al., *Compulsive Eating*, 2–3.

21 **suffered many of obesity's:** Wells, "After 12 Years of Reviewing Restaurants, I'm Leaving the Table."

21 **including brain imaging:** Cottone et al., *Compulsive Eating*, 6.

21 **development of the Yale:** Cottone et al., *Compulsive Eating*, 7.

21 **"the three points of the compass":** Kessler, *The End of Overeating*.

21 **"a continuum of addiction":** Tatarsky, "Demystifying Harm Reduction."

22 **pre-addiction:** McLellan, "Pre-addiction."

22 **two to five symptoms:** McLellan, "Pre-addiction."

22 **a human process:** I would like to again acknowledge the late Dr. Edward Khantzian for the phrase, which was the title of his book *Treating Addiction as a Human Process*.

22 **85% in fact:** Hughes et al., "Changing the Narrative Around Obesity in the UK."

23 **addiction and eating disorder worlds:** Author interview with Wilcox, April 2024.

23 **intergenerationally:** Author interview with Cywes, April 2024.

23 **diabetic crisis:** Author interview with McArthur, April 2024.

23 **"While I was asking":** Author interview with Kalayjian, May 2024.

24 **variability in glucose:** Author interview with Leduc, April 2024.

25 **its kind in French:** Arbour, "You Are Not Alone!"

25 **"what I imagine":** Author interview with Dennis, September 2024.

26 **"controlled by brain":** Institute of Medicine, *Pathways of Addiction*.

26 **"countervailing":** Institute of Medicine, *Pathways of Addiction*.

3: Betrayed by Our Own Biology

Sources
Works Referenced

Anguah, K. O., M. M. Syed-Abdul, Q. Hu, M. Jacome-Sosa, C. Heimowitz, V. Cox, and E. J. Parks. "Changes in Food Cravings and Eating Behavior After a Dietary Carbohydrate Restriction Intervention Trial." *Nutrients* 12, no. 1 (December 24, 2019): 52. doi: 10.3390/nu12010052. PMID: 31878131; PMCID: PMC7019570.

Bae, Jae Hyun. "The Expanding Role of CGM in Wellness: From Glycemic Control to Holistic Health." Lecture presented at International Congress on Obesity and Metabolic Syndrome (ICOMES), Seoul, Republic of Korea, September 5–7, 2024.

Bai Ling, Nilla Sivakumar, Shenliang Yu, Sheyda Mesgarzadeh, et al. "Enteroendocrine Cell Types That Drive Food Reward and Aversion." *eLife* 11, (2022): e74964. doi: 10.7554/eLife.74964.

Bechara, A., K. C. Berridge, W. K. Bickel, J. A. Morón, S. B. Williams, and J. S. Stein. "A Neurobehavioral Approach to Addiction: Implications for the Opioid Epidemic and the Psychology of Addiction." *Psychol Sci Public Interest* 20, no. 2 (October 2019): 96–127. https://doi.org/10.1177/1529100619860513.

Bechara, A., H. Damasio, and A. R. Damasio. "Emotion, Decision Making and the Orbitofrontal Cortex." *Cerebral Cortex* 10, no. 3 (March 2000): 295–307. https://doi.org/10.1093/cercor/10.3.295.

Belfort De Aguiar, R., D. Seo, C. Lacadie, S. Naik, C. Schmidt, W. Lam, J. Hwang, T. Constable, R. Sinha, and R. S. Sherwin. "Humans with Obesity Have Disordered Brain Responses to Food Images During Physiological Hyperglycemia." *Am J Physiol Endocrinol Metab* 314, no. 5 (May 1, 2018): E522–E529. doi: 10.1152/ajpendo.00335.2017.

Berntson, G. G., G. J. Norman, A. Bechara, J. Bruss, D. Tranel, and J. T. Cacioppo. "The Insula and Evaluative Processes." *Psychol Sci* 22, no. 1 (January 2011): 80–86. https://doi .org/10.1177/0956797610391097.

Berridge, Kent C., and Morten L. Kringelbach. "Pleasure Systems in the Brain." *Neuron* 86, no. 3 (2015): 646–64. DOI: 10.1016/j.neuron.2015.02.018.

Berthoud, Hans-Rudolf, Vance L. Albaugh, and Winfried L. Neuhuber. "Gut-Brain Communication and Obesity: Understanding Functions of the Vagus Nerve." *J Clin Invest* 131, no. 10 (May 17, 2021): e143770. https://doi.org/10.1172/JCI143770.

Chan, O., and R. Sherwin. "Influence of VMH Fuel Sensing on Hypoglycemic Responses." *Trends Endocrinol Metab* 24, no. 12 (December 2013): 616–24. doi: 10.1016/j.tem.2013.08.005. Epub September 21, 2013.

Chandler-Laney, P. C., S. A. Morrison, L. L. Goree, et al. "Return of Hunger Following a Relatively High Carbohydrate Breakfast Is Associated with Earlier Recorded Glucose Peak and Nadir." *Appetite* 80 (September 2014): 236–41. https://doi.org/10.1016/j.appet .2014.04.031.

Cleveland Clinic. "Dopamine." March 23, 2022. https://my.clevelandclinic.org/health /articles/22581-dopamine.

Cleveland Clinic. "Duodenum." May 24, 2024. https://my.clevelandclinic.org/health /body/duodenum.

Cleveland Clinic. "Small Intestine." October 14, 2024. https://my.clevelandclinic.org /health/body/22135-small-intestine.

DeFronzo, R. "Keynote 2: New Horizons for T2D Treatment." Keynote lecture presented at the Achieve Targets in Diabetes Care (ATDC) conference, Keystone, CO, July 10–13, 2024.

Demeke, S., K. Rohde, L. Chollet-Hinton, C. Sutton, K. L. Kong, and T. L. Fazzino. "Change in Hyper-palatable Food Availability in the US Food System over 30 Years: 1988–2018." *Public Health Nutr* 26, no. 1 (January 2023): 182–89. https://doi.org/10.1017 /s1368980022001227.

Dilsaver, D., K. Rohde, L. Chollet-Hinton, and T. L. Fazzino. "Hyper-palatable Foods in Elementary School Lunches: Availability and Contributing Factors in a National Sample of US Public Schools." *PLOS One* 18, no. 2 (2023): e0281448. https://doi.org/10.1371 /journal.pone.0281448.

Drayer, Lisa. "Why Is Bacon So Addictive?" CNN Health, March 6, 2019. https://www .cnn.com/2019/03/02/health/bacon-addictive-food-drayer/index.html.

Droutman, V., S. J. Read, and A. Bechara. "Revisiting the Role of the Insula in Addiction." *Trends Cogn Sci* 19, no. 7 (July 2015): 414–20. https://doi.org/10.1016/j.tics.2015.05 .005.

Fang, Lisa Z., Josué A. Lily Vidal, Oishi Hawlader, and Michiru Hirasawa. "High-Fat Diet-Induced Elevation of Body Weight Set Point in Male Mice." *Obesity* 31, no. 4 (2023): 1000–1010. doi:10.1002/oby.23650.

Farr, Olivia M., Chiang-shan R. Li, and Christos S. Mantzoros. "Central Nervous System Regulation of Eating: Insights from Human Brain Imaging." *Metab Clinical Exp* 65, no. 5 (2016): 699–713. DOI: 10.1016/j.metabol.2016.02.002.

Fazzino, T. L., A. B. Courville, J. Guo, and K. D. Hall. "Ad Libitum Meal Energy Intake Is Positively Influenced by Energy Density, Eating Rate, and Hyper-palatable Food Across Four Dietary Patterns." *Nat Food* 4, no. 2 (February 2023): 144–47. https://doi .org/10.1038/s43016-022-00688-4.

Fazzino, T. L., K. Rohde, and D. K. Sullivan. "Hyper-palatable Foods: Development of a Quantitative Definition and Application to the US Food System Database." *Obesity* (Silver Spring, MD) 27, no. 11 (November 2019): 1761–68. https://doi.org/10.1002/oby.22639.

Fazzino, Tera. "Crossing Fields to Make Scientific Connections: Reinforcement Processes in Addiction, Binge Eating, and Obesity." Presented at VCBH Lecture Series, May 18, 2022. https://www.youtube.com/watch?v=CKaMVTZUG-E&ab_channel=Vermont CenteronBehaviorandHealth.

Goodman, J., and M. G. Packard. "Memory Systems and the Addicted Brain." *Front Psychiatry* 7 (2016): 24. https://doi.org/10.3389/fpsyt.2016.00024.

Groves, Melissa. "Sucrose vs. Glucose vs. Fructose: What's the Difference?" Healthline. October 19, 2022. https://www.healthline.com/nutrition/sucrose-glucose-fructose.

Hawks, Z. W., E. D. Beck, L. Jung, et al. "Dynamic Associations Between Glucose and Ecological Momentary Cognition in Type 1 Diabetes." *NPJ Digit Med* 7, no. 1 (March 18, 2024): 59. https://doi.org/10.1038/s41746-024-01036-5.

Huberman, Andrew. "Dr. Anna Lembke: Understanding and Treating Addiction." Huberman Lab, August 15, 2021. https://www.hubermanlab.com/episode/dr-anna -lembke-understanding-and-treating-addiction.

Inchauspe, Jessie. *Glucose Revolution: The Life-Changing Power of Balancing Your Blood Sugar.* Simon and Schuster, 2022.

Jewett, Benjamin, and E. Sandeep Sharma. *Physiology, GABA.* StatPearls, 2024. https:// www.ncbi.nlm.nih.gov/books/NBK513311/.

Kaelberer, M. M., K. L. Buchanan, M. E. Klein, et al. "A Gut-Brain Neural Circuit for Nutrient Sensory Transduction." *Science* 361, no. 6408 (September 21, 2018). https://doi .org/10.1126/science.aat5236.

Kaelberer, M. M., L. E. Rupprecht, W. W. Liu, P. Weng, and D. V. Bohórquez. "Neuropod Cells: The Emerging Biology of Gut-Brain Sensory Transduction." *Annu Rev Neurosci* 43 (July 8, 2020): 337–53. https://doi.org/10.1146/annurev-neuro-091619-022657.

Kaplan, R. J., C. E. Greenwood, G. Winocour, and T. M. Wolever. "Cognitive Performance Is Associated with Glucose Regulation in Healthy Elderly Persons and Can Be Enhanced with Glucose and Dietary Carbohydrates." *Am J Clin Nutr* 72, no. 3 (2000): 825–36. doi:10.1093/ajcn/72.3.825.

Kessler, David. *The End of Overeating: Taking Control of the Insatiable American Diet.* Rodale, 2010.

Kessler, D. *A Question of Intent: A Great American Battle with a Deadly Industry.* PublicAffairs, 2002. https://books.google.com/books?id=FGx-tjk30dMC.

Klaassen, Tim, and Daniel Keszthelyi. "Satiation or Satiety? More Than Mere Semantics." *Lancet* 397, no. 10279 (2021): 1060–61. https://www.thelancet.com/journals/lancet /article/PIIS0140–6736(21)00245–2/fulltext.

Konanur, V. R., S. J. Hurh, T. M. Hsu, and M. F. Roitman. "Dopamine Neuron Activity Evoked by Sucrose and Sucrose-Predictive Cues Is Augmented by Peripheral and Central Manipulations of Glucose Availability." *Eur J Neurosci* 59, no. 10 (May 2024): 2419–35. https://doi.org/10.1111/ejn.16214.

Krause, M., P. W. German, S. A. Taha, and H. L. Fields. "A Pause in Nucleus Accumbens

Neuron Firing Is Required to Initiate and Maintain Feeding." *J Neurosci* 30, no. 13 (March 31, 2010): 4746–56. https://doi.org/10.1523/jneurosci.0197-10.2010.

Kullmann, S., A. Kleinridders, D. M. Small, A. Fritsche, H. U. Häring, H. Preissl, and M. Heni. "Central Nervous Pathways of Insulin Action in the Control of Metabolism and Food Intake." *Lancet Diabetes Endocrinol* 8, no. 6 (June 2020): 524–34. doi: 10.1016 /S2213-8587(20)30113-3. PMID: 32445739.

Kwechansky Marketing Research. *Project 16.* Report for Imperial Tobacco. October 18, 1977.

Kwechansky Marketing Research. *Project 16.* Report for Imperial Tobacco. May 7, 1982. RJR ID 502987357-68.

Lembke, A. "From Dopamine Nation to Dopamine Planet." Lecture presented at the International Food Addiction Consensus Conference (IFACC), London, UK, May 17, 2024.

Lennerz, B. S., D. C. Alsop, L. M. Holsen, et al. "Effects of Dietary Glycemic Index on Brain Regions Related to Reward and Craving in Men." *Am J Clin Nutr* 98, no. 3 (September 2013): 641–47. https://doi.org/10.3945/ajcn.113.064113.

Lennerz, B., and J. K. Lennerz. "Food Addiction, High-Glycemic-Index Carbohydrates, and Obesity." *Clin Chem* 64, no. 1 (January 2018): 64–71. https://doi.org/10.1373 /clinchem.2017.273532.

Lin, G., R. Siddiqui, Z. Lin, et al. "Blood Glucose Variance Measured by Continuous Glucose Monitors Across the Menstrual Cycle." *NPJ Digit Med* 6, no. 1 (August 11, 2023): 140. https://doi.org/10.1038/s41746-023-00884-x.

Liu, S., A. K. Globa, F. Mills, et al. "Consumption of Palatable Food Primes Food Approach Behavior by Rapidly Increasing Synaptic Density in the VTA." *Proc Natl Acad Sci USA* 113, no. 9 (March 1, 2016): 2520–25. https://doi.org/10.1073/pnas.1515724113.

Mason, A. E., K. Jhaveri, S. Schleicher, et al. "Sweet Cognition: The Differential Effects of Glucose Consumption on Attentional Food Bias in Individuals of Lean and Obese Status." *Physiol Behav* 206 (July 1, 2019): 264–73. https://doi.org/10.1016/j.physbeh.2019 .04.014.

McDougle, Molly, Alan de Araujo, Arashdeep Singh, et al. "Separate Gut-Brain Circuits for Fat and Sugar Reinforcement Combine to Promote Overeating." *Cell Metabolism* 36, no. 2 (2024): 393–407.e7. https://doi.org/10.1016/j.cmet.2023.12.014.

Moon, Jun Sung. "Current Evidence of CGM Use in Weight Management—Possibilities and Concerns." Lecture presented at International Congress on Obesity and Metabolic Syndrome (ICOMES), Seoul, Republic of Korea, September 5–7, 2024.

Naleid, A. M., J. W. Grimm, D. A. Kessler, et al. "Deconstructing the Vanilla Milkshake: The Dominant Effect of Sucrose on Self-administration of Nutrient-Flavor Mixtures." *Appetite* 50, no. 1 (January 2008): 128–38. https://doi.org/10.1016/j.appet.2007.06.011.

Naqvi, N. H., and A. Bechara. "The Hidden Island of Addiction: The Insula." *Trends Neurosci* 32, no. 1 (January 2009): 56–67. https://doi.org/10.1016/j.tins.2008.09.009.

Naqvi, N. H., and A. Bechara. "The Insula and Drug Addiction: An Interoceptive View of Pleasure, Urges, and Decision-Making." *Brain Struct Funct* 214, no. 5–6 (June 2010): 435–50. https://doi.org/10.1007/s00429-010-0268-7.

Naqvi, N. H., N. Gaznick, D. Tranel, and A. Bechara. "The Insula: A Critical Neural Substrate for Craving and Drug Seeking Under Conflict and Risk." *Ann NY Acad Sci* 1316 (May 2014): 53–70. https://doi.org/10.1111/nyas.12415.

Nicola, S. M., S. A. Taha, S. W. Kim, and H. L. Fields. "Nucleus Accumbens Dopamine

Release Is Necessary and Sufficient to Promote the Behavioral Response to Reward-Predictive Cues." *Neuroscience* 135, no. 4 (2005): 1025–33. https://doi.org/10.1016/j.neuroscience.2005.06.088.

Noël, X., D. Brevers, and A. Bechara. "A Neurocognitive Approach to Understanding the Neurobiology of Addiction." *Curr Opin Neurobiol* 23, no. 4 (August 2013): 632–38. https://doi.org/10.1016/j.conb.2013.01.018.

Noël, X., D. Brevers, and A. Bechara. "A Triadic Neurocognitive Approach to Addiction for Clinical Interventions." *Front Psychiatry* 4 (December 2013): 179. https://doi.org/10.3389/fpsyt.2013.00179.

O'Connor, Sarah, and Iwona Rudkowska. "Energy Intake." *Dietary Fatty Acids and the Metabolic Syndrome: A Personalized Nutrition Approach* 87 (2019): 43–146. https://doi.org/10.1016/bs.afnr.2018.07.004.

Page, K. A., J. Arora, M. Qiu, R. Relwani, R. T. Constable, and R. S. Sherwin. "Small Decrements in Systemic Glucose Provoke Increases in Hypothalamic Blood Flow Prior to the Release of Counterregulatory Hormones." *Diabetes* 58, no. 2 (February 2009): 448–52. https://doi.org/10.2337/db08–1224.

Page, Kathleen A., Dongju Seo, Renata Belfort De Aguiar, et al. "Circulating Glucose Levels Modulate Neural Control of Desire for High-Calorie Foods in Humans." *J Clin Investig* 121, no. 10 (2011): 4161–19. doi:10.1172/JCI57873.

Perez, Catalina, François Lucas, and Anthony Sclafani. "Increased Flavor Acceptance and Preference Conditioned by the Postingestive Actions of Glucose." *Physiol Behav* 64, no. 4 (1998): 483–92. https://doi.org/10.1016/S0031–9384(98)00104–8.

Ranganath, C. *Why We Remember: Unlocking Memory's Power to Hold On to What Matters.* Knopf Doubleday, 2024. https://books.google.com/books?id=Mda_EAAAQBAJ.

Reasoner, B. D., A. D. Boes, and J. C. Geerling. "Sustained, Effortless Weight Loss After Damage to the Left Frontoinsular Cortex: A Case Report." *Case Rep Neurol* 15, no. 1 (March 28, 2023): 63–68. https://doi.org/10.1159/000529533.

Robinson, Mike J. F., Terry E. Robinson, and Kent C. Berridge. "Chapter 39: Incentive Salience and the Transition to Addiction." In *Biological Research on Addiction*, vol. 2. Ed. Peter M. Miller. Academic Press, 2013.

Schiff, S. "What Have I Learned from Bariatric Patients About Their Mind and Behaviours?" Lecture presented at the International Federation for Surgery of Obesity and Metabolic Disorders, Naples, Italy, August 31, 2023.

Sclafani, A. "Gut-Brain Nutrient Signaling: Appetition vs. Satiation." *Appetite* 71 (December 2013): 454–58. https://doi.org/10.1016/j.appet.2012.05.024.

Sclafani, A. "How Food Preferences Are Learned: Laboratory Animal Models." *Proc Nutr Soc* 54, no. 2 (July 1995): 419–27. https://doi.org/10.1079/pns19950011.

Sclafani, A., and K. Ackroff. "Flavor Preferences Conditioned by Intragastric Glucose but Not Fructose or Galactose in C57BL/6J Mice." *Physiol Behav* 106, no. 4 (June 25, 2012): 457–61. doi: 10.1016/j.physbeh.2012.03.008. Epub March 14, 2012. PMID: 22445944; PMCID: PMC3349008.

Sclafani, A., and K. Ackroff. "Nutrient-Conditioned Intake Stimulation Does Not Require a Distinctive Flavor Cue in Rats." *Appetite* 154 (November 1, 2020): 104793. https://doi.org/10.1016/j.appet.2020.104793.

Shamanna, Paramesh. "Digital Twin (DT) Technology in Type 2 Diabetes Remission and Glycemic Improvement: Eighteen Months Results from a Randomized Controlled

Trial." Lecture presented at the American Diabetic Association 84th Scientific Sessions Program, Orlando, FL, June 21–24, 2024.

Sharma, A. "Heterogeneous Drivers of Obesity: Emotions, Hormones, and Habits, Oh My!" Lecture presented at Thirty-First European Congress on Obesity (ECO), Venice, Italy, May 12, 2024.

Smith, Dana G. "Who Should Be Tracking Their Glucose?" *New York Times*, July 12, 2023. https://www.nytimes.com/2023/07/12/well/eat/glucose-blood-sugar-monitors.html.

Speakman, John R., David A. Levitsky, David B. Allison, et al. "Set Points, Settling Points and Some Alternative Models: Theoretical Options to Understand How Genes and Environments Combine to Regulate Body Adiposity." *Dis Model Mech* 4, no. 6 (2011): 733–45. DOI: 10.1242/dmm.008698.

Sutton, C. A., A. M. L'Insalata, and T. L. Fazzino. "Reward Sensitivity, Eating Behavior, and Obesity-Related Outcomes: A Systematic Review." *Physiol Behav* 252 (August 1, 2022): 113843. https://doi.org/10.1016/j.physbeh.2022.113843.

Taha, S. A., and H. L. Fields. "Encoding of Palatability and Appetitive Behaviors by Distinct Neuronal Populations in the Nucleus Accumbens." *J Neurosci* 25, no. 5 (February 2, 2005): 1193–202. https://doi.org/10.1523/jneurosci.3975–04.2005.

Taha, S. A., and H. L. Fields. "Inhibitions of Nucleus Accumbens Neurons Encode a Gating Signal for Reward-Directed Behavior." *J Neurosci* 26, no. 1 (January 4, 2006): 217–22. https://doi.org/10.1523/jneurosci.3227 05.2006.

Taha, S. A., S. M. Nicola, and H. L. Fields. "Cue-Evoked Encoding of Movement Planning and Execution in the Rat Nucleus Accumbens." *J Physiol* 584, no. 3 (November 1, 2007): 801–18. https://doi.org/10.1113/jphysiol.2007.140236.

Taha, S. A., E. Norsted, L. S. Lee, et al. "Endogenous Opioids Encode Relative Taste Preference." *Eur J Neurosci* 24, no. 4 (August 2006): 1220–26. https://doi.org/10.1111/j .1460–9568.2006.04987.x.

Terauchi, Akiko, and Hisashi Umemori. "How Are Dopaminergic Circuits Established?" Harvard Brain Science Initiative, 2023. https://brain.harvard.edu/hbi_news/how-are -dopaminergic-circuits-established.

Touzani, Khalid, Richard J. Bodnar, and Anthony Sclafani. "Acquisition of Glucose-Conditioned Flavor Preference Requires the Activation of Dopamine D1-Like Receptors Within the Medial Prefrontal Cortex in Rats." *Neurobiol Learn Mem* 94, no. 2 (2010): 214–19. DOI: 10.1016/j.nlm.2010.05.009.

Townsend, Jeremy R., Trevor O. Kirby, Philip A. Sapp, Adam M. Gonzalez, Tess M. Marshall, and Ralph Esposito. "Nutrient Synergy: Definition, Evidence, and Future Directions." *Front Nutr* 10 (2023): 1279925. DOI: 10.3389/fnut.2023.1279925.

Turel, O., Q. He, L. Wei, and A. Bechara. "The Role of the Insula in Internet Gaming Disorder." *Addict Biol* 26, no. 2 (March 2021): e12894. https://doi.org/10.1111/adb.12894.

Wei, L., S. Zhang, O. Turel, A. Bechara, and Q. He. "A Tripartite Neurocognitive Model of Internet Gaming Disorder." *Front Psychiatry* 8 (2017): 285. https://doi.org/10.3389 /fpsyt.2017.00285.

Wise, Roy A. "Roles for Nigrostriatal—Not Just Mesocorticolimbic—Dopamine in Reward and Addiction." *Trends Neurosci* 32, no. 10 (2009): 517–24. DOI: 10.1016/j.tins.2009.06.004.

Woolley, J. D., B. S. Lee, S. A. Taha, and H. L. Fields. "Nucleus Accumbens Opioid Signaling Conditions Short-Term Flavor Preferences." *Neuroscience* 146, no. 1 (April 25, 2007): 19–30. https://doi.org/10.1016/j.neuroscience.2007.01.005.

Wyatt, P., S. E. Berry, G. Finlayson, et al. "Postprandial Glycaemic Dips Predict Appetite and Energy Intake in Healthy Individuals." *Nat Metab* 3, no. 4 (April 2021): 523–29. https://doi.org/10.1038/s42255-021-00383-x.

Interviews and Correspondence with the Author

Belfort De Aguiar, Renata (January 2024; April 2024).

Berridge, Kent (October 2024).

Civille, Gail (September 2024).

de Araujo, Ivan (August 2024).

Elbaraby, Nancy Samir (June 2024).

Fazzino, Tera (September 2024).

Germine, Laura Thi (August 2024).

Koob, George (February 2024; May 2024).

Levine, Allen (August 2024).

Page, Kathleen (May 2024).

Roitman, Mitchell (May 2024).

Sclafani, Anthony (May 2024).

Small, Dana (February 2024; March 2024; July 2024).

Wise, Roy (May 2024).

Zorrilla, Eric (January 2024; February 2024).

Notes

27   **homeostatic and hedonic systems:** Sharma, "Heterogeneous Drivers of Obesity."

28   **Evolutionary psychologists:** Berridge and Kringelbach, "Pleasure Systems in the Brain."

29   **"pleasure, physical reward, emotion":** Sharma, "Heterogeneous Drivers of Obesity."

29   **"not eaten all day":** Sharma, "Heterogeneous Drivers of Obesity."

30   **"lifestyle and behavioral interventions":** Sharma, "Heterogeneous Drivers of Obesity."

30   **beyond its starring role:** Cleveland Clinic, "Dopamine."

30   **incentive salience:** Author interview with Berridge, October 2024.

31   **strengthens the neurocircuits:** Author interview with Wise, May 2024.

31   **"target to pin":** Author interview with Berridge, October 2024.

31   **"big reward":** Ranganath, *Why We Remember*.

31   **"Dopamine activity ramps up":** Ranganath, *Why We Remember*.

31   **"based largely on your expectations from past experiences":** Ranganath, *Why We Remember*.

32   **"It could be mild dysphoria":** Author interview with Koob, May 2024.

32   **"as certain neurons":** Author interview with Zorrilla, January 2024.

32   **"What happens right after":** Huberman, "Dr. Anna Lembke."

32   **"immediately compensate":** Lembke, "From Dopamine Nation to Dopamine Planet."

33   **"'baseline'":** Author interview with Roitman, May 2024.

33   **three systems involved:** Noël et al., "A Triadic Neurocognitive Approach to Addiction for Clinical Interventions."

33   **benign brain tumor:** Reasoner et al., "Sustained, Effortless Weight Loss After Damage to the Left Frontoinsular Cortex."

34   **subtle difference between:** Speakman et al., "Set Points, Settling Points and Some Alternative Models."

34   **"settling point":** Speakman et al., "Set Points, Settling Points and Some Alternative Models."

35   **Bearing this history in mind:** Naleid et al., "Deconstructing the Vanilla Milkshake."

35   **undertook experiments:** Naleid et al., "Deconstructing the Vanilla Milkshake."

35   **table sugar:** Groves, "Sucrose vs. Glucose vs. Fructose."

35   **greater physiological effect:** Townsend et al., "Nutrient Synergy."

36   **substantial reinforcer:** Author interview with Sclafani, May 2024.

36   **senior food industry designer:** Kessler, *End of Overeating*.

36   **"The poison":** Author interview with Fazzino, September 2024.

36   **sought a data-driven:** Fazzino, "Crossing Fields to Make Scientific Connections"; Fazzino et al., "Hyper-palatable Foods."

37   **"The ultimate food":** Author interview with Civille, September 2024.

38   **"if a neuron encodes":** Kessler, *End of Overeating*, 35–36.

38   **body's preferred carb-based:** Groves, "Sucrose vs. Glucose vs. Fructose."

38   **as well as others:** Berthoud et al., "Gut-Brain Communication and Obesity."

38   **specifically, the duodenum:** Cleveland Clinic, "Duodenum."

38   **mice and rats:** Sclafani and Ackroff, "Flavor Preferences Conditioned by Intragastric Glucose."

39   **these cells are critical:** Bai Ling et al., "Enteroendocrine Cell Types That Drive Food Reward and Aversion."

39   **"Most people are eating":** Author interview with Roitman, May 2024.

39   **which regulates appetite:** Farr et al., "Central Nervous System Regulation of Eating."

39   **"When dopamine":** Author interview with de Araujo, August 2024.

40   **"fatigue-related":** Author interview with Germine, August 2024; Hawks et al., "Dynamic Associations Between Glucose and Ecological Momentary Cognition in Type 1 Diabetes."

41   **greater energy intake:** O'Connor and Rudkowska, "Energy Intake."

41   **glucose drops before meals:** Belfort De Aguiar et al., "Humans with Obesity Have Disordered Brain Responses to Food Images during Physiological Hyperglycemia"; author interviews with Belfort De Aguiar, January 2024, April 2024.

41   **"Changes in sweet cravings":** Anguah et al., "Changes in Food Cravings and Eating Behavior."

42   **high insulin levels:** Kullmann et al., "Central Nervous Pathways of Insulin Action in the Control of Metabolism and Food Intake."

4: Sensitivity and Susceptibility

Sources
Works Referenced

Bessesen, Dan. "Regulation of Body Weight: Relevance to Obesity." Lecture presented at the Research and Innovation Conference, Denver, CO, January 17, 2023.

Brownell, Kelly D., and Mark S. Gold, eds. *Food and Addiction: A Comprehensive Handbook.* Oxford University Press, 2012.

Edwin Thanarajah, S., A. G. DiFeliceantonio, K. Albus, et al. "Habitual Daily Intake of a Sweet and Fatty Snack Modulates Reward Processing in Humans." *Cell Metab* 35, no. 4 (April 4, 2023): 571–84.e6. https://doi.org/10.1016/j.cmet.2023.02.015.

Epel, E. S., A. J. Tomiyama, A. E. Mason, et al. "The Reward-Based Eating Drive Scale: A Self-report Index of Reward-Based Eating." *PLOS One* 9, no. 6 (2014): e101350. https://doi.org/10.1371/journal.pone.0101350.

Harris, Richard. "How Helpful Would a Genetic Test for Obesity Risk Be?" NPR, May 6, 2019. https://www.npr.org/sections/health-shots/2019/05/06/719558715/how-useful-would-a-genetic-test-for-obesity-risk-be.

Horvath, Tamas. "Obesity Pathophysiology: Treating the Chronic Disease of Obesity." Lecture presented at 2023 Columbia Cornell Obesity: Etiology, Prevention, and Treatment, New York, May 3–6, 2023.

Kessler, D. A. *The End of Overeating: Taking Control of the Insatiable American Appetite.* Harmony/Rodale, 2010. https://books.google.com/books?id=QFR1M3Vwe1wC.

Kessler, D. *A Question of Intent: A Great American Battle with a Deadly Industry.* PublicAffairs, 2002. https://books.google.com/books?id=FGx-tjk30dMC.

Leibel, R. "Genetics of Obesity (Gene x Development & Environment)." Lecture presented at 2024 Columbia Cornell Obesity Medicine, New York, May 1–4, 2024.

Roberts, Carl. "Current and Emerging Obesity Medications: Behavioural Mechanisms of Action—What We Know and What We Don't." Lecture presented at the Thirty-First European Congress on Obesity (ECO), Venice, Italy, May 12, 2024.

Roberts, Carl A., Paul Christiansen, and Jason C. G. Halford. "Tailoring Pharmacotherapy to Specific Eating Behaviours in Obesity: Can Recommendations for Personalised Therapy Be Made from the Current Data?" *Acta Diabetologica* 54, no. 8 (2017): 715–25. DOI: 10.1007/s00592-017-0994-x.

Sanyaolu, Adekunle, Chuku Okorie, Xiaohua Qi, Jennifer Locke, and Saif Rehman. "Childhood and Adolescent Obesity in the United States: A Public Health Concern." *Glob Pediatr Health* 6 (2019). DOI: 10.1177/2333794X19891305.

Stunkard, Albert J., Jennifer R. Harris, Nancy L. Pedersen, and Gerald E. McClearn. "The Body-Mass Index of Twins Who Have Been Reared Apart." *N Eng J Med* 322, no. 21 (1990): 1483–87. DOI: 10.1056/NEJM199005243222102.

Interviews and Correspondence with the Author

Risch, Neil (December 2023).

Notes

44   **"now I hate it":** Kessler, *A Question of Intent.*

44   **give up ultraformulated:** Epel et al., "The Reward-Based Eating Drive Scale: A Self-report Index of Reward-Based Eating."

45   **"prevalence of childhood obesity":** Sanyaolu et al., "Childhood and Adolescent Obesity in the United States."

45   **eating behaviors formed:** Brownell and Gold, eds., *Food and Addiction*, 10.

45   **"reduces preference for low-fat food":** Edwin Thanarajah et al., "Habitual Daily Intake of a Sweet and Fatty Snack Modulates Reward Processing."

45   **detail the components:** Roberts, "Current and Emerging Obesity Medications."

46   **people who struggle:** Kessler, *The End of Overeating*.

46   **"biological vulnerability":** Roberts, "Current and Emerging Obesity Medications."

46   **Dr. Daniel Bessesen:** Bessesen, "Regulation of Body Weight: Relevance to Obesity."

47   *still* **a higher degree:** Stunkard et al., "The Body-Mass Index of Twins Who Have Been Reared Apart."

47   **in an environment:** Leibel, "Genetics of Obesity (Gene x Development & Environment)."

48   **"organisms that were developed":** Leibel, "Genetics of Obesity."

48   **"Our default":** Horvath, "Obesity Pathophysiology."

5: The Legacy of Obesity

Sources
Works Referenced

ABC News. "The Fight Against Childhood Obesity: Two Kids' Stories." ABC News, May 14, 2010. https://abcnews.go.com/Nightline/childhood-obesity-pediatric-weight-management-clinic/story?id=10650793.

BBC News. "Childhood Obesity: 10 of Your Stories." BBC News, October 2, 2012. https://www.bbc.com/news/magazine-19743173.

Dinkevich, Eugene. "An Ounce of Prevention: A Brief Family-Centered Approach to the Obesity Counseling in Pediatric Primary Care." Lecture presented at 2024 Columbia Cornell Obesity: Etiology, Prevention, and Treatment, Columbia University, New York, May 1–4, 2024.

Ducharme, Jamie. "Teens Are Taking Wegovy for Weight Loss. But Doctors Have a Lot to Learn." *Time*, June 6, 2023. https://time.com/6285055/wegovy-teenagers-weight-loss-risks/.

Fox, Claudia, and Aaron Kelly. "Pharmacotherapy for Obesity in Youth." Lecture presented at 2024 Columbia Cornell Obesity: Etiology, Prevention, and Treatment, Columbia University, New York, May 1–4, 2024.

González, Irene, Albert Lecube, Miguel Ángel Rubio, and Pedro Pablo García-Luna. "Pregnancy After Bariatric Surgery: Improving Outcomes for Mother and Child." *Int J Women's Health* 8 (2016): 721–29. DOI: 10.2147/IJWH.S99970.

Hampl, S. E., S. G. Hassink, A. C. Skinner, S. C. Armstrong, S. E. Barlow, C. F. Bolling, K. C. Avila Edwards, et al. "Clinical Practice Guideline for the Evaluation and Treatment of Children and Adolescents with Obesity." *Pediatrics* 151, no. 2 (February 1, 2023): e2022060640. doi: 10.1542/peds.2022-060640. Erratum in *Pediatrics* 153, no. 1 (January 1, 2024): e2023064612. doi: 10.1542/peds.2023-064612. PMID: 36622115.

Hilts, Philip J. "F.D.A. Head Calls Smoking a Pediatric Disease." *New York Times*, March

9, 1995. https://www.nytimes.com/1995/03/09/us/fda-head-calls-smoking-a-pediatric
-disease.html.

Kolata, Gina. "Being Sugar-Deprived Had Major Effects on These Children's Health."
New York Times, October 31, 2024.

Lovelace, Berkely, Jr., Kori Lynch, and Anne Thompson. "What Happens When You
Stop Taking a Weight Loss Drug? Many People Gain the Weight Back." Today.com,
January 19, 2023. https://www.today.com/health/diet-fitness/s-happens-stop-taking
-weight-loss-drug-wegovy-rcna66489.

Miller, Lisa. "An American Girlhood in the Ozempic Era." *The Cut*, December 19, 2023.
https://www.thecut.com/article/weight-loss-drugs-ozempic-kids-childhood-obesity
.html.

Nicholson, Wanda. Interviewed in Elizabeth Cooney, "To Treat Obesity in Children,
Task Force Favors Behavioral Therapy over Drugs Like Wegovy." *Stat News*, June 18,
2024. https://www.statnews.com/2024/06/18/children-obesity-behavioral-therapy-weg
ovy-recommendations/.

Ohlsson, C., M. Bygdell, M. Nethander, A. Rosengren, and J. M. Kindblom. "BMI Change
During Puberty Is an Important Determinant of Adult Type 2 Diabetes Risk in Men."
J Clin Endocrinol Metab 104, no. 5 (May 1, 2019): 1823–32. doi: 10.1210/jc.2018-01339.
PMID: 30517677; PMCID: PMC6456008.

Singhal, Vibha. Interviewed in Vanessa Villafuerte, "Are GLP-1 Drugs Safe for Children? Doctors Say Despite High Use Among Youth, No Unique Health Risks Detected."
UCLA Health, July 10, 2024. https://www.uclahealth.org/news/release/are-glp-1-drugs
-safe-children-doctors-say-despite-high-use.

Sole-Smith, Virginia. Interviewed in Erica Schwiegershausen, "What If You Weren't
Scared of Your Kid Being Fat?" *New York Magazine*, April 20, 2023. https://www.thecut
.com/article/interview-virginia-sole-smith-parenting-fatphobia.html?origSession=D24
12170n3hNnyk5TCNXHqVuOUYBczocaRDvroPZ6sCvoe5fPc%3D.

Sole-Smith, Virginia. "Why the New Obesity Guidelines for Kids Terrify Me." *New York
Times*, January 26, 2023. https://www.nytimes.com/2023/01/26/opinion/aap-obesity
-guidelines-bmi-wegovy-ozempic.html.

Interviews and Correspondence with the Author

Fox, Claudia (December 2024).

Rosenbaum, Michael (September 2024).

Notes

49   **one idea about:** Author interview with Rosenbaum, September 2024.

49   **"laying the metabolic groundwork":** Author interview with Rosenbaum, Sep-
      tember 2024.

50   **as a fifteen-year-old:** Fox and Kelly, "Pharmacotherapy for Obesity in Youth."
      The facts of this case were changed. I want to acknowledge Dr. Claudia Fox for her
      assistance and permission.

50   **In 2023, reporter:** Miller, "An American Girlhood in the Ozempic Era."

50   **In another story:** BBC News, "Childhood Obesity."

50   **released new guidelines:** Hampl et al., "Clinical Practice Guideline for the Eval-
      uation and Treatment of Children and Adolescents with Obesity."

51   **to study people living:** Author interview with Rosenbaum, September 2024.

51   **"Primary care gets":** Dinkevich, "An Ounce of Prevention."

52   **overweight at age eight:** Ohlsson et al., "BMI Change During Puberty Is an Important Determinant of Adult Type 2 Diabetes Risk in Men."

52   **Recent research from:** Kolata, "Being Sugar-Deprived Had Major Effects on These Children's Health."

52   **In March 1995**: Hilts, "F.D.A. Head Calls Smoking a Pediatric Disease."

6: Regain as Relapse

Sources
Works Referenced

Anderson, J. W., E. C. Konz, R. C. Frederich, and C. L. Wood. "Long-term Weight-Loss Maintenance: A Meta-analysis of US Studies." *Am J Clin Nutr* 74, no. 5 (2001): 579–84. DOI: 10.1093/ajcn/74.5.579.

Hall, K. "Calories, Carbs, or Quality: What Matters Most for Body Weight?" Lecture presented at 2024 Columbia Cornell Obesity, New York, May 1–4, 2024.

Hall, Kevin D., and Scott Kahan. "Maintenance of Lost Weight and Long-term Management of Obesity." *Med Clin N Am* 102, no. 1 (2018): 183–97. DOI: 10.1016/j.mcna.2017.08.012.

Koob, George. "Hyperkatifeia and Negative Reinforcement as a Driving Force in Addiction-Like Overeating." Lecture presented at the American Psychiatric Association, San Francisco, CA, May 23, 2023.

Leibel, R. L., M. Rosenbaum, and J. Hirsch. "Changes in Energy Expenditure Resulting from Altered Body Weight." *N Engl J Med* 332, no. 10 (1995): 621–28. https://doi.org/10.1056/nejm199503093321001.

MacLean, P. "Physiology of the Weight Reduced State: From Mechanisms to Clinical Application." Lecture presented at Obesity Week 2022 by the Obesity Society, San Diego, CA, November 1–4, 2022.

Martins, C. "Metabolic Adaption and Increased Drive to Eat as Drivers of Weight Regain in Individuals with Obesity: Myth or Reality? An Exercise in Adversarial Collaboration." Lecture presented at Nutrition 2023, Boston, MA, July 22–25, 2023.

Rosenbaum, M. "The Physiology of the Weight Reduced State: Factors Opposing Weight Loss Maintenance." Lecture presented at Obesity Week 2023 by the Obesity Society, Dallas, TX, October 14–17, 2023.

Rosenbaum, M. "Why Is It So Hard to Keep Weight Off?" Lecture presented at 2024 Columbia Cornell Obesity: Etiology, Prevention, and Treatment, May 1–4, 2024.

Schiff, S. "What Have I Learned from Bariatric Patients About Their Mind and Behaviors?" Lecture presented at the International Federation for Surgery of Obesity and Metabolic Disorders, Naples, Italy, August 31, 2023.

Sharma, A. "Heterogeneous Drivers of Obesity: Emotions, Hormones, and Habits, Oh My!" Lecture presented at Thirty-First European Congress on Obesity (ECO), Venice, Italy, May 12, 2024.

Interviews and Correspondence with the Author

Berridge, Kent (March 2024).

Koob, George (February 2024; May 2024).

Martins, Catia (April 2024).

Rosenbaum, Michael (September 2024).

Schiff, Sami (May 2024).

Notes

53 **"The minute you reduce":** Sharma, "Heterogeneous Drivers of Obesity."

53 **meta-analysis of the propensity:** Anderson et al., "Long-term Weight-Loss Maintenance."

53 **"weight comes back":** MacLean, "Physiology of the Weight Reduced State."

53 **"in the plastic surgery":** Author interview with Rosenbaum, September 2024; MacLean, "Physiology of the Weight Reduced State"; Rosenbaum, "Why Is It So Hard to Keep Weight Off?"

54 **"Weight regain":** Martins, "Metabolic Adaption and Increased Drive to Eat as Drivers of Weight Regain in Individuals with Obesity."

54 **"There would be no forces":** Author interview with Rosenbaum, September 2024.

54 **"what the body is expending":** MacLean, "Physiology of the Weight Reduced State."

54 **fed people:** Leibel et al., "Changes in Energy Expenditure Resulting from Altered Body Weight."

55 **for every kilogram:** Hall, "Calories, Carbs, or Quality."

56 **"argued years ago":** Author interviews with Koob, February 2024 and May 2024; Koob, "Hyperkatifeia and Negative Reinforcement as a Driving Force in Addiction-Like Overeating."

56 **alternating periods:** Author interview with Schiff, May 2024.

7: Body Positivity, Health Positivity

Sources
Works Referenced

Aune, D., S. Schlesinger, T. Norat, and E. Riboli. "Body Mass Index, Abdominal Fatness, and the Risk of Sudden Cardiac Death: A Systematic Review and Dose-Response Meta-analysis of Prospective Studies." *Eur J Epidemiol* 33, no. 8 (2018): 711–22. DOI: 10.1007/s10654-017-0353-9.

Baker, Katie J. M. "They Promoted Body Positivity. Then They Lost Weight." *New York Times*, February 26, 2024. https://www.nytimes.com/2024/02/26/style/body-positive-influencers-weight-loss.html.

Bays, Harold E. "Adiposopathy: Is 'Sick Fat' a Cardiovascular Disease?" *J Am Coll Cardiol* 57, no. 25 (2011): 2461–73. DOI: 10.1016/j.jacc.2011.02.038.

Beuther, David A., and E. Rand Sutherland. "Overweight, Obesity, and Incident Asthma." *Am J Respir Crit Care Med* 175, no. 7 (2006): 661–66. https://doi.org/10.1164/rccm.200611-1717OC.

Bhaskaran, K., I. Dos Santos Silva, D. A. Leon, I. J. Douglas, and L. Smeeth. "Association of BMI with Overall and Cause-Specific Mortality: A Population-Based Cohort Study of 3.6 Million Adults in the UK." *Lancet Diabetes Endocrinol* 6, no. 12 (December 2018): 944–53. https://doi.org/10.1016/S2213–8587(18)30288–2.

Bjerregaard, Lise G., Britt W. Jensen, Lars Ängquist, Merete Osler, Thorkild I. A. Sørensen, and Jennifer L. Baker. "Change in Overweight from Childhood to Early Adulthood and Risk of Type 2 Diabetes." *N Engl J Med* 378, no. 14 (2018): 1302–12.

Blüher, Matthias. "Metabolically Healthy Obesity." *Endoc Rev* 41, no. 3 (2020): bnaa004. DOI: 10.1210/endrev/bnaa004.

Blüher, Matthias. "Metabolically Healthy Obesity: Fact or Fiction?" Lecture presented at the Fifty-Ninth Annual Meeting of the EASD (European Association for the Study of Diabetes), Hamburg, Germany, October 2–6, 2023.

Caleyachetty, R., G. N. Thomas, K. A. Toulis, et al. "Metabolically Healthy Obese and Incident Cardiovascular Disease Events Among 3.5 Million Men and Women." *J Am Coll Cardiol* 70, no. 12 (2017): 1429–37. https://doi.org/10.1016/j.jacc.2017.07.763.

Deanfield, John, Subodh Verma, Benjamin Scirica, et al. "Semaglutide and Cardiovascular Outcomes in Patients with Obesity and Prevalent Heart Failure: A Prespecified Analysis of the SELECT Trial." *Lancet* 404 (2024): 773–86. DOI: 10.1016/S0140–6736(24)01498–3.

DeFronzo, R. "Keynote 2: New Horizons for T2D Treatment." Keynote lecture presented at the Achieve Targets in Diabetes Care (ATDC) conference, Keystone, CO, July 10–13, 2024.

Després, Jean-Pierre. "Abdominal Obesity: The Most Prevalent Cause of the Metabolic Syndrome and Related Cardiometabolic Risk." *EHJ-S* 8, no. suppl_B (2006): B4–B12. https://doi.org/10.1093/eurheartj/sul002.

Després, J.-P., S. Moorjani, P. J. Lupien, A. Tremblay, A. Nadeau, and C. Bouchard. "Regional Distribution of Body Fat, Plasma Lipoproteins, and Cardiovascular Disease." *Arterioscler* 10, no. 4 (July–August 1990): 497–511. https://doi.org/10.1161/01.atv.10.4.497.

deVos, Kelly. "The Problem with Body Positivity." *New York Times*, May 29, 2018. https://www.nytimes.com/2018/05/29/opinion/weight-loss-body-positivity.html.

Di Angelantonio, Emanuele, Shilpa N. Bhupathiraju, David Wormser, et al. "Body-Mass Index and All-Cause Mortality: Individual-Participant-Data Meta-Analysis of 239 Prospective Studies in Four Continents." *Lancet* 388, no. 10046 (2016): 776–86. https://doi.org/10.1016/S0140–6736(16)30175–1.

Dicker, Dror. "Obesity as a Disease: A Controversial Idea." Lecture presented at Thirty-First European Congress on Obesity (ECO), Venice, Italy, May 12–15, 2024.

Echouffo-Tcheugui, J. B., Meghan I. Short, Vanessa Xanthakis, et al. "Natural History of Obesity Subphenotypes: Dynamic Changes over Two Decades and Prognosis in the Framingham Heart Study." *J Clin Endocrinol Metab* 104, no. 3 (2019): 738–52. https://pubmed.ncbi.nlm.nih.gov/30339231/.

Fairburn, Christopher G. *Overcoming Binge Eating: The Proven Program to Learn Why You Binge and How You Can Stop*. Second ed. Guilford Press, 2013.

Farrell, Amy Erdman. *Fat Shame: Stigma and the Fat Body in American Culture*. NYU Press, 2011.

Fernandez-Aranda, F. "Management of Eating Disorders and Obesity from Transdiagnostic Perspective." Lecture presented at Thirty-First European Congress on Obesity (ECO), Venice, Italy, May 12–15, 2024.

Ferrante, A. "Obesity and Comorbidities." Lecture presented at 2023 Columbia Cornell Obesity: Etiology, Prevention, and Treatment, New York, May 3–6, 2023.

Ferrante, A. "Obesity and Comorbidities." Lecture presented at 2024 Columbia Cornell Obesity: Etiology, Prevention, and Treatment, New York, May 1–4, 2024.

Field, A. E., E. H. Coakley, A. Must, et al. "Impact of Overweight on the Risk of Developing Common Chronic Diseases During a 10-Year Period." *Arch Intern Med* 161, no. 13 (July 9, 2001): 1581–86. https://doi.org/10.1001/archinte.161.13.1581.

Fingeret, M., P. Marques-Vidal, and P. Vollenweider. "Incidence of Type 2 Diabetes, Hypertension, and Dyslipidemia in Metabolically Healthy Obese and Non-obese." *Nutr Metab Cardiovasc Dis* 28, no. 10 (2018): 1036–44. DOI: 10.1016/j.numecd.2018.06.011.

Fuller, Cheryl. *The Fat Lady Sings: A Psychological Exploration of the Cultural Fat Complex and Its Effects.* Routledge, 2017.

Goossens, Gijs H. "Sexual Dimorphism in Cardiometabolic Health: The Role of Adipose Tissue and Skeletal Muscle." Lecture presented at Thirty-First European Congress on Obesity (ECO), Venice, Italy, May 12, 2024.

Hampel, Howard, Neena S. Abraham, and Hashem B. El-Serag. "Meta-analysis: Obesity and the Risk for Gastroesophageal Reflux Disease and Its Complications." *Annals of Internal Medicine* 143, no. 3 (August 2, 2005): 199–211.

Herman, C. P., and D. Mack. "Restrained and Unrestrained Eating." *J Pers* 43, no. 4 (December 1975): 647–60. https://doi.org/10.1111/j.1467–6494.1975.tb00727.x.

Hill, A. "Programme-Fed and Focused Interventions for Eating Disorders." Lecture presented at Thirty-First European Congress on Obesity (ECO), Venice, Italy, May 12, 2024.

Kenchaiah S., J. C. Evans, D. Levy, et al. "Obesity and the Risk of Heart Failure." *N Engl J Med* 347 (2002): 305–13. https//doi.org/10.1056/NEJMoa020245.

Kilpatrick, Eric S., Alan S. Rigby, and Stephen L. Atkin. "The Effect of Glucose Variability on the Risk of Microvascular Complications in Type 1 Diabetes." *Diabetes Care* 29, no. 7 (2006): 1486–90. https://doi.org/10.2337/dc06–0293.

Lauby-Secretan, Beatrice, Chiara Scoccianti, Dana Loomis, Yann Grosse, Franca Bianchini, and Kurt Straif. "Body Fatness and Cancer—Viewpoint of the IARC Working Group." *N Engl J Med* 375, no. 8 (August 25, 2016): 794–98. DOI: 10.1056/NEJMsr1606602.

Leone, A. "Adherence to the Mediterranean Diet and Risk of Anxiety and Depression in People with Obesity: A Cross-Sectional Analysis." Lecture presented at Thirty-First European Congress on Obesity (ECO), Venice, Italy, May 12, 2024.

Lincoff, A. M. "Semaglutide and Cardiovascular Outcomes in Patients with Overweight or Obesity Who Do Not Have Diabetes: The SELECT Trial." Lecture presented at American Heart Association Scientific Sessions 2023, Philadelphia, PA, November 11–13, 2023.

Lincoff, A. M., Kristine Brown-Frandsen, Helen M. Colhoun, et al., and SELECT trial investigators. "Semaglutide and Cardiovascular Outcomes in Obesity Without Diabetes." *N Engl J Med* 389, no. 24 (2023): 2221–32. DOI: 10.1056/NEJMoa2307563.

Look AHEAD Research Group. "Cardiovascular Effects of Intensive Lifestyle Intervention in Type 2 Diabetes." *N Engl J Med* 369, no. 2 (2013): 145–54. https://www.nejm.org/doi/full/10.1056/NEJMoa1212914.

Look AHEAD Research Group. "Effect of a Long-Term Behavioural Weight Loss Intervention on Nephropathy in Overweight or Obese Adults with Type 2 Diabetes: A

Secondary Analysis of the Look AHEAD Randomised Clinical Trial." *Lancet Diabetes Endocrinol* 2, no. 10 (October 2014): 801–9. DOI:10.1016/S2213–8587(14)70156–1.

Look AHEAD Research Group. "Eight-Year Weight Losses with an Intensive Lifestyle Intervention: The Look AHEAD Study." *Obesity* (Silver Spring, MD) 22, no. 1 (2014): 5–13. https://pubmed.ncbi.nlm.nih.gov/24307184/.

Look AHEAD Research Group, Xavier Pi-Sunyer, George Blackburn, Frederick L. Brancati, et al. "Reduction in Weight and Cardiovascular Disease Risk Factors in Individuals with Type 2 Diabetes: One-Year Results of the Look AHEAD Trial." *Diabetes Care* 30, no. 6 (2007): 1374–83. https://pubmed.ncbi.nlm.nih.gov/17363746/.

Look AHEAD Research Group, Thomas A. Wadden, Delia S. West, Linda Delahanty, et al. "The Look AHEAD Study: A Description of the Lifestyle Intervention and the Evidence Supporting It." *Obesity* (Silver Spring, MD) 14, no. 5 (2006): 737–52. https://pubmed.ncbi.nlm.nih.gov/16855180/.

Lundgren, H., C. Bengtsson, G. Blohme, L. Lapidus, and L. Sjöström. "Adiposity and Adipose Tissue Distribution in Relation to Incidence of Diabetes in Women: Results from a Prospective Population Study in Gothenburg, Sweden." *Int J Obes* 13, no. 4 (1989): 413–23.

Morrison, Rebecca. "I'm Fat. Here's Why I'm Not Taking a Weight Loss Drug." *Washington Post*, September 28, 2024. https://www.washingtonpost.com/wellness/2024/09/28/why-im-not-taking-a-weight-loss-drug/.

Nissen, Steven N. "Metabolic Surgery vs. Pharmacotherapy for Treatment of Obesity." Lecture presented at the Practical Ways to Achieve Targets in Diabetes Care Keystone Conference in Keystone, CO, July 12–16, 2023.

Nunes-Silva, Jose. "Is There Such a Thing as Metabolically Healthy Obesity?" Lecture presented at the International Congress on Obesity (ICO), São Paulo, Brazil, June 26–29, 2024.

The Nutrition Source. "Intuitive Eating." Harvard T. H. Chan School of Public Health, November 2023. https://nutritionsource.hsph.harvard.edu/intuitive-eating/.

The Original Intuitive Eating Pros. "10 Principles of Intuitive Eating." 2019. https://www.intuitiveeating.org/about-us/10-principles-of-intuitive-eating/.

Perreault, Leigh. "Treating Obesity to Treat Type 2 Diabetes." Lecture presented at the Boston Course in Obesity Medicine, Boston, MA, June 13–16, 2023.

Petrov, M. S., and R. Taylor. "Intra-Pancreatic Fat Deposition: Bringing Hidden Fat to the Fore." *Nat Rev Gastroenterol Hepatol* 19, no. 3 (March 2022): 153–68. https://doi.org/10.1038/s41575-021-00551-0.

Piché, Marie-Eve, André Tchernof, and Jean-Pierre Després. "Obesity Phenotypes, Diabetes, and Cardiovascular Diseases." *Circ Res* 126, no. 11 (2020): 1477–500.

Reaven, Gerald M. *Clinician's Guide to Non-insulin-dependent Diabetes Mellitus: Pathogenesis and Treatment.* Marcel Dekker, 1989.

Reaven, Gerald M. "Role of Insulin Resistance in Human Disease." *Diabetes* 37, no. 12 (1988): 1595–607. https://doi.org/10.2337/diab.37.12.1595.

Rickman, Amy D., Donald A. Williamson, Corby K. Martin, et al. "The CALERIE Study: Design and Methods of an Innovative 25% Caloric Restriction Intervention." *Contemp Clin Trials* 32, no. 6 (2011): 874–81. DOI: 10.1016/j.cct.2011.07.002.

Rios, J. M., M. K. Berg, and A. N. Gearhardt. "Evaluating Bidirectional Predictive Pathways Between Dietary Restraint and Food Addiction in Adolescents." *Nutrients* 15, no. 13 (June 30, 2023). https://doi.org/10.3390/nu15132977.

Ruiz, Michelle. "They Rejected Diet Culture 30 Years Ago. Then They Went Main-stream." *New York Times*, January 18, 2023. https://www.nytimes.com/2023/01/18/well /intuitive-eating.html.

Salvia, Meg G. "The Look AHEAD Trial: Translating Lessons Learned into Clinical Practice and Further Study." *Diabetes Spectr* 30, no. 3 (2017): 166–70. DOI: 10.2337 /ds17–0016.

Sattar, N. "Mechanisms Linking Adiposity and Cardiovascular Disease." Lecture presented at Thirty-First European Congress on Obesity (ECO), Venice, Italy, May 12, 2024.

Schachter, S. "Obesity and Eating: Internal and External Cues Differentially Affect the Eating Behavior of Obese and Normal Subjects." *Science* 161, no. 3843 (August 23, 1968): 751–56. https://doi.org/10.1126/science.161.3843.751.

Schachter, S. "Some Extraordinary Facts About Obese Humans and Rats." *Am Psychol* 26, no. 2 (February 1971): 129–44. https://doi.org/10.1037/h0030817.

Smith, Gordon, Bettina Mittendorfer, and Samuel Klein. "Metabolically Healthy Obesity: Facts and Fantasies." *J Clin Invest* 129, no. 10 (2019): 3978–89. DOI: 10.1172 /JCI129186.

Squires, Sally. "Holding Fast for a Change." *Washington Post*, January 20, 2003. https:// www.washingtonpost.com/archive/lifestyle/wellness/2003/01/21/holding-fast-for-a -change/d514c957–5da6–41b3–81c8–5be852c03027/.

Stewart, T. M., C. K. Martin, and D. A. Williamson. "The Complicated Relationship Between Dieting, Dietary Restraint, Caloric Restriction, and Eating Disorders: Is a Shift in Public Health Messaging Warranted?" *Int J Environ Res Public Health* 19, no. 1 (January 3, 2022). https://doi.org/10.3390/ijerph19010491.

Strings, Sabrina. *Fearing the Black Body: The Racial Origins of Fat Phobia.* NYU Press, 2019.

Taylor, R. "Newly Diagnosed Type 2 Diabetes—What Should Be the Focus of Management in 2024?" Lecture presented at the American Diabetic Association Eighty-Fourth Scientific Sessions Program, Orlando, FL, June 21–24, 2024.

Taylor, R. "Type 2 Diabetes and Remission: Practical Management Guided by Pathophysiology." *J Intern Med* 289, no. 6 (June 2021): 754–70. https://doi.org/10.1111/joim .13214.

Taylor, R. "Understanding the Cause of Type 2 Diabetes." *Lancet Diabetes Endocrinol* 12, no. 9 (2024): 664–73. https://doi.org/10.1016/s2213–8587(24)00157–8.

Taylor, R. "What We Learned from the DiRECT Trial and Related Studies." Lecture presented at Thirty-First European Congress on Obesity (ECO), Venice, Italy, May 12, 2024.

Taylor, R., A. Ramachandran, W. S. Yancy Jr., and N. G. Forouhi. "Nutritional Basis of Type 2 Diabetes Remission." *BMJ* 374 (July 7, 2021): n1449. https://doi.org/10.1136/bmj .n1449.

Tribole, Evelyn. "Principle 8: Respect Your Body." Evelyn Tribole: The Original Intuitive Eating Pro, February 27, 2019. https://www.evelyntribole.com/principle-8-respect -your-body/.

Tribole, Evelyn, and Elyse Resch. *The Intuitive Eating Workbook: 10 Principles for Nourishing a Healthy Relationship with Food.* A New Harbinger Self-Help Workbook, 2017.

Twig, Gilad, Gal Yaniv, Hagai Levine, et al. "Body-Mass Index in 2.3 Million Adolescents and Cardiovascular Death in Adulthood." *New Eng J Med* 374, no. 25 (2016): 2430–40.

Vague, J. "La différenciation sexuelle: Facteur déterminant des formes de l'obésité" [Sexual differentiation: Determining factor in forms of obesity]. *Presse Med (1893)* 55, no. 30 (May 24, 1947): 339.

van Vliet-Ostaptchouk, J. V., M. L. Nuotio, S. N. Slagter, D. Doiron, K. Fischer, L. Foco, A. Gaye, et al. "The Prevalence of Metabolic Syndrome and Metabolically Healthy Obesity in Europe: A Collaborative Analysis of Ten Large Cohort Studies." *BMC Endocr Disord* 14 (2014): 9. https://doi.org/10.1186/1472–6823–14–9.

Wong, C. X., T. Sullivan, M. T. Sun, et al. "Obesity and the Risk of Incident, Postoperative, and Post-ablation Atrial Fibrillation: A Meta-analysis of 626,603 Individuals in 51 Studies." *JACC Clin Electrophysiol* 1 (2015): 139–52. DOI: 10.1016/j.jacep.2015.04.004.

Interviews and Correspondence with the Author

Bays, Harold (November 2024).

Flegal, Katherine (November 2024).

Schiff, Sami (May 2024).

Stunkard, Mickey (2005).

Taylor, Roy (May 2024).

Tribole, Evelyn (March 2024).

Notes

57 **"What would the freedom":** Tribole, "Principle 8."

58 **practice of intuitive eating:** Ruiz, "They Rejected Diet Culture 30 Years Ago."

58 **practice offers ten principles:** The Original Intuitive Eating Pros, "10 Principles of Intuitive Eating."

58 **"Think about what steps":** Author interview with Tribole, March 2024.

58 **But our views diverged:** Author interview with Tribole, March 2024.

59 **"It's an interesting way":** Hill, "Programme-Fed and Focused Interventions for Eating Disorders."

59 **Make Peace with Food:** The Original Intuitive Eating Pros, "10 Principles of Intuitive Eating."

59 **Schachter theorized:** Schachter, "Obesity and Eating"; Schachter, "Some Extraordinary Facts About Obese Humans and Rats."

59 **hypothesize that the cultural:** Squires, "Holding Fast for a Change."

60 **"restrained eating":** Herman and Mack, "Restrained and Unrestrained Eating."

60 **dietary restraint:** Rios et al., "Evaluating Bidirectional Predictive Pathways Between Dietary Restraint and Food Addiction in Adolescents."

60 **most definitive one:** Rickman et al., "The CALERIE Study."

60 **"food addiction significantly predicted":** Rios et al., "Evaluating Bidirectional Predictive Pathways Between Dietary Restraint and Food Addiction in Adolescents."

61 **obesity and eating disorders:** Fernandez-Aranda, "Management of Eating Disorders and Obesity from Transdiagnostic Perspective."

61 **"mesolimbic dopaminergic system":** Author interview with Schiff, May 2024.

62 **late Dr. Gerald Reaven:** Reaven, "Role of Insulin Resistance in Human Disease."

62 **the accumulation of:** Lundgren et al., "Adiposity and Adipose Tissue Distribution in Relation to Incidence of Diabetes in Women."

63 **The apple shape:** Vague, "La différenciation sexuelle."

63 **specifically the visceral:** Després et al., "Abdominal Obesity."; Després et al., "Regional Distribution of Body Fat, Plasma Lipoproteins, and Cardiovascular Disease."

63 **"We know that efficiency":** Ferrante, "Obesity and Comorbidities."

63 **more fat inside:** Author interview with Taylor, May 2024; Taylor, "What We Learned from the DiRECT Trial and Related Studies"; Taylor, "Newly Diagnosed Type 2 Diabetes."

64 **"As you carry more weight":** Sattar, "Mechanisms Linking Adiposity and Cardiovascular Disease."

65 **29% increase in cardiovascular:** Dicker, "Obesity as a Disease"; Bhaskaran et al., "Association of BMI with Overall and Cause-Specific Mortality."

65 **every BMI unit above 25:** Dicker, "Obesity as a Disease"; Field et al., "Impact of Overweight on the Risk of Developing Common Chronic Diseases During a 10-Year Period"; Kilpatrick et al., "The Effect of Glucose Variability on the Risk of Microvascular Complications in Type 1 Diabetes."

65 **The following chart:** I would like to acknowledge Dr. Anthony Ferrante for enumerating the risks associated with many of these diseases and conditions in his 2023 and 2024 lectures at the Columbia Cornell Obesity conferences, and Dr. Dror Dicker for his lecture, also enumerating these risks, at the 2024 European Congress on Obesity.

66 **focused on a triumvirate:** DeFronzo, "Keynote 2: New Horizons for T2D Treatment."

66 **"driving the diabetes":** DeFronzo, "Keynote 2: New Horizons for T2D Treatment."

66 **uses the term "sick fat":** Author interview with Bays, November 2024; Bays, "Adiposopathy: Is 'Sick Fat' a Cardiovascular Disease?"

66 **"people facing multiple conditions":** Sattar, "Mechanisms Linking Adiposity and Cardiovascular Disease."

67 **one of the largest and longest:** Look AHEAD Research Group, Pi-Sunyer et al., "Reduction in Weight"; Look AHEAD Research Group, "Effect of a Long-Term Behavioural Weight Loss Intervention on Nephropathy in Overweight or Obese Adults with Type 2 Diabetes."

67 **An even larger 2023 trial:** Lincoff et al., "Semaglutide and Cardiovascular Outcomes in Patients with Overweight or Obesity Who Do Not Have Diabetes"; Deanfield et al., "Semaglutide and Cardiovascular Outcomes in Patients with Obesity and Prevalent Heart Failure."

67 **percentage of men who have:** Blüher, "Metabolically Healthy Obesity."

68 **"If you store fat":** Goossens, "Sexual Dimorphism in Cardiometabolic Health."

68 **"when BMI is the same":** Goossens, "Sexual Dimorphism in Cardiometabolic Health."

69 **the excess fat mass:** Echouffo-Tcheugui et al., "Natural History of Obesity Subphenotypes."

8: The Journey

Sources
Works Referenced

Ahmad, F. A., and S. Mahmud. "Acute Pancreatitis Following Orlistat Therapy: Report of Two Cases." *JOP Journal of the Pancreas* 11, no. 1 (2010): 61–63.

Bays, Harold. "Excessive Weight Reduction with Highly Effective Anti-obesity Medications: A Roundtable Discussion." Lecture presented at the Spring Obesity Summit, New York, April 21–23, 2023.

Bello, N. T. "Update on Drug Safety Evaluation of Naltrexone/Bupropion for the Treatment of Obesity." *Expert Opin Drug Saf* 18, no. 7 (2019): 549–52.

Boyd, S. T., and B. A. Fremming. "Rimonabant—A Selective CB1 Antagonist." *Ann Pharmacother* 39, no. 4 (2005): 684–90.

Bray, G. A., and J. Q. Purnell. "An Historical Review of Steps and Missteps in the Discovery of Anti-obesity Drugs." In *Endotext*, ed. K. R. Feingold, B. Anawalt, M. R. Blackman, et al. MDText.com, July 10, 2022. https://www.ncbi.nlm.nih.gov/books/NBK581942/.

Colman, E. "Anorectics on Trial: A Half Century of Federal Regulation of Prescription Appetite Suppressants." *Ann Intern Med* 143, no. 5 (2005): 380–85.

Cosentino, G., A. O. Conrad, and G. I. Uwaifo. "Phentermine and Topiramate for the Management of Obesity: A Review." *Drug Des Dev Ther* 7 (April 5, 2011): 267–78. DOI: 10.2147/DDDT.S31443.

Dilliraj, L. N., G. Schiuma, D. Lara, et al. "The Evolution of Ketosis: Potential Impact on Clinical Conditions." *Nutrients* 14, no. 17 (2022): 3613.

Drew, B. S., A. F. Dixon, and J. B. Dixon. "Obesity Management: Update on Orlistat." *Vasc Health Risk Manag* 3, no. 6 (2007): 817–21.

Drucker, D. J., J. F. Habener, and J. J. Holst. "Discovery, Characterization, and Clinical Development of the Glucagon-Like Peptides." *J Clin Invest* 127, no. 12 (2017): 4217–27.

Drucker, Daniel. "The Obesity Society Keynote Speaker." Lecture presented at Obesity Week 2018 by the Obesity Society, Nashville, TN, November 11–15, 2018.

Farr, O. M., R. L. Chiang-shan, and C. S. Mantzoros. "Central Nervous System Regulation of Eating: Insights from Human Brain Imaging." *Metab* 65, no. 5 (2016): 699–713.

FDA Approved Labeling Text. "NDA 020505-S-050 Topamax (topiramate) oral tablets (25mg, 50mg, 100mg and 200mg); NDA 020844-S-041 Topamax (topiramate) sprinkle capsules (15mg and 25mg)." October 2012. https://www.accessdata.fda.gov/drugsatfda_docs/label/2012/020844s041lbl.pdf.

Flemyng, M. *A Discourse on the Nature, Causes, and Cure of Corpulency. Illustrated by a Remarkable Case, Read Before the Royal Society, November 1757. And Now First Published, by Malcolm Flemyng, MD*. L. Davis and C. Reymers, 1760.

Flier, J. S. "Drug Development Failure: How GLP-1 Development Was Abandoned in 1990." *Perspect Biol Med* 67, no. 3 (Summer 2024): 325–36. https://dx.doi.org/10.1353/pbm.2024.a936213.

GlobalData. "GLP1 Agonists Set to Become the Best-Selling Drugs in 2024, Says GlobalData." March 15, 2024. https://www.globaldata.com/media/pharma/glp1-agonists-set-to-become-the-best-selling-drugs-in-2024-says-globaldata/?utm_source=chatgpt.com.

Hamed, K., M. N. Alosaimi, B. A. Ali, et al. "Glucagon-Like Peptide-1 (GLP-1) Receptor Agonists: Exploring Their Impact on Diabetes, Obesity, and Cardiovascular Health Through a Comprehensive Literature Review." *Cureus* 16, no. 9 (September 1, 2024): e68390. DOI: 10.7759/cureus.68390.

Holst, J. J., and C. F. Deacon. "Inhibition of the Activity of Dipeptidyl-Peptidase IV as a Treatment for Type 2 Diabetes." *J Diabetes* 47, no. 11 (1998): 1663–70.

Horn, Deborah B. "Informing Treatment Decisions: Predictors of Response in Incretin-Based Therapies." Lecture presented at the International Congress on Obesity (ICO), São Paulo, Brazil, June 26–29, 2024.

Jastreboff, A. M. "Nutrient-Stimulated Hormones-Based Therapies for the Treatment of Obesity: Sparks from the Pipeline." Lecture presented at 2024 Columbia Cornell Obesity: Etiology, Prevention, and Treatment, May 1–4, 2024.

Jastreboff, A. M., L. M. Kaplan, J. P. Frías, et al. "Triple-Hormone-Receptor Agonist Retatrutide for Obesity—A Phase 2 Trial." *N Eng J Med* 389, no. 6 (2023): 514–26.

Kahan, Scott. "One Size Does Not Fit All: Evolving Approaches to Optimize Obesity Pharmacotherapy." Lecture presented at Obesity Week 2023 by the Obesity Society, Dallas, TX, October 14–17, 2023.

Korner, Judith. "Advances in Obesity Pharmacotherapy over the Past 60+ Years." Lecture presented at Seminar on Appetitive Behaviors, Columbia University, New York, May 30, 2024.

Lowe, Michael. "Self-Control as the Mediator of Change in the Behavioral Treatment of Obesity: Has It Outlived Its Usefulness?" Lecture presented at the Association for the Study of Obesity (virtual), September 30, 2021.

Montero, Alex, Grace Sparks, Marley Presiado, and Liz Hamel. "KFF Health Tracking Poll May 2024: The Public's Use and Views of GLP-1 Drugs." KFF, May 10, 2024. https://www.kff.org/health-costs/poll-finding/kff-health-tracking-poll-may-2024-the-publics-use-and-views-of-glp-1-drugs/.

Nadkarni, P., O. G. Chepurny, and G. G. Holz. "Regulation of Glucose Homeostasis by GLP-1." *Prog Mol Biol Transl Sci* 121 (2014): 23–65.

Nissen, Steven N. "Metabolic Surgery vs. Pharmacotherapy for Treatment of Obesity." Lecture presented at the Practical Ways to Achieve Targets in Diabetes Care Keystone Conference in Keystone, CO, July 12–16, 2023.

Novo Nordisk Foundation. "Episode 1: A Diabetes Doctor's Dream," from *The Story of GLP-1*, directed by Morten Busch (Colorbone Media, 2021), YouTube, November 27, 2022. https://www.youtube.com/watch?v=nrh5WAMfW3w.

Onakpoya, I. J., C. J. Heneghan, and J. K. Aronson. "Post-marketing Withdrawal of Anti-obesity Medicinal Products Because of Adverse Drug Reactions: A Systematic Review." *BMC Med* 14 (2016): 1–11.

Papavramidou, N., and H. Christopoulou-Aletra. "Management of Obesity in the Writings of Soranus of Ephesus and Caelius Aurelianus." *Obesity Surg* 18 (2008): 763–65.

Reuters. "FDA Advisory Committee Did Not Recommend Approval of Rimonabant (ZIMULTI) for Use in Obese and Overweight Patients with Associated Risk Factors." August 9, 2007. https://www.reuters.com/article/world/fda-advisory-committee-did-not-recommend-approval-of-rimonabant-zimulti-for-us-idUSIN20070613182621SNY/.

Richards, Jesse. "Excessive Weight Reduction with Highly Effective Anti-obesity Medications: A Roundtable Discussion." Lecture presented at the Spring Obesity Summit, New York, April 21–23, 2023.

Tang-Christensen, M., P. Larsen, R. Goke, et al. "Central Administration of GLP-1-(7–36) Amide Inhibits Food and Water Intake in Rats." *Am J Physiol Regul Integr Comp Physiol* 271, no. 4 (1996): R848–R856.

US Food and Drug Administration. "FDA Approved Labeling Text, NDA 020505-S-050 Topamax (Topiramate) Oral Tablets, NDA 020844-S-041 Topamax (Topiramate) Sprinkle Capsules." 2012.

US Food and Drug Administration. "FDA Requests the Withdrawal of the Weight-Loss Drug Belviq, Belviq XR (Lorcaserin) from the Market. Potential Risk of Cancer Outweighs the Benefits." FDA Drug Safety Communication, February 13, 2020.

van Dijk, G., T. Thiele, R. Seeley, S. Woods, and I. Bernstein. "Glucagon-Like Peptide-1 and Satiety." *Nat* 385, no. 6613: 214.

Wei, Y., and S. Mojsov. "Distribution of GLP-1 and PACAP Receptors in Human Tissues." *Acta Physiol* 157, no. 3 (1996): 355–57.

Zhu, H., D. Bi, Y. Zhang, et al. "Ketogenic Diet for Human Diseases: The Underlying Mechanisms and Potential for Clinical Implementations." *Signal Transduct Target Ther* 7, no. 1 (2022): 11.

Interviews and Correspondence with the Author

Drucker, Daniel (May 2024).

Flier, Jeffrey (August 2024).

Notes

76   **Eating is a complex biological activity:** Farr, "Central Nervous System Regulation of Eating."

76   **recommended a treatment:** Bray and Purnell, "An Historical Review of Steps and Missteps."

76   **two dozen other weight-loss drugs:** Onakpoya et al., "Post-marketing Withdrawal of Anti-obesity Medicinal Products Because of Adverse Drug Reactions."

76   **lorcaserin was withdrawn:** US Food and Drug Administration, "FDA Requests the Withdrawal of the Weight-Loss Drug Belviq, Belviq XR (Lorcaserin) from the Market."

76   **Rimonabant is what's known as a CB1 antagonist:** Boyd, "Rimonabant—A Selective CB1."

77   **Phentermine was cleared by the FDA:** Colman, "Anorectics on Trial."

77   **Topiramate can cause fetal harm:** US Food and Drug Administration, "FDA Approved Labeling Text."

78   **special warning box:** Bello, "Update on Drug Safety Evaluation of Naltrexone/Bupropion for the Treatment of Obesity."

78   **lead to pancreatitis and severe liver injury:** Ahmad, "Acute Pancreatitis Following Orlistat Therapy."

79   **GLP-1 drugs are actually:** Drucker, "Discovery, Characterization, and Clinical Development of the Glucagon-Like Peptides."

79   **stimulates insulin production:** Nadkarni et al., "Regulation of Glucose Homeostasis by GLP-1."

80   **brain injections of a GLP-1 agonist:** van Dijk et al., "Glucagon-Like Peptide-1 and Satiety."

80   **"hundreds of peptides":** Drucker, "The Obesity Society Keynote Speaker."

80   **said Dr. Lotte Bjerre Knudsen:** Novo Nordisk Foundation, "Episode 1: A Diabetes Doctor's Dream."

80   **could reach areas of the brain:** Tang-Christensen et al., "Central Administration of GLP-1."

80   **promoted feelings of satiety:** Holst and Deacon, "Inhibition of the Activity of Dipeptidyl-Peptidase IV as a Treatment for Type 2 Diabetes."

81   **"It's light-years from":** Bays, "Excessive Weight Reduction with Highly Effective Anti-Obesity Medications."

82   **"data from the SURMOUNT-1":** Richards, "Excessive Weight Reduction with Highly Effective Anti-Obesity Medications."

82   **"even if your patient":** Richards, "Excessive Weight Reduction with Highly Effective Anti-obesity Medications."

82   **$40 billion:** GlobalData, "GLP1 Agonists Set to Become the Best-Selling Drugs in 2024, Says GlobalData."

82   **one in eight:** Montero et al., "KFF Health Tracking Poll May 2024: The Public's Use and Views of GLP-1 Drugs."

83   **"The self-control theory":** Lowe, "Self-Control as the Mediator of Change in the Behavioral Treatment of Obesity."

83   **"an unmitigated disaster":** Nissen, "Metabolic Surgery vs. Pharmacotherapy for Treatment of Obesity."

83   **"They had coaches":** Nissen, "Metabolic Surgery vs. Pharmacotherapy for Treatment of Obesity."

9: The Biological Forces That Oppose Weight Loss

Sources
Works Referenced

Aronne, Louis J. "Leveraging Incretin Hormones for Weight Loss in Individuals with Obesity: Tirzepatide and Retatrutide: SURMOUNT and TRIUMPH Trial Series." Lecture presented at Seminar on Appetitive Behaviors, Columbia University, New York, May 30, 2024.

Hall, Kevin. "The Calculus of Calories: Quantifying Body Weight Regulation in Humans." Virtual lecture presented at Obesity Medicine 2023 by Obesity Medicine Association, May 2023.

Hall, Kevin. "Carbs, Calories, or Quality: What Matters Most for Body Weight." Virtual lecture presented at 2023 Columbia Cornell Obesity: Etiology, Prevention, and Treatment, New York, May 3–6, 2023.

Hall, Kevin. "Diet Wars: Unveiling the Carbohydrate-Insulin Model and Energy Balance Model." Lecture presented at the International Congress on Obesity (ICO), São Paulo, Brazil, June 26–29, 2024.

Hall, Kevin. "Physiology of the Weight Loss Plateau in Response to Lifestyle Intervention, Novel Pharmacological Therapy and Bariatric Surgery." Lecture presented at the International Congress on Obesity (ICO), São Paulo, Brazil, June 26–29, 2024.

Kushner, Robert. "Beyond Medication: The Role of Behavior Change." Lecture presented at Obesity Medicine 2024 by Obesity Medicine Association Academy, Denver, CO, May 2024.

Lam, Y. Y., and E. Ravussin. "Indirect Calorimetry: An Indispensable Tool to Understand and Predict Obesity." *Eur J Clin Nutr* 71, no. 3 (2017): 318–22. doi:10.1038/ejcn.2016.220.

Leibel, R. L., M. Rosenbaum, and J. Hirsch. "Changes in Energy Expenditure Resulting from Altered Body Weight." *N Engl J Med* 332, no. 10 (March 9, 1995): 621–28. https://doi.org/10.1056/nejm199503093321001.

Le Roux, Carel. "State of Obesity in 2023." Lecture presented at the 2023 Blackburn Course in Obesity Medicine: Treating Obesity, by Harvard Medical School, Cambridge, MA, June 5–8, 2023.

National Institute of Diabetes and Digestive and Kidney Diseases. "Body Weight Planner." US Department of Health and Human Services—National Institutes of Health. https://www.niddk.nih.gov/bwp.

Pontzer, Herman. *Burn: New Research Blows the Lid Off How We Really Burn Calories, Stay Healthy, and Lose Weight.* Penguin, 2022.

Wadden, T. A., R. H. Neiberg, R. R. Wing, et al. "Four-Year Weight Losses in the Look AHEAD Study: Factors Associated with Long-Term Success." *Obesity* (Silver Spring, MD) 19, no. 10 (2011): 1987–98. https://doi.org/10.1038/oby.2011.230.

Interviews and Correspondence with the Author

Aronne, Louis (May 2024).

Wyatt, Holly (January 2024).

Notes

85 **"a pair of negative feedback loops":** Hall, "Physiology of the Weight Loss Plateau in Response to Lifestyle Intervention, Novel Pharmacological Therapy and Bariatric Surgery."

86 **you can always tell:** Le Roux, "State of Obesity in 2023."

87 **to successfully *maintain* weight loss:** Wadden et al., "Four-Year Weight Losses in the Look AHEAD Study."

87 **Seminar on Appetitive Behavior:** Aronne, "Leveraging Incretin Hormones for Weight Loss in Individuals with Obesity."

10: How to Determine Your Healthy Weight Goal

Sources
Works Referenced

Abraham, Tobin M., et al. "Association Between Visceral and Subcutaneous Adipose Depots and Incident Cardiovascular Disease Risk Factors." *Circ* 132, no. 17 (October 27, 2015): 1639–47. DOI: 10.1161/CIRCULATIONAHA.114.015000.

Allerton, Timothy D., Elvis A. Carnero, Christopher Bock, Karen D. Corbin, et al. "Reliability of Measurements of Energy Expenditure and Substrate Oxidation Using Whole-Room Indirect Calorimetry." *Obesity* (Silver Spring, MD) 29, no. 9 (2021): 1508–15. DOI: 10.1002/oby.23226.

Anthanont, Pimjai, and Michael D. Jensen. "Does Basal Metabolic Rate Predict Weight Gain?" *Am J Clin Nutr* 104, no. 4 (2016): 959–63. DOI:10.3945/ajcn.116.134965.

Bertz, F., C. R. Pacanowski, and D. A. Levitsky. "Frequent Self-Weighing with Electronic Graphic Feedback to Prevent Age-Related Weight Gain in Young Adults." *Obesity* (Silver Spring, MD) 23, no. 10 (October 2015): 2009–14. DOI: 10.1002/oby.21211.

Borga, Magnus, et al. "Advanced Body Composition Assessment: From Body Mass Index to Body Composition Profiling." *J Invest Med* 66, no. 5 (2018): 1–9. DOI: 10.1136/jim -2018–000722.

Busetto, Luca. "The Difficulties in Obesity Definition in Terms of Anthropometric Measures." Lecture presented at the Sixtieth Annual Meeting of the EASD (European Association for the Study of Diabetes), Madrid, Spain, September 10–13, 2024.

Busetto, Luca, et al. "A New Framework for the Diagnosis, Staging and Management of Obesity in Adults." *Nature Med* 30, no. 9 (2024): 2395–99. DOI:10.1038/s41591-024 -03095-3.

Busetto, Luca, Volker Schnecke, Maria Overvad, et al. "Changes in Visceral Adiposity Modify the Impact of Weight Loss on the 10-Year Risk of Obesity-Related Complications: A Population-Based Cohort Study." Lecture presented at the Thirty-First European Congress on Obesity (ECO), Venice, Italy, May 12–15, 2024.

Deanfield, John, Subodh Verma, Benjamin Scirica, et al. "Semaglutide and Cardiovascular Outcomes in Patients with Obesity and Prevalent Heart Failure: A Prespecified Analysis of the SELECT Trial." *Lancet* 404 (2024): 773–86. DOI: 10.1016/S0140– 6736(24)01498–3.

Dulloo, A. G., and J.-P. Montani. "Pathways from Dieting to Weight Regain, to Obesity and to the Metabolic Syndrome: An Overview." *Obes Rev* 16, Suppl. 1 (2015): 1–6. DOI: 10.1111/obr.12250.

Eknoyan, Garabed. "Adolphe Quetelet (1796–1874)—The Average Man and Indices of Obesity." *Nephrol Dial Transplant* 23, no. 1 (2008): 47–51. https://doi.org/10.1093/ndt/gfm517.

Flegal, Katherine M. "How Body Size Became a Disease." In *Routledge Handbook of Critical Obesity Studies*. Ed. Michael Gard, Darren Powell, and Jose Tenorio. Taylor and Francis Group, 2022.

Flegal, Katherine M. "Use and Misuse of BMI Categories." *AMA J Ethics* 25, no. 7 (July 2023): E550–E558. DOI: 10.1001/amajethics.2023.550.

Fontana, L., and H. B. Hu. "Optimal Body Weight for Health and Longevity: Bridging Basic, Clinical, and Population Research." *Aging Cell* 13, no. 3 (June 2014): 391400. DOI: 10.1111/acel.12207. Epub March 14, 2014. PMID: 24628815; PMCID: PMC4032609.

Fothergill, Erin, Juen Guo, Lilian Howard, et al. "Persistent Metabolic Adaptation 6 Years After 'The Biggest Loser' Competition." *Obesity* (Silver Spring, MD) 24, no. 8 (2016): 1612–19. DOI: 10.1002/oby.21538.

Frankenfield, David, Lori Roth-Yousey, and Charlene Compher. "Comparison of Predictive Equations for Resting Metabolic Rate in Healthy Nonobese and Obese Adults: A Systematic Review." *J Am Diet Assoc* 105, no. 5 (2005): 775–89. DOI: 10.1016/j. jada.2005.02.005.

Godman, Heidi. "Lessons from 'The Biggest Loser.'" Harvard Health Publishing, January 24, 2018. https://www.health.harvard.edu/diet-and-weight-loss/lessons-from-the -biggest-loser.

Gribble, Fiona M., and Frank Reimann. "Metabolic Messengers: Glucagon-Like Peptide 1." *Nat Metab* 3, no. 2 (2021): 142–48. DOI: 10.1038/s42255-020-00327-x.

Hall, Kevin. "Calories, Carbs, or Quality: What Matters Most for Body Weight?" Lecture presented at 2024 Columbia Cornell Obesity Medicine, New York, May 3, 2024.

Hall, Kevin D. "Diet versus Exercise in 'The Biggest Loser' Weight Loss Competition." *Obesity* (Silver Spring, MD) 21, no. 5 (2013): 957–59. DOI: 10.1002/oby.20065.

Johannsen, Darcy L., Nicolas D. Knuth, Robert Huizenga, et al. "Metabolic Slowing with Massive Weight Loss Despite Preservation of Fat-Free Mass." *J Clin Endocrinol Metab* 97, no. 7 (2012): 2489–96. DOI: 10.1210/jc.2012–1444. Erratum in *J Clin Endocrinol Metab* 101, no. 5 (2016): 2266. DOI: 10.1210/jc.2016–1651.

Kenny, Glen P., Sean R. Notley, and Daniel Gagnon. "Direct Calorimetry: A Brief Historical Review of Its Use in the Study of Human Metabolism and Thermoregulation." *Eur J Appl Physiol* 117, no. 9 (2017): 1765–85. DOI: 10.1007/s00421-017-3670-5.

Keys, Ancel, Flaminio Fidanza, Martti J. Karvonen, Noburu Kimura, and Henry L. Taylor. "Indices of Relative Weight and Obesity." *Int J Epidemiol* 43, no. 3 (2014): 655–65. https://doi.org/10.1093/ije/dyu058.

Keys, Ancel, A. Menotti, C. Aravanis, et al. "The Seven Countries Study: 2,289 Deaths in 15 Years." *Prev Med* 13, no. 2 (1984): 141–54. DOI: 10.1016/0091–7435(84)90047–1.

Klein, Samuel. "Comparing GLP-1 Agonists and Their Effect on Weight Loss." Lecture presented at the Endocrine Society's 2023 Annual Meeting, Chicago, IL, June 15–18, 2023.

Knuth, Nicholas D., Darcy L. Johannsen, Robyn A. Tamboli, et al. "Metabolic Adaptation Following Massive Weight Loss Is Related to the Degree of Energy Imbalance and Changes in Circulating Leptin." *Obesity* 22, no. 12 (2014): 2563–69. DOI: 10.1002/oby.20900.

Koenen, Mascha, Michael A. Hill, Paul Cohen, and James R. Sowers. "Obesity, Adipose Tissue and Vascular Dysfunction." *Circ Res* 128, no. 7 (2021): 951–68. DOI: 10.1161 /CIRCRESAHA.121.318093.

Kruschiz, Renate, Sandra J. Wallner-Liebmann, Michael J. Hamlin, et al. "Detecting Body Fat—A Weighty Problem: BMI versus Subcutaneous Fat Patterns in Athletes and Non-athletes." *PLOS One* 8, no. 8 (2013): e72002. DOI: 10.1371/journal.pone.0072002.

Lam, Y. Y., and E. Ravussin. "Indirect Calorimetry: An Indispensable Tool to Understand and Predict Obesity." *Eur J Clin Nutr* 71, no. 3 (2017): 318–22. DOI: 10.1038/ejcn.2016.220.

Lincoff, A. M. "Semaglutide and Cardiovascular Outcomes in Patients with Overweight or Obesity Who Do Not Have Diabetes: The SELECT Trial." Lecture presented at American Heart Association Scientific Sessions 2023, Philadelphia, PA, November 11–13, 2023.

Lincoff, A. M., Kristine Brown-Frandsen, Helen M. Colhoun, et al., and SELECT trial investigators. "Semaglutide and Cardiovascular Outcomes in Obesity Without Diabetes." *N Engl J Med* 389, no. 24 (2023): 2221–32. DOI: 10.1056/NEJMoa2307563.

Martin, Alyce M., Emily W. Sun, and Damien J. Keating. "Mechanisms Controlling Hormone Secretion in the Human Gut and Its Relevance to Metabolism." *J Endocrinol* 244, no. 1 (2019): R1–R15. DOI: 10.1530/JOE-19–0399.

Mitchell, Lachlan, Silvia Bel-Serrat, Mirjam Heinen, et al. "Waist Circumference-to-Height Ratio and Body Mass Index for Obesity Classification in Irish Children." *Acta Paediatr* 110, no. 5 (2021): 1541–47. DOI: 10.1111/apa.15724.

National Heart, Lung, and Blood Institute. "Calculate Your BMI." NHLBI, n.d. https:// www.nhlbi.nih.gov/health/educational/lose_wt/BMI/bmicalc.htm.

Nevill, Alan M., Tim Olds, Arthur D. Stewart, and Michael J. Duncan. "A New Waist-to-Height Ratio Predicts Abdominal Adiposity in Adults." *Res Sports Med* 28, no. 1 (2020): 15–26. DOI: 10.1080/15438627.2018.1502183.

Nordqvist, Christian. "Why BMI Is Inaccurate and Misleading." Medical News Today, January 20, 2022. https://www.medicalnewstoday.com/.

Palmer, Bill F., and Deborah J. Clegg. "The Sexual Dimorphism of Obesity." *Mol Cell Endocrinol* 402 (2015): 113–19. DOI: 10.1016/j.mce.2014.11.029.

Pappas, Stephanie. "'The Biggest Loser' Has Big Problems, Health Experts Say." Live Science, February 21, 2010. https://www.livescience.com/9820-biggest-loser-big-problems-health-experts.html.

Piaggi, Paolo. "Metabolic Determinants of Weight Gain in Humans." *Obesity* 27, no. 5 (2019): 691–99. DOI: 10.1002/oby.22456.

Plucker, Andrew, Diana M. Thomas, Nick Broskey, et al. "Adult Energy Requirements Predicted from Doubly Labeled Water." *Int J Obes* 42, no. 8 (2018): 1515–23. DOI: 10.1038/s41366-018-0168-0.

Pray, Rachel, and Suzanne Riskin. "The History and Faults of the Body Mass Index and Where to Look Next: A Literature Review." *Cureus* 15, no. 11 (2023): e48230. DOI: 10.7759/cureus.48230.

Qi, Xingyun, Nancy J. Rusch, Jiaojiao Fan, et al. "Mitochondrial Proton Leak in Cardiac Aging." *GeroScience* 45, no. 4 (2023): 2135–43. DOI: 10.1007/s11357-023-00757-x.

Quetelet, Adolphe. *Physique sociale, ou essai sur le développement des facultés de l'homme* [Social physics, or an essay on the development of human faculties]. Muquardt, 1869.

Ravussin E., I. T. Harper, R. Rising, and C. Bogardus. "Energy Expenditure by Doubly Labeled Water: Validation in Lean and Obese Subjects." *Am J Physiol* 261, no. 3, part 1 (1991): E402–E409. DOI: 10.1152/ajpendo.1991.261.3.E402.

Rising, Russel, Kathryn Whyte, Jeanine Albu, and Xavier Pi-Sunyer. "Evaluation of a New Whole Room Indirect Calorimeter Specific for Measurement of Resting Metabolic Rate." *Nutr Metab* 12 (2015): 46. DOI: 10.1186/s12986-015-0043-0.

Salans, Lester B., E. S. Horton, and E. A. Sims. "Experimental Obesity in Man: Cellular Character of the Adipose Tissue." *J Clin Invest* 50, no. 5 (1971): 1005–11. DOI: 10.1172/JCI106570.

Stanford, Fatima C. "Healthcare Disparities in Obesity Treatment." Lecture presented at the Boston Course in Obesity Medicine, Cambridge, MA, June 13–16, 2023.

Tataranni, P. A., I. T. Harper, S. Snitker, et al. "Body Weight Gain in Free-Living Pima Indians: Effect of Energy Intake vs. Expenditure." *Int J Obes Relat Metab Dis* 27, no. 12 (2003): 1578–83. DOI: 10.1038/sj.ijo.0802469.

Zhang Fu-Liang, Jia-Xin Ren, Peng Zhang, et al. "Strong Association of Waist Circumference (WC), Body Mass Index (BMI), Waist-to-Height Ratio (WHtR), and Waist-to-Hip Ratio (WHR) with Diabetes: A Population-Based Cross-Sectional Study in Jilin Province, China." *J Diab Res* 2021 (May 14, 2021): 8812431. DOI: 10.1155/2021/8812431.

Zong Xin'nan, Roya Kelishadi, Young Mi Hong, et al. "Establishing International Optimal Cut-Offs of Waist-to-Height Ratio for Predicting Cardiometabolic Risk in Children and Adolescents Aged 6–18 Years." *BMC Med* 21, no. 1 (2023): 442. DOI: 10.1186/s12916-023-03169-y.

Interviews and Correspondence with the Author

Busetto, Luca (September 2024).

Flegal, Katherine (November 2024).

Krakoff, Jon (July 2023).

Stanford, Fatima (November 2024).

Notes

89 **healthy metabolism should adjust:** Piaggi, "Metabolic Determinants of Weight Gain in Humans."

89 **inmates in a Vermont prison:** Salans et al., "Experimental Obesity in Man."

90 **studied the contestants:** Johannsen et al., "Metabolic Slowing with Massive Weight Loss Despite Preservation of Fat-Free Mass"; Fothergill et al., "Persistent Metabolic Adaptation 6 Years After 'The Biggest Loser' Competition"; Hall, "Diet versus Exercise in 'The Biggest Loser' Weight Loss Competition."

90 **heat the body generates:** Kenny, "Direct Calorimetry."

91 **"doubly labeled water":** Plucker et al., "Adult Energy Requirements Predicted from Doubly Labeled Water."

92 **relatively low energy expenditure:** Lam and Ravussin, "Indirect Calorimetry"; Ravussin et al., "Energy Expenditure by Doubly Labeled Water"; Allerton et al., "Reliability of Measurements of Energy Expenditure and Substrate Oxidation Using Whole-Room Indirect Calorimetry"; Tataranni et al., "Body Weight Gain in Free-Living Pima Indians."

92 **how much visceral fat:** Abraham, "Association Between Visceral and Subcutaneous Adipose Depots and Incident Cardiovascular Disease Risk Factors."

92 **person on a scale of classifications:** National Heart, Lung, and Blood Institute, "Calculate Your BMI."

92 **distribution of fat:** Nordqvist, "Why BMI Is Inaccurate and Misleading."

93 **a relatively poor predictor:** Koenen et al., "Obesity, Adipose Tissue and Vascular Dysfunction."

93 **measurement was first suggested:** Eknoyan, "Adolphe Quetelet (1796–1874)"; Quetelet, *Physique sociale.*

93 **Seven Countries Study:** Keys, "The Seven Countries Study."

93 **variable in children and adolescents:** Eknoyan, "Adolphe Quetelet (1796–1874)."

93 **the ratio is most relevant:** Pray and Riskin, "History and Faults."

93 **half or less than:** Nevill et al., "A New Waist-to-Height Ratio Predicts Abdominal Adiposity in Adults."

94 **ratio of less than 0.53:** Busetto et al., "Changes in Visceral Adiposity."

94 **"Progressive amounts of weight loss":** Klein, "Comparing GLP-1 Agonists and Their Effect on Weight Loss."

95 **The SELECT trial:** Lincoff, "Semaglutide and Cardiovascular Outcomes in Patients with Overweight or Obesity Who Do Not Have Diabetes"; Lincoff et al., "Semaglutide and Cardiovascular Outcomes in Obesity Without Diabetes"; Deanfield et al., "Semaglutide and Cardiovascular Outcomes in Patients with Obesity and Prevalent Heart Failure."

95 **variety of increased health risks:** Fontana and Hu, "Optimal Body Weight for Health and Longevity."

95 **suggests a target BMI:** Busetto et al., "Changes in Visceral Adiposity Modify the Impact of Weight Loss on the 10-Year Risk of Obesity-Related Complications"; Busetto, "The Difficulties in Obesity Definition in Terms of Anthropometric Measures."

95 **tool for maintaining weight:** Bertz et al., "Frequent Self-Weighing with Electronic Graphic Feedback to Prevent Age-Related Weight Gain in Young Adults."

11: Toxic Fat

Sources
Works Referenced

Bray, G. A., and C. Bouchard. "The Biology of Human Overfeeding: A Systematic Review." *Obes Rev* 21, no. 9 (September 2020): e13040. https://doi.org/10.1111/obr.13040.

Browning, Jeffrey. "Fate of Acetyl CoA Determines Metabolic Health." Lecture presented at Obesity Week 2024 by the Obesity Society, Atlanta, GA, November 4–7, 2024.

Cuevas, Ada. "Menopause: A Fat-Driven Cardiometabolic Transition." Lecture presented at International Congress on Obesity, São Paulo, Brazil, June 26–29, 2024.

Cushman, Mary, Christina M. Shay, Virginia J. Howard, et al. "Ten-Year Differences in Women's Awareness Related to Coronary Heart Disease: Results of the 2019 American Heart Association National Survey: A Special Report from the American Heart Association." *Circ* 143, no. 7 (2021): e239–e248. DOI: 10.1161/CIR.0000000000000907.

Dhawan, Shivani, May Bakir, Erika Jones, et al. "Sex and Gender Medicine in Physician Clinical Training: Results of a Large, Single-Center Survey." *Biol Sex Differ* 7 (Suppl. 1), no. 37 (2016): 43–46. https://doi.org/10.1186/s13293-016-0096-4.

Dilliraj, L. N., G. Schiuma, D. Lara, et al. "The Evolution of Ketosis: Potential Impact on Clinical Conditions." *Nutrients* 14, no. 17 (2022): 3613.

El Khoudary, Samar R., Brooke Aggarwal, Theresa M. Beckie, et al. "Menopause Transition and Cardiovascular Disease Risk: Implications for Timing of Early Prevention: A Scientific Statement from the American Heart Association." *JAHA* 142, no. 25 (2020): e506–e532. https://doi.org/10.1161/CIR.0000000000000912.

El Khoudary, Samar R., Gail Greendale, Sybil L. Crawford, Nancy E. Avis, et al. "The Menopause Transition and Women's Health at Midlife: A Progress Report from the Study of Women's Health Across the Nation (SWAN)." *Menopause* (New York) 26, no. 10 (2019): 1213–27. DOI: 10.1097/GME.0000000000001424.

Gambacciani, M., M. Ciaponi, B. Cappagali, et al. "Body Weight, Body Fat Distribution, and Hormonal Replacement Therapy in Early Postmenopausal Women." *J Clin Endocrinol Metab* 82, no. 2 (1997): 414–17. DOI: 10.1210/jcem.82.2.3735.

Genazzani, Alessandro D., Tabatha Petrillo, Elisa Semprini, et al. "Metabolic Syndrome, Insulin Resistance and Menopause: The Changes in Body Structure and the Therapeutic Approach." *GREM* 4, no. 2–3 (2024): 086–091. DOI: 10.53260/grem.234026.

Gower, Barbara. "Beneficial Effects of Carbohydrate Restriction in Patients with Type 2 Diabetes Can Be Traced to Changes in Hepatic Metabolism." Lecture presented at Nutrition 2024 by the American Society for Nutrition, Chicago, IL, June 29–July 2, 2024.

Gower, Barbara. "Hepatic Ketone Production as the Governing Factor in Determining Fatty Liver and Type 2 Diabetes." Lecture presented at Nutrition 2024 by the American Society for Nutrition, Chicago, IL, June 29–July 2, 2024.

Hodis, Howard N., and Wendy J. Mack. "Menopausal Hormone Replacement Therapy and Reduction of All-Cause Mortality and Cardiovascular Disease: It Is About Time and Timing." *Cancer Journal* (Sudbury, MA) 28, no. 3 (2022): 208–23. DOI: 10.1097/PPO.0000000000000591.

Hurtado Andrade, Maria D. "Navigating Midlife: Menopause's Impact on Obesity." Lecture presented at Obesity Medicine 2024: A New Path Forward, Denver, CO, April 25–28, 2024.

Hurtado Andrade, Maria D., Mariam Saadedine, Ekta Kapoor, et al. "Weight Gain in Midlife Women." *Curr Obes Rep* 13, no. 2 (2024): 352–63. DOI: 10.1007/s13679-024-00555-2.

Hurtado Andrade, Maria D., Elif Tama, Sima Fansa, et al. "Weight Loss Response to Semaglutide in Postmenopausal Women With and Without Hormone Therapy Use." *Menopause* (New York) 31, no. 4 (2024): 266–74. DOI: 10.1097/GME.0000000000002310.

Isakadze, Nino, Puj K. Mehta, Karen Law, et al. "Addressing the Gap in Physician Preparedness to Assess Cardiovascular Risk in Women: A Comprehensive Approach to Cardiovascular Risk Assessment in Women." *Curr Treat Opt Cardiovasc Med* 21, no. 9 (2019): 47. DOI: 10.1007/s11936-019-0753-0.

Iyer, Tara K., and Heather Hirsch. "Clinical Impact of 2020 American Heart Association Statement on Menopause and Cardiovascular Disease Risk." *Cleve Clin J Med* 89, no. 1 (2022): 13–17. DOI: 10.3949/ccjm.89a.21031.

Iyer, Tara K., and JoAnn E. Manson. "Recent Trends in Menopausal Hormone Therapy Use in the US: Insights, Disparities, and Implications for Practice." *JAMA Health Forum* 5, no. 9 (2024): e243135. DOI: 10.1001/jamahealthforum.2024.3135.

Kahn, Darcy, Emily Macias, Simona Zarini, et al. "Exploring Visceral and Subcutaneous Adipose Tissue Secretomes in Human Obesity: Implications for Metabolic Disease." *Endocrinol* 163, no. 11 (2022): bqac140. DOI: 10.1210/endocr/bqac140.

Karvonen-Gutierrez, Carrie, and Catherine Kim. "Association of Mid-life Changes in Body Size, Body Composition and Obesity Status with the Menopausal Transition." *Healthcare* (Basel, Switzerland) 4, no. 42 (2016): 1–16. DOI: 10.3390/healthcare4030042.

Kodoth, Varna, Samantha Scaccia, and Brooke Aggarwal. "Adverse Changes in Body Composition During the Menopausal Transition and Relation to Cardiovascular Risk: A Contemporary Review." *Women's Health Reports* (New Rochelle, NY) 3, no. 1 (2022): 573–81. DOI: 10.1089/whr.2021.0119.

Kumar, Rekha. "Women's Health and Obesity." Lecture presented at 2024 Columbia Cornell Obesity: Etiology, Prevention, and Treatment, Columbia University, New York, May 2, 2024.

Lee, Jane J., Alison Pedley, Udo Hoffmann, et al. "Association of Changes in Abdominal Fat Quantity and Quality with Incident Cardiovascular Disease Risk Factors." *J Am Coll Cardiol* 68, no. 14 (2016): 1509–21. DOI: 10.1016/j.jacc.2016.06.067.

Libby, Peter. "The Changing Landscape of Atherosclerosis." *Nat* 592 (2021): 524–33. https://doi.org/10.1038/s41586-021-03392-8.

Libby, Peter. "Mechanisms of Acute Coronary Syndromes and Their Implications for Therapy." *N Engl J Med* 368, no. 21 (2013): 2004–13. DOI: 10.1056/NEJMra1216063.

Lo, Justin, Susan J. Melhorn, Sarah Kee, et al. "Hypothalamic Gliosis Is Associated with Multiple Cardiovascular Disease Risk Factors." *medRxiv* [preprint] (2024). DOI: 10.1101/2024.09.19.24313914.

Lovell, Tammy. "HRT Prescribing Increased by Almost Half in One Year, NHS Figures Show." *Pharm J* (October 30, 2023). https://pharmaceutical-journal.com/article/news/hrt-prescribing-increased-by-almost-half-in-one-year-nhs-figures-show.

Lundblad, Marie W., Bjarne K. Jacobsen, Jonas Johansson, et al. "Reference Values for DXA-Derived Visceral Adipose Tissue in Adults 40 Years and Older from a European Population: The Tromsø Study 2015–2016." *J Obes* 2021 (2021). https://doi.org/10.1155/2021/6634536.

Research News. "North American Menopause Society Updates Position Statement on Hormone Therapy, Says Benefits Outweigh Risks for Some Women." Breastcancer.org, July 7, 2017. https://www.breastcancer.org/research-news/nams-updates-hrt-position -statement.

Sewaybricker, Leticia E., Alyssa Huang, Suchitra Chandrasekaran, et al. "The Significance of Hypothalamic Inflammation and Gliosis for the Pathogenesis of Obesity in Humans." *Endocr Rev* 44, no. 2 (2023): 281–96. DOI: 10.1210/endrev/bnac023.

Takaya, Junji, Hirohiko Higashino, and Yohnosuke Kobayashi. "Intracellular Magnesium and Insulin Resistance." *Magnesium Res* 17, no. 2 (2004): 126–36. https://pubmed .ncbi.nlm.nih.gov/15319146/.

Tariq, Bisma, Samantha Phillips, Rina Biswakarma, et al. "Women's Knowledge and Attitudes to the Menopause: A Comparison of Women over 40 Who Were in the Perimenopause, Post Menopause and Those Not in the Peri or Post Menopause." *BMC Women's Health* 23, no. 460 (2023): 1–16. DOI: 10.1186/s12905-023-02424-x.

Westman, Eric. "The Evidence For and Against the Carbohydrate-Insulin Model of Obesity." Lecture presented at the Overcoming Obesity 2022 Conference by Obesity Medicine Association, Anaheim, CA, October 12–16, 2022.

Wong, Kate. "Women's Fat Deposits Help Offset Load Imposed by Pregnancy." *Sci Am*, September 26, 2001. https://www.scientificamerican.com/article/womens-fat-deposits-help/.

Interviews and Correspondence with the Author

Baker, Christian (September 2024).

Browning, Jeffrey (August 2024).

Fox, Caroline (December 2024).

Westman, Eric (April 2024).

Notes

97   **"always been about the calories":** Author interview with Westman, April 2024.

97   **close to 90% correlation:** Bray and Bouchard, "The Biology of Human Overfeeding."

97   **having one pound or less:** Author interview with Fox, December 2024.

98   **visceral adipose tissue (VAT):** Kahn et al., "Exploring Visceral and Subcutaneous Adipose Tissue Secretomes in Human Obesity."

98   **"a fire within":** Libby, "The Changing Landscape of Atherosclerosis."

98   **inflammation impacts both:** Sewaybricker et al., "The Significance of Hypothalamic Inflammation and Gliosis for the Pathogenesis of Obesity in Humans."

98   **"needed to lose visceral adiposity":** Browning, "Fate of Acetyl CoA Determines Metabolic Health"; author interview with Browning, August 2024.

100   **a state:** Dilliraj et al., "The Evolution of Ketosis."

100   **restriction without reducing calories:** Gower, "Beneficial Effects of Carbohydrate Restriction in Patients with Type 2 Diabetes Can Be Traced to Changes in Hepatic Metabolism."

101   **the American Heart Association:** El Khoudary et al., "The Menopause Transition and Women's Health at Midlife."

101   **that 60 to 70%:** Kodoth et al., "Adverse Changes in Body Composition During the Menopausal Transition and Relation to Cardiovascular Risk."

101   **But weight gain:** Hurtado Andrade et al., "Weight Gain in Midlife Women."

101   **One longitudinal study:** Gambacciani et al., "Body Weight, Body Fat Distribution, and Hormonal Replacement Therapy in Early Postmenopausal Women."

102   **progesterone and estrogen wane:** Hurtado Andrade et al., "Weight Gain in Midlife Women."

102   **Scientists have theorized:** Wong, "Women's Fat Deposits Help Offset Load Imposed by Pregnancy."

102   **Visceral fat accounts:** Karvonen-Gutierrez and Kim, "Association of Mid-life Changes in Body Size, Body Composition and Obesity Status with the Menopausal Transition."

102   **This fat is also:** Genazzani et al., "Metabolic Syndrome, Insulin Resistance and Menopause."

102   **"particularly deleterious":** El Khoudary et al., "The Menopause Transition and Women's Health at Midlife."

102   **"What people often don't":** Kumar, "Women's Health and Obesity."

103   **The prevalence of metabolic:** Hurtado Andrade et al., "Weight Gain in Midlife Women."

103   **"In women, we should":** Cuevas, "Menopause."

103   **"Currently, there is":** Iyer and Hirsch, "Clinical Impact of 2020 American Heart Association Statement on Menopause and Cardiovascular Disease Risk."

103   **In 2009, 65% of women:** Cushman et al., "Ten-Year Differences in Women's Awareness Related to Coronary Heart Disease."

103   **only 22% of primary:** Isakadze et al., "Addressing the Gap in Physician Preparedness to Assess Cardiovascular Risk in Women."

103   **women rely largely:** Tariq et al., "Women's Knowledge and Attitudes to the Menopause."

103   **70% said they received:** Dhawan et al., "Sex and Gender Medicine in Physician Clinical Training."

104   **The use of hormone therapy:** Iyer and Manson, "Recent Trends in Menopausal Hormone Therapy Use in the US."

104   **But subsequent research:** Research News, "North American Menopause Society Updates Position Statement on Hormone Therapy."

104   **shown a 30 to 50%:** Hodis and Mack, "Menopausal Hormone Replacement Therapy and Reduction of All-Cause Mortality and Cardiovascular Disease."

104   **She followed 106 women:** Hurtado Andrade et al., "Weight Loss Response to Semaglutide in Postmenopausal Women With and Without Hormone Therapy Use."

12: Resetting Body Weight

Sources
Works Referenced

Aronne, Louis. "Overcoming Barriers to Initiating Anti-obesity Medications." Lecture presented at the Spring Obesity Summit, New York, April 21–23, 2023.

Gribble, Fiona M., and Frank Reimann. "Metabolic Messengers: Glucagon-like Peptide 1." *Nat Metab* 3, no. 2 (2021): 142–48. DOI: 10.1038/s42255-020-00327-x.

Horvath, Tamas. "Obesity Pathophysiology: Treating the Chronic Disease of Obesity."

Lecture presented at 2023 Columbia Cornell Obesity: Etiology, Prevention, and Treatment, New York, May 3–6, 2023.

Martin, Alyce M., Emily W. Sun, and Damien J. Keating. "Mechanisms Controlling Hormone Secretion in Human Gut and Its Relevance to Metabolism." *J Endocrinol* 244, no. 1 (2019): R1–R15. DOI: 10.1530/JOE-19–0399.

Seeley, Randy. "Body Weight Set Points: What Are They, Can They Be Changed and What Does It Mean for Successful Treatment Strategies?" Lecture presented at Novel Therapies for Type 2 Diabetes and Obesity Summit, Boston, MA, May 31–June 1, 2023.

Sumithran, Priya, Luke Prendergast, Elizabeth Delbridge, et al. "Long-Term Persistence of Hormonal Adaptations to Weight Loss." *N Engl J Med* 365, no. 17 (2011): 1597–604. DOI: 10.1056/NEJMoa1105816.

Interviews and Correspondence with the Author

Friedman, Jeffrey (September 2024).

Hu, Frank (December 2023).

Roitman, Mitchell (May 2024).

Seeley, Randy (December 2023).

Sumithran, Priya (January 2024).

Notes

106 **"Consider seeing a light":** Author interview with Seeley, December 2023.

107 **"simplest conceptualization":** Author interview with Friedman, September 2024.

108 **"dynamic and subject to change":** Author interview with Roitman, May 2024.

108 **overweight and obese participants:** Sumithran et al., "Long-Term Persistence of Hormonal Adaptations to Weight Loss."

109 **slide with two columns:** Aronne, "Overcoming Barriers to Initiating Antiobesity Medications."

109 **did not clarify how:** Author interview with Sumithran, January 2024.

109 **"fundamental flaw":** Horvath, "Obesity Pathophysiology."

13: A New Era

Sources
Works Referenced

Ahmad, F. A., and S. Mahmud. "Acute Pancreatitis Following Orlistat Therapy: Report of Two Cases." *JOP Journal of the Pancreas* 11, no. 1 (2010): 61–63.

Aldhaleei, W. A., T. M. Abegaz, and A. S. Bhagavathula. "Glucagon-Like Peptide-1 Receptor Agonists Associated Gastrointestinal Adverse Events: A Cross-Sectional Analysis of the National Institutes of Health All of Us Cohort." *Pharmaceuticals* (Basel, Switzerland) 17, no. 2 (February 2024): 199. DOI: 10.3390/ph17020199. PMID: 38399414; PMCID: PMC10891568.

Alhadeff, Amber L. "If You Give a Mouse Ozempic." Lecture presented at Seminar on Appetitive Behaviors, Columbia University, New York, May 30, 2024.

Alhadeff, Amber L., Laura E. Rupprecht, and Matthew R. Hayes. "GLP-1 Neurons in the Nucleus of the Solitary Tract Project Directly to the Ventral Tegmental Area and

Nucleus Accumbens to Control for Food Intake." *Endocrinology* 153, no. 2 (2012): 647–58. https://doi.org/10.1210/en.2011-1443.

Aranäs, C., C. E. Edvardsson, O. T. Shevchouk, et al. "Semaglutide Reduces Alcohol Intake and Relapse-Like Drinking in Male and Female Rats." *EBioMedicine* 93 (July 2023): 104642. https://doi.org/10.1016/j.ebiom.2023.104642.

Ard, Jamy. "SURMOUNT-3: Safety Results." Lecture presented at Obesity Week 2023 by the Obesity Society, Dallas, TX, October 14–17, 2023.

Aronne, L. J., N. Sattar, D. B. Horn, et al. "Continued Treatment with Tirzepatide for Maintenance of Weight Reduction in Adults with Obesity: The SURMOUNT-4 Randomized Clinical Trial." *JAMA* 331, no. 1 (2024): 38–48.

Aronne, Louis J. "SURMOUNT-4: Study Efficacy and Safety Results." Lecture presented at the Fifty-Ninth Annual Meeting of the EASD (European Association for the Study of Diabetes), Hamburg, Germany, October 2–6, 2023.

Astrup, Arne. "Precision Dietary Management of Obesity and Type 2 Diabetes." Lecture presented at Jean Mayer USDA Human Nutrition Research Center on Aging (virtual), February 13, 2023.

Astrup, Arne. "Reflections on the Discovery of GLP-1 as a Satiety Hormone: Implications for Obesity Therapy and Future Directions." *Eur J Clin Nutri* 78 (2024): 551–56. https://doi.org/10.1038/s41430-024-01460-6.

Bello, N. T. "Update on Drug Safety Evaluation of Naltrexone/Bupropion for the Treatment of Obesity." *Expert Opin Drug Saf* 18, no. 7 (2019): 549–52.

Blundell J., G. Finlayson, M. Axelsen, et al. "Effects of Once-Weekly Semaglutide on Appetite, Energy Intake, Control of Eating, Food Preference and Body Weight in Subjects with Obesity." *Diabetes Obes Metab* 19, no. 9 (September 2017): 1242–51. DOI: 10.1111/dom.12932. Epub 2017 May 5. PMID: 28266779; PMCID: PMC5573908.

Boyd, S. T., and B. A. Fremming. "Rimonabant—A Selective CB1 Antagonist." *Ann Pharmacother* 39, no. 4 (2005): 684–90.

Bray, George A., and Donna H. Ryan. "Evidence-Based Weight Loss Interventions: Individualized Treatment Options to Maximize Patient Outcomes." *Diab Obes Metab* 23, Suppl. 1 (2021): 50–62. DOI: 10.1111/dom.14200.

Camilleri, Michael. "Definite Benefits of GLP-1 Receptor Agonists: What Is the Risk of Gastroparesis and Lung Aspiration?" *Gut* (e-pub August 17, 2024). DOI: 10.1136/gutjnl-2024-333036.

Camilleri, Michael. "Incretin Impact on Gastric Function in Obesity: Physiology, and Pharmacological, Surgical and Endoscopic Treatments." *J Physiol* (November 23, 2024). https://doi.org/10.1113/JP287535.

Camilleri, Michael, Paula Carlson, and Saam Dilmaghani. "Prevalence and Variations in Gastric-Emptying Delay in Response to GLP-1 Receptor Agonist Liraglutide." *Obesity* 32, no. 2 (2024): 232–33.

Chen, Xinda, Peiyi Zhao, Weihao Wang, et al. "The Antidepressant Effects of GLP-1 Receptor Agonists: A Systematic Review and Meta-analysis." *Am J Geriatr Psychiatry* 32, no. 1 (2024): 117–27. https://www.ajgponline.org/article/S1064-7481(23)00394-9/fulltext.

Chomko, Maureen. "Protocol in Practice—Standing Orders for RD/RN Management of GLP-1/GIP Receptor Agonist." Lecture presented at the Eighty-Fourth Annual Scientific Session of the American Diabetes Association, Orlando, FL, June 21–24, 2024.

Chuong, V., M. Farokhnia, S. Khom, et al. "The Glucagon-Like Peptide-1 (GLP-1) Analogue Semaglutide Reduces Alcohol Drinking and Modulates Central GABA

Neurotransmission." *JCI Insight* 8, no. 12 (June 22, 2023): e170671. DOI: 10.1172/jci.insight.170671.

Colman, E. "Anorectics on Trial: A Half Century of Federal Regulation of Prescription Appetite Suppressants." *Ann Intern Med* 143, no. 5 (2005): 380–85.

Colvin, Kayla J., Henry S. Killen, Maxwell J. Kanter, et al. "Brain Site-Specific Inhibitory Effects of the GLP-1 Analogue Exendin-4 on Alcohol Intake and Operant Responding for Palatable Food." *Int J Mol Sci* 21, no. 24 (2020): 9710. https://doi.org/10.3390/ijms21249710.

Cosentino, G., A. O. Conrad, and G. I. Uwaifo. "Phentermine and Topiramate for the Management of Obesity: A Review." *Drug Des Devel Ther* (2011): 267–78.

Dawkins, Colleen. "Is Weight Loss Everything? Nutrition and Lifestyle Are Missing Puzzle Pieces." Lecture presented at the Eighty-Fourth Annual Scientific Session of the American Diabetes Association, Orlando, FL, June 21–24, 2024.

Dickson, Suzanne L., Rozita H. Shirazi, Caroline Hansson, et al. "The Glucagon-Like Peptide 1 (GLP-1) Analogue, Exendin-4, Decreases the Rewarding Value of Food: A New Role for Mesolimbic GLP-1 Receptors." *J Neurosci* 32, no. 14 (2012): 4812–20. DOI: 10.1523/JNEUROSCI.6326–11.2012.

Dilliraj, L. N., G. Schiuma, D. Lara, et al. "The Evolution of Ketosis: Potential Impact on Clinical Conditions." *Nutrients* 14, no. 17 (2022): 3613.

Drew, B. S., A. F. Dixon, and J. B. Dixon. "Obesity Management: Update on Orlistat." *Vasc Health Risk Manag* 3, no. 6 (2007): 817–21.

Drucker, Daniel. "The Obesity Society Keynote Speaker." Lecture presented at Obesity Week 2018 by the Obesity Society, Nashville, TN, November 11–15, 2018.

Drucker, D. J., J. F. Habener, and J. J. Holst. "Discovery, Characterization, and Clinical Development of the Glucagon-Like Peptides." *J Clin Invest* 127, no. 12 (2017): 4217–27.

Eli Lilly and Company. "Lilly's Zepbound® (Tirzepatide) Superior to Wegovy® (Semaglutide) in Head-to-Head Trial Showing an Average Weight Loss of 20.2% vs. 13.7%." Eli Lilly, December 4, 2024. https://investor.lilly.com/news-releases/news-release-details/lillys-zepboundr-tirzepatide-superior-wegovyr-semaglutide-head.

Farr, O. M., R. L. Chiang-shan, and C. S. Mantzoros. "Central Nervous System Regulation of Eating: Insights from Human Brain Imaging." *Metab* 65, no. 5 (2016): 699–713.

Fink-Jensen, A., G. Wörtwein, M. K. Klausen, et al. "Effect of the Glucagon-Like Peptide-1 (GLP-1) Receptor Agonist Semaglutide on Alcohol Consumption in Alcohol-Preferring Male Vervet Monkeys." *Psychopharmacology* (2024): 1–8. https://doi.org/10.1007/s00213-024-06637-2.

Flemyng, M. *A Discourse on the Nature, Causes, and Cure of Corpulency. Illustrated by a Remarkable Case, Read before the Royal Society, November 1757. And Now First Published, by Malcolm Flemyng, MD.* L. Davis and C. Reymers, 1760.

Flier, Jeffrey S. "Drug Development Failure: How GLP-1 Development Was Abandoned in 1990." *Perspect Biol Med* 67, no. 3 (2024): 325–36. https://dx.doi.org/10.1353/pbm.2024.a936213.

Fullin, Kerianne, Anne Thorndike, and Layla Abushamat. "A Weighty Debate: Surgery, Drugs, Lifestyle, Paradox." Lecture presented at the American Heart Association Scientific Sessions, Philadelphia, PA, November 10–13, 2023.

Gamble, John-Michael. "Suicide Risk." Lecture presented at the Eighty-Fourth Annual Scientific Session of the American Diabetes Association, Orlando, FL, June 21–24, 2024.

Gaudiani, Jennifer L. *Sick Enough: A Guide to the Medical Complications of Eating Disorders.* Routledge, 2018.

Gleason, Patrick P., Benjamin Y. Urick, Landon Z. Marshall, Nicholas Friedlander, Yang Qiu, and R. Scott Leslie. "Real-World Persistence and Adherence to Glucagon-Like Peptide-1 Receptor Agonists Among Obese Commercially Insured Adults Without Diabetes." *J Manag Care Spec Pharm* 30, no. 8 (August 2024): 860–67. DOI: 10.18553/jmcp.2024.23332.

Goodman, Christopher W. "More Data on the Association of GLP-1 Agonists with Severe Depression." Journal Watch, September 12, 2024. https://www.jwatch.org/na57915/2024/09/12/more-data-association-glp-1-agonists-with-severe.

Hamed, K., M. N. Alosaimi, B. A. Ali, et al. "Glucagon-Like Peptide-1 (GLP-1) Receptor Agonists: Exploring Their Impact on Diabetes, Obesity, and Cardiovascular Health Through a Comprehensive Literature Review." *Cureus* 16, no. 9 (2024): e68390. DOI: 10.7759/cureus.68390.

Hayes, Matthew R. "Back to Basics: Incretin Neurobiology." Lecture presented at Obesity Week 2023 by the Obesity Society, Dallas, TX, October 14–17, 2023.

Hjerpsted, Julie B., Anne Flint, Ashley Brooks, et al. "Semaglutide Improves Postprandial Glucose and Lipid Metabolism, and Delays First-Hour Gastric Emptying in Subjects with Obesity." *Diabetes Obes Metab* 20, no. 3 (2018): 610–19. DOI: 10.1111/dom.13120.

Holst, Jens Juul. "Comments: The SURMOUNT-4 Trial." Lecture presented at the Fifty-Ninth Annual Meeting of the EASD (European Association for the Study of Diabetes), Hamburg, Germany, October 2–6, 2023.

Holst, Jens Juul. "From the Incretin Concept and the Discovery of GLP-1 to Today's Diabetes Therapy." *Front Endocrin* 10, no. 260 (2019): 1–10. DOI: 10.3389/fendo.2019.00260.

Holst, J. J., and C. F. Deacon. "Inhibition of the Activity of Dipeptidyl-Peptidase IV as a Treatment for Type 2 Diabetes." *Diabetes* 47, no. 11 (1998): 1663–70.

Horn, Deborah B. "Informing Treatment Decisions: Predictors of Response in Incretin-Based Therapies." Lecture presented at the International Congress on Obesity (ICO), São Paulo, Brazil, June 26–29, 2024.

Howell, E., H. M. Baumgartner, L. J. Zallar, J. A. Selva, L. Engel, and P. J. Currie. "Glucagon-Like Peptide-1 (GLP-1) and 5-Hydroxytryptamine 2c (5-HT2c) Receptor Agonists in the Ventral Tegmental Area (VTA) Inhibit Ghrelin-Stimulated Appetitive Reward." *Int J Molec Sci* 20, no. 4 (2019): 889. DOI: 10.3390/ijms20040889.

Jalleh, Ryan J., Chris K. Rayner, Trygve Hausken, et al. "Gastrointestinal Effects of GLP-1 Receptor Agonists: Mechanisms, Management, and Future Directions." *Lancet Gastroenterol and Hepatol* 9, no. 10 (2024): 957–64.

Jastreboff, Ania M. "Nutrient-Stimulated Hormone-Based Therapies for the Treatment of Obesity: Sparks from the Pipeline." Lecture presented at 2024 Columbia Cornell Obesity: Etiology, Prevention, and Treatment, May 1–4, 2024.

Jastreboff, Ania M., Louis J. Aronne, Nadia N. Ahmad, et al., for the SURMOUNT-1 Investigators. "Tirzepatide Once Weekly for the Treatment of Obesity." *New Eng J Med* 387, no. 3 (2022): 205–16. DOI: 10.1056/NEJMoa2206038.

Jastreboff, A. M., L. M. Kaplan, J. P. Frías, et al. "Triple-Hormone-Receptor Agonist Retatrutide for Obesity—A Phase 2 Trial." *New Eng J Med* 389, no. 6 (2023): 514–26.

Jastreboff, Ania M., Lee M. Kaplan, Juan P. Frías, et al., and Retatrutide Phase 2 Obesity Trial Investigators. "Triple-Hormone-Receptor Agonist Retatrutide for Obesity—A Phase 2 Trial." *New Eng J Med* 389, no. 6 (2023): 514–26. DOI: 10.1056/NEJMoa2301972.

Jenkins, William, Mahmoud Nassar, and Husam Ghanim. "#1704366 Gastroparesis Incidence Post-initiation of Semaglutide vs. Sitagliptin in Type 2 Diabetes: A Retrospective Trinetx Database Analysis." *Endocr Pract* 30, no. 5 (2024): S35–S36. https://doi.org/10.1016/j.eprac.2024.03.189.

Jensterle, M., S. Ferjan, L. Ležaič, et al. "Semaglutide Delays 4-Hour Gastric Emptying in Women with Polycystic Ovary Syndrome and Obesity." *Diabetes Obes Metab* 25, no. 4 (2023): 975–84. DOI: 10.1111/dom.14944.

Kahan, Scott. "One Size *Does Not* Fit All: Evolving Approaches to Optimize Obesity Pharmacotherapy." Lecture presented at Obesity Week 2023 by the Obesity Society, Dallas, TX, October 14–17, 2023.

Kanu, E. O. "Euglycemic Ketoacidosis After the Addition of Glucagon-Like Peptide-1 Receptor Agonist: A Case Report." *Ann Intern Med Clin Cases* 3, no. 6 (2024): e230565.

Karaivazoglou, Katerina, Ioanna Aggeletopoulou, and Christos Triantos. "The Contribution of the Brain-Gut Axis to the Human Reward System." *Biomedicines* 12, no. 8 (2024): 1861–73. DOI: 10.3390/biomedicines12081861.

Keys, Ancel. *The Biology of Human Starvation*. University of Minnesota Press, 1950.

Korner, Judith. "Advances in Obesity Pharmacotherapy over the Past 60+ Years." Lecture presented at Seminar on Appetitive Behaviors, Columbia University, New York, May 30, 2024.

Korner, Judith. "Side Effects of Pharmacologic Treatment and Their Management." Lecture presented at 2024 Columbia Cornell Obesity: Etiology, Prevention, and Treatment, May 1–4, 2024.

Lähteenvuo, Markku, Jari Tiihonen, Anssi Solismaa, et al. "Repurposing Semaglutide and Liraglutide for Alcohol Use Disorder." *JAMA Psychiatry* 82, no. 1 (2025): 94–98. DOI:10.1001/jamapsychiatry.2024.3599.

Leggio, Lorenzo. "GLP-1RA in Alcohol Use Disorder." Lecture presented at the Eighty-Fourth Annual Scientific Session of the American Diabetes Association, Orlando, FL, June 21–24, 2024.

Lilly, a Medicine Company. "Mounjaro." https://mounjaro.lilly.com/.

Lilly, a Medicine Company. "Zepbound." https://zepbound.lilly.com/.

Lincoff, A. M., K. Brown-Frandsen, H. M. Colhoun, et al., for the SELECT Trial Investigators. "Semaglutide and Cardiovascular Outcomes in Obesity Without Diabetes." *N Engl J Med* 389, no. 24 (December 14, 2023): 2221–32. DOI: 10.1056/NEJMoa2307563. Epub November 11, 2023. PMID: 37952131.

Love, Shayla. "Understanding Desire in the Age of Ozempic." *The Atlantic*, September 30, 2024. https://www.theatlantic.com/health/archive/2024/09/ozempic-glp1-desire-buddhism/680088/.

Marathe, C. S., C. K. Rayner, K. L. Jones, and M. Horowitz. "Effects of GLP-1 and Incretin-Based Therapies on Gastrointestinal Motor Function." *J Diab Res* 2011, no. 1 (2011): 279530. DOI: 10.1155/2011/279530.

Maselli, Daniel, Jessica Atieh, Matthew M. Clark, et al. "Effects of Liraglutide on Gastrointestinal Functions and Weight in Obesity: A Randomized Clinical and Pharmacogenomic Trial." *Obesity* (Silver Spring, MD) 30, no. 8 (2022): 1608–20. DOI: 10.1002/oby.23481.

Mesgun, Sami, Adily Elmi, Jaime Perez, et al. "Sa1961 Increased Risk of De Novo Gastroparesis in Non-diabetic Obese Patients on GLP-1 Receptor Agonists for Weight Loss: A Multi-network Study." *Gastroenterol* 166, no. 5 (2024): S-596.

Nadkarni, P., O. G. Chepurny, and G. G. Holz. "Regulation of Glucose Homeostasis by GLP-1." *Prog Mol Biol Transl Sci* 121 (2014): 23–65.

Nathani, Piyush, Madhav Desai, Harsh K. Patel, et al. "Incidence of Gastrointestinal Side Effects in Patients Prescribed Glucagon-Like Peptide-1 (GLP-1) Analogs: Real-World Evidence." *Gastroenterol* 166, no. 5 (2024): S-598.

Novo Nordisk. "See Information Below for the Only FDA-Approved Medicines Containing Semaglutide." n.d. https://tinyurl.com/425zha7b.

Novo Nordisk Foundation. "The Story of GLP-1." YouTube, November 7, 2022. https://www.youtube.com/watch?v=nrh5WAMfW3w.

Onakpoya, I. J., C. J. Heneghan, and J. K. Aronson. "Post-marketing Withdrawal of Anti-obesity Medicinal Products Because of Adverse Drug Reactions: A Systematic Review." *BMC Med* 14 (2016): 1–11.

Papavramidou, N., and H. Christopoulou-Aletra. "Management of Obesity in the Writings of Soranus of Ephesus and Caelius Aurelianus." *Obes Surg* 18 (2008): 763–65.

Pasqualotto, E., R. O. M. Ferreira, M. P. Chavez, et al. "Effects of Once-Weekly Subcutaneous Retatrutide on Weight and Metabolic Markers: A Systematic Review and Meta-analysis of Randomized Controlled Trials." *Metab Open* (2024): 100321. DOI: 10.1016/j.metop.2024.100321.

Qapaja, Thabet, Osama Hamid, Mohammed Abu-Rumaileh, Gizem Kaya, Sherif Saleh, and Samita Garg. "877 Gastroparesis Risk in Patients with Type 2 Diabetes Prescribed GLP-1 Receptor Agonists." *Gastroenterol* 166, no. 5 (2024): S-204. https://doi.org/10.1016/S0016–5085(24)00962–4.

Qeadan, F., A. McCunn, and B. Tingey. "The Association Between Glucose-Dependent Insulinotropic Polypeptide and/or Glucagon-Like Peptide-1 Receptor Agonist Prescriptions and Substance-Related Outcomes in Patients with Opioid and Alcohol Use Disorders: A Real-World Data Analysis." *Addiction* (October 16, 2024). DOI: 10.1111/add.16679. Epub ahead of print. PMID: 39415416.

Reuters. "FDA Advisory Committee Did Not Recommend Approval of Rimonabant (Zimulti®) for Use in Obese and Overweight Patients with Associated Risk Factors." Reuters, 2007.

Richards, Jesse, et al. "Successful Treatment of Binge Eating Disorder with the GLP-1 Agonist Semaglutide: A Retrospective Cohort Study." *Obes Pillars* 7 (July 20, 2023): 100080. DOI:10.1016/j.obpill.2023.100080.

Schoretsanitis, Georgios, Stefan Weiler, Corrado Barbui, et al. "Disproportionality Analysis from World Health Organization Data on Semaglutide, Liraglutide, and Suicidality." *JAMA Netw Open* 7, no. 8 (2024): e2423385. DOI: 10.1001/jamanetworkopen.2024.23385.

Shirazi, Rozita H., Suzanne L. Dickson, and Karolina P. Skibicka. "Gut Peptide GLP-1 and Its Analogue, Exendin-4, Decrease Alcohol Intake and Reward." *PLOS One* 8, no. 4 (2013): e61965. https://doi.org/10.1371/journal.pone.0061965.

Sodhi, Mohit, Ramin Rezaeianzadeh, Abbas Kezouh, and Mahyar Etminan. "Risk of Gastrointestinal Adverse Events Associated with Glucagon-Like Peptide-1 Receptor Agonists for Weight Loss." *JAMA* 330, no. 18 (2023): 1795–97.

The SURMOUNT-4 Investigators. "Treatment with Tirzepatide for Maintenance of Weight Reduction in Adults with Obesity: The SURMOUNT-4 Randomized Clinical Trial." *JAMA* 331, no. 1 (2024): 38–48. DOI: 10.1001/jama.2023.24945.

Tang-Christensen, M., P. Larsen, R. Goke, et al. "Central Administration of GLP-1-(7–36) Amide Inhibits Food and Water Intake in Rats." *Am J Physiol Regul Integr Comp Physiol* 271, no. 4 (1996): R848–R856.

Terhune, Chad. "Exclusive: Most Patients Stop Using Wegovy, Ozempic for Weight Loss Within Two Years." Reuters, July 10, 2024. https://www.reuters.com/business/healthcare-pharmaceuticals/most-patients-stop-using-wegovy-ozempic-weight-loss-within-two-years-analysis-2024-07-10/.

"Tides Are Changing for Obesity." Session presented at the Endocrine Society's 2023 Annual Meeting, Chicago, IL, June 15–18, 2023.

Tucker, Todd. *The Great Starvation Experiment: Ancel Keys and the Men Who Starved for Science.* University of Minnesota Press, 2007.

Ueda, Peter, Jonas Söderling, Viktor Wintzell, et al. "GLP-1 Receptor Agonist Use and Risk of Suicide Death." *JAMA Int Med* 184, no. 11 (2024): 1301–12. DOI: 10.1001/jamainternmed.2024.4369.

US Food and Drug Administration. "FDA Approved Labeling Text, NDA 020505-S-050 Topamax (Topiramate) Oral Tablets, NDA 020844-S-041 Topamax (Topiramate) Sprinkle Capsules." US FDA, 2012.

US Food and Drug Administration. "2–13–2020 FDA Drug Safety Communication: FDA Requests the Withdrawal of the Weight-Loss Drug Belviq, Belviq XR (Lorcaserin) from the Market. Potential Risk of Cancer Outweighs the Benefits." US FDA, February 13, 2020. fda.gov2020.

van Dijk, G., T. Thiele, R. Seeley, S. Woods, and I. Bernstein. "Glucagon-Like Peptide-1 and Satiety." *Nature* 385, no. 6613 (1997): 214.

Van Rijswijk, A.-S., N. van Olst, W. Schats, D. L. van der Peet, and A. W. van de Laar. "What Is Weight Loss After Bariatric Surgery Expressed in Percentage Total Weight Loss (% TWL)? A Systematic Review." *Obes Surg* 31, no. 8 (2021): 3833–47.

Wadden, Thomas A., Gregory K. Brown, Christina Egebjerg, et al. "Psychiatric Safety of Semaglutide for Weight Management in People Without Known Major Psychopathology: Post Hoc Analysis of the STEP 1, 2, 3, and 5 Trials." *JAMA Int Med* 184, no. 11 (2024): 1290–1300. DOI: 10.1001/jamainternmed.2024.4346.

Wadden, Thomas A., Ariana M. Chao, Sriram Machineni, et al. "Tirzepatide After Intensive Lifestyle Intervention in Adults with Overweight or Obesity: The SUR-MOUNT-3 Phase 3 Trial." *Nat Med* 29, no. 11 (2023): 2909–18. DOI: 10.1038/s41591-023-02597-w.

Wang, W., N. D. Volkow, N. A. Berger, P. B. Davis, D. C. Kaelber, and R. Xu. "Associations of Semaglutide with Incidence and Recurrence of Alcohol Use Disorder in Real-World Population." *Nat Commun* 15, no. 1 (2024): 4548. DOI: 10.1038/s41467-024-48780-6.

Wang, Xue-Feng, Jing-Jing Liu, Julia Xia, et al. "Endogenous Glucagon-Like Peptide-1 Suppresses High-Fat Food Intake by Reducing Synaptic Drive onto Mesolimbic Dopamine Neurons." *Cell Rep* 12, no. 5 (2015): 726–33.

Wei, Y., and S. Mojsov. "Distribution of GLP-1 and PACAP Receptors in Human Tissues." *Acta Physiol Scand* 157, no. 3 (1996): 355–57.

Wilding, John P. H., Rachel L. Batterham, Salvatore Calanna, et al., STEP 1 Study Group. "Once-Weekly Semaglutide in Adults with Overweight or Obesity." *New Eng J Med* 384, no. 11 (2021): 989–1002. DOI: 10.1056/NEJMoa2032183.

Zhu, H., D. Bi, Y. Zhang, et al. "Ketogenic Diet for Human Diseases: The Underlying

Mechanisms and Potential for Clinical Implementations." *Signal Transduct Targ Ther* 7, no. 11 (2022): 11.

Interviews and Correspondence with the Author

Alhadeff, Amber (May 2024).

Batterham, Rachel (August 2023).

Berridge, Kent (May 2024).

Blundell, John (September 2024).

Borner, Tito (August 2024).

Camilleri, Michael (September 2024).

Davis, Kim (September 2024).

Drucker, Daniel (May 2024).

Gaudiani, Jennifer (August 2024).

Grill, Harvey (August 2023; July 2024; October 2024).

Hayes, Matthew (July 2024).

Holst, Jens (September 2024).

Lutz, Thomas (May 2024).

Manejwala, Omar (July 2024).

Ryan, Donna (May 2023).

Skibicka, Karolina (August 2024).

Notes

114 **"People don't stop eating":** Author interview with Blundell, September 2024.

115 **head-to-head clinical trial:** Eli Lilly and Company, "Lilly's Zepbound® (Tirzepatide) Superior to Wegovy® (Semaglutide) in Head-to-Head Trial Showing an Average Weight Loss of 20.2% vs. 13.7%."

115 **believe that GIP masks:** Author interview with Borner, August 2024; author interview with Hayes, July 2024.

115 **emphasizes that the averages:** Kahan, "One Size *Does Not* Fit All."

116 **investigated why some individuals:** Horn, "Informing Treatment Decisions."

116 **"in the long run":** Horn, "Informing Treatment Decisions."

116 **a new drug called retatrutide:** Jastreboff, "Nutrient-Stimulated Hormone-Based Therapies for the Treatment of Obesity."

117 **work on these compounds:** Drucker, "The Obesity Society Keynote Speaker."

118 **"no question that these drugs":** Author interview with Borner, August 2024.

118 **"very clear evidence":** Author interview with Lutz, May 2024.

118 **GLP-1s can trigger:** Alhadeff, "If You Give a Mouse Ozempic."

118 **both seemed equally:** Author interview with Alhadeff, May 2024.

118 **aversive symptoms exist:** Author interview with Borner, August 2024; author interview with Hayes, July 2024; "Back to Basics."

119 **points out that:** Author interview with Borner, August 2024.

120 **taste aversion conditioning:** Author interviews with Grill, August 2023, July 2024, and October 2024.

121 **satiety increases when:** Astrup, "Precision Dietary Management of Obesity and Type 2 Diabetes."

121 **infused GLP-1 drugs:** Allison, "Reflections on the Discovery of GLP-1 as a Satiety Hormone and Implications for Management of Obesity"; Astrup, "Reflections on the Discovery of GLP-1 as a Satiety Hormone."

122 **Animal tests support:** Author interview with Skibicka, August 2024.

122 **Injecting a GLP-1 agonist:** Howell et al., "Glucagon-Like Peptide-1 (GLP-1) and 5-Hydroxytryptamine 2c (5-HT2c) Receptor Agonists . . ."

122 **particularly for "high responders":** Dickson et al., "The Glucagon-Like Peptide 1."

122 **been searching for:** Leggio, "GLP-1RA in Alcohol Use Disorder."

122 **place preference in rodents:** Chuong et al., "The Glucagon-Like Peptide-1 (GLP-1) Analogue Semaglutide Reduces Alcohol Drinking and Modulates Central GABA Neurotransmission."

122 **and nonhuman primates:** Fink-Jensen et al., "Effect of the Glucagon-Like Peptide-1 (GLP-1) Receptor Agonist Semaglutide on Alcohol Consumption in Alcohol-Preferring Male Vervet Monkeys."

122 **significantly reduced alcohol:** Aranäs et al., "Semaglutide Reduces Alcohol Intake and Relapse-Like Drinking in Male and Female Rats."

123 **several recent cohort studies:** Wang et al., "Associations of Semaglutide with Incidence and Recurrence of Alcohol Use Disorder in Real-World Population"; Lähteenvuo et al., "Repurposing Semaglutide and Liraglutide for Alcohol Use Disorder"; Qeadan et al., "The Association Between Glucose-Dependent Insulinotropic Polypeptide . . ."

123 **"naturally occurring hormones":** Karaivazoglou et al., "The Contribution of the Brain-Gut Axis to the Human Reward System."

123 **reduces appetite even more:** Pasqualotto et al., "Effects of Once-Weekly Subcutaneous Retatrutide on Weight and Metabolic Markers."

124 **"Semaglutide does not cause":** Author interview with Ryan, May 2023.

125 **"GLP-1s and severe depression":** Chen et al., "The Antidepressant Effects of GLP-1 Receptor Agonists"; Gamble, "Suicide Risk"; Goodman, "More Data on the Association of GLP-1 Agonists with Severe Depression"; Ueda et al., "GLP-1 Receptor Agonist Use"; Wadden et al., "Psychiatric Safety of Semaglutide for Weight Management in People Without Known Major Psychopathology."

125 **for a person accustomed:** Love, "Understanding Desire in the Age of Ozempic."

126 **slowing the passage of food:** Marathe et al., "Effects of GLP-1 and Incretin-Based Therapies on Gastrointestinal Motor Function."

126 **radioactive tracer:** The radioactive tracer containing technetium-99m.

126 **81% of the patients:** Aronne et al., "Continued Treatment with Tirzepatide for Maintenance of Weight Reduction in Adults with Obesity."

126 **only 7% of the patients:** Aronne, "SURMOUNT-4."

127 **SELECT trial:** Lincoff et al., "Semaglutide and Cardiovascular Outcomes in Obesity Without Diabetes."

127 **39.7% of patients:** Ard, "SURMOUNT-3."

127 **"don't have any side effects":** "Tides Are Changing for Obesity."

127 **digging into the data:** A study by Dr. Mohit Sodhi at the University of British Columbia indicated that these drugs have a hazard ratio of 3.67 for developing

gastroparesis, that is, more than triple the risk compared to other obesity treatments. Dr. William Jenkins from the University of Buffalo found no increased risk documented in electronic health records. However, Dr. S. Mesgun at the Cleveland Clinic reported a 52% increase in new gastroparesis cases among patients taking GLP-1s. Dr. Piyush Nathani at the University of Kansas found a 79% higher risk of gastroparesis for GLP-1 users. Dr. Thabet Qapaja, an internist affiliated with the Cleveland Clinic, observed a 24% rise in new diagnoses at twelve and twenty-four months. FDA data showed that 15.8% of 15,399 reported gastrointestinal events with GLP-1s involved delayed gastric emptying. Lastly, a 2024 study by Dr. Wafa Aldhaleei at the Mayo Clinic in Rochester, Minnesota, revealed that 5.1% of patients in a real-world cohort on GLP-1 drugs had gastroparesis.

127 **I contacted Novo Nordisk:** The company, in a letter dated June 27, 2023, stated, "Delay in gastric emptying may be considered a potential mechanism by which Ozempic® reduces food intake; however, it does not appear to be the primary mode of action in reducing appetite and body weight. Based on data from a 12-week, randomized, double-blind crossover study, which assessed gastric emptying via an absorption test with acetaminophen, gastric emptying during the first hour was delayed with Ozempic® compared to placebo, however, no statistical difference between Ozempic® and placebo was observed in the overall rate of postprandial gastric emptying (0–5 hours)." Hjerpsted et al., "Semaglutide Improves Postprandial Glucose and Lipid Metabolism, and Delays First-Hour Gastric Emptying in Subjects with Obesity."

127 **randomized controlled trial of patients without diabetes:** Using the gold standard (a technetium-99m scan); author interview with Camilleri, September 2024.

127 **significantly delayed gastric emptying:** Camilleri, "Definite Benefits of GLP-1 Receptor Agonists." Note: This study did not record symptoms. Nausea is a common symptom of GLP-1s.

127 **Data published in the journal:** Camilleri et al., "Prevalence and Variations in Gastric Emptying Delay in Response to GLP-1 Receptor Agonist Liraglutide."

127 **We don't know:** Author interview with Camilleri, September 2024.

127 **A 2023 study:** This study was carried out in women with polycystic ovary syndrome and obesity. Jensterle et al., "Semaglutide Delays 4-Hour Gastric Emptying in Women with Polycystic Ovary Syndrome and Obesity."

128 **starvation and gastroparesis:** Gaudiani, *Sick Enough.*

128 **"Pure calorie restriction":** Author interview with Gaudiani, August 2024.

14: Using the Anti-Obesity Drugs

Sources
Works Referenced

Adams, Ted D., Tapan S. Mehta, Lance E. Davidson, and Steven C. Hunt. "All-Cause and Cause-Specific Mortality Associated with Bariatric Surgery: A Review." *Curr Atheroscler Rep* 17 (2005): 74. DOI: 10.1007/s11883-015-0551-4.

Adams, T. D., A. M. Stroup, R. E. Gress, K. F. Adams, E. E. Calle, S. C. Smith, R. C. Halverson, S. C. Simper, P. N. Hopkins, and S. C. Hunt. "Cancer Incidence and Mortality after Gastric Bypass Surgery." *Obesity* (Silver Spring, MD) 17, no. 4 (April 2009): 796–802. doi: 10.1038/oby.2008.610. Epub Jan 15, 2009. PMID: 19148123; PMCID: PMC2859193.

Albrechtsen, N. J. W., R. Albrechtsen, L. Bremholm, et al. "Glucagon-Like Peptide 1 Receptor Signaling in Acinar Cells Causes Growth-Dependent Release of Pancreatic Enzymes." *Cell Rep* 17, no. 11 (2016): 2845–56.

Aldawsari, M., F. A. Almadani, N. Almuhammadi, S. Algabsani, Y. Alamro, and M. Aldhwayan. "The Efficacy of GLP-1 Analogues on Appetite Parameters, Gastric Emptying, Food Preference and Taste Among Adults with Obesity: Systematic Review of Randomized Controlled Trials." *Diabetes Metab Syndr Obes* 16 (March 2, 2023): 575–95. DOI: 10.2147/DMSO.S387116. PMID: 36890965; PMCID: PMC9987242.

Alduraibi, R. K., Y. M. Alrebdi, and Y. F. Altowayan. "Euglycemic Diabetic Ketoacidosis After the Initiation of Dulaglutide in Patient with Type 2 Diabetes." *Medicine* (Baltimore) 102, no. 23 (2023): e34027. https://www.ncbi.nlm.nih.gov/pmc/articles/PMC10256347/.

Alfaris, Nasreen, Stephanie Waldrop, Veronica Johnson, Brunna Boaventura, Karla Kendrick, and Fatima Cody Stanford. "GLP-1 Single, Dual, and Triple Receptor Agonists for Treating Type 2 Diabetes and Obesity: A Narrative Review." *EClinicalMedicine* 75 (2024). https://www.thelancet.com/journals/eclinm/article/PIIS2589-5370(24)00361-4/fulltext.

Al Oweidat, Khaled, Ahmad A. Toubasi, Raya B. Abu Tawileh, Hind B. Abu Tawileh, and Manar M. Hasuneh. "Bariatric Surgery and Obstructive Sleep Apnea: A Systematic Review and Meta-analysis." *Sleep Breath* 27, no. 6 (2023): 2283–94. DOI: 10.1007/s11325-023-02840-1.

Ballsmider, L. A., A. C. Vaughn, M. David, A. Hajnal, P. M. Di Lorenzo, and K. Czaja. "Sleeve Gastrectomy and Roux-en-Y Gastric Bypass Alter the Gut-Brain Communication." *Neural Plast* (2015): 601985. DOI: 10.1155/2015/601985.

Batterham, Rachel. "Do Post-surgical Changes in Gut Hormones Help Control Food Intake and Regulate Energy Balance?" Lecture presented at the IFSO World Congress XXVI, Naples, Italy, August 30, 2023.

Blue Health Intelligence. *Real-World Trends in GLP-1 Treatment Persistence and Prescribing for Weight Management.* Issue Brief. May 2024. https://www.bcbs.com/media/pdf/BHI_Issue_Brief_GLP1_Trends.pdf.

Bonora, B. M., A. Avogaro, and G. P. Fadini. "Euglycemic Ketoacidosis." *Curr Diab Rep* 20 (2020): 1–7.

Christensen, S., K. Robinson, S. Thomas, and D. R. Williams. "Dietary Intake by Patients Taking GLP-1 and Dual GIP/GLP-1 Receptor Agonists: A Narrative Review and Discussion of Research Needs." *Obes Pillars* (2024): 100121.

Chumakova-Orin, Maryna, Carolina Vanetta, Dimitrios P. Moris, and Alfredo D. Guerron. "Diabetes Remission After Bariatric Surgery." *World J Diabetes* 12, no. 7 (2021): 1093–1101. DOI: 10.4239/wjd.v12.i7.1093.

Cleveland Clinic. "Duodenal Switch." April 6, 2022. https://my.clevelandclinic.org/health/treatments/22725-duodenal-switch.

Cleveland Clinic. "The Gut-Brain Connection." September 9, 2023. https://my.cleveland clinic.org/health/body/the-gut-brain-connection.

Cooney, Elizabeth. "To Treat Obesity in Children, Task Force Favors Behavioral Therapy over Drugs Like Wegovy." *STAT,* June 18, 2024. https://www.statnews.com/2024/06/18/children-obesity-behavioral-therapy-wegovy-recommendations/#:~:text=%E2%80%9CWe%20believe%20we%20need%20more,per%20medication%20from%20our%20review.

Cummings, David E., David S. Weigle, R. Scott Frayo, Patricia A. Breen, Marina K. Ma, E. Patchen Dellinger, and Jonathan Q. Purnell. "Plasma Ghrelin Levels After Diet-Induced Weight Loss or Gastric Bypass Surgery." *N Eng J Med* 346, no. 21 (2002): 1623–30. DOI: 10.1056/NEJMoa012908.

Del Olmo-Garcia, M. I., and J. F. Merino-Torres. "GLP-1 Receptor Agonists and Cardiovascular Disease in Patients with Type 2 Diabetes." *J Diabetes Res* 2018 (April 2, 2018): 4020492. DOI: 10.1155/2018/4020492. PMID: 29805980; PMCID: PMC5902002.

Dicker, Dror, Yael Wolff Sagy, Noga Ramot, et al. "Bariatric Metabolic Surgery vs. Glucagon-Like Peptide-1 Receptor Agonists and Mortality." *JAMA Netw Open* 7, no. 6 (2024): e2415392. DOI: 10.1001/jamanetworkopen.2024.15392.

Doran, G. T. "There's a S.M.A.R.T. Way to Write Management's Goals and Objectives." *Management Review* 70 (1981): 35–36.

Drucker, Daniel. "The Benefits of GLP-1 Drugs Beyond Obesity." *Science* 385, no. 6706 (July 18, 2024): 258–60.

Drucker, Daniel J. "GLP-1 Physiology Informs the Pharmacotherapy of Obesity." *Mol Metab* 57 (2022): 101351. DOI: 10.1016/j.molmet.2021.101351.

Eisenberg, Dan, Scott A. Shikora, Edo Aarts, et al. "2022 American Society for Metabolic and Bariatric Surgery (ASMBS) and International Federation for the Surgery of Obesity and Metabolic Disorders (IFSO): Indications for Metabolic and Bariatric Surgery." *Surg Obes Relat Dis* 18, no. 12 (2022): 1345–56. DOI: 10.1016/j.soard.2022.08.013.

Elder, Katherine A., and Bruce M. Wolfe. "Bariatric Surgery: A Review of Procedures and Outcomes." *J Gastroenterol* 132, no. 6 (2007): 2253–71. DOI: 10.1053/j.gastro.2007.03.057.

Eli Lilly. "How Much Should I Expect to Pay for Mounjaro® (Tirzepatide)?" Accessed January 4, 2025. https://pricinginfo.lilly.com/mounjaro.

Felsenreich, Daniel M., Felix B. Langer, Ronald Kefurt, et al. "Weight Loss, Weight Regain, and Conversions to Roux-en-Y Gastric Bypass: 10-Year Results of Laparoscopic Sleeve Gastrectomy." *Surg Obes Relat Dis* 12, no. 9 (2016): 1655–62. DOI: 10.1016/j.soard.2016.02.021.

Fox, Claudia, and Aaron Kelly. "Pharmacotherapy for Obesity in Youth." Lecture presented at 2024 Columbia Cornell Obesity: Etiology, Prevention, and Treatment, May 1–4, 2024.

Frazer, Monica, Caroline Swife, Noelle N. Gronroos, et al. "Real-World Hemoglobin Ac1 Changes, Prescribing Provider Types, and Medication Dose Among Patients with Type 2 Diabetes Mellitus Initiating Treatment with Oral Semaglutide." *Adv Ther* 40, no. 11 (November 2023): 5102–114.

Friedrichsen, M., A. Breitschaft, S. Tadayon, A. Wizert, and D. Skovgaard. "The Effect of Semaglutide 2.4 mg Once Weekly on Energy Intake, Appetite, Control of Eating, and Gastric Emptying in Adults with Obesity." *Diab Obes Metab* 23, no. 3 (2021): 754–62.

Gaffney, Theresa. "Could New Childhood Obesity Guidelines Fuel Eating Disorders?" *Stat News*, September 16, 2024. https://www.statnews.com/2024/09/16/could-new-childhood-obesity-guidelines-fuel-eating-disorders/.

Gautron, Laurent. "The Phantom Satiation Hypothesis of Bariatric Surgery." *Front Neurosci* 15 (2021): 626085. DOI: 10.3389/fnins.2021.626085.

Gawdat, Khaled. "Shocking Sleeve Dilemmas (Equally Unfavorable or Unsatisfactory) Revision Choices After Sleeve Gastrectomy Explain the Higher Revision Rates Than in Gastric Bypass Patients." Lecture presented at IFSO Melbourne 2024, September 3–6, 2024.

Gawdat, Khaled. "Sleeve Gastrectomy Is Doomed to Fail as a Stand-Alone Procedure." Lecture presented at the International Federation for Surgery of Obesity and Metabolic Disorders (IFSO), Napoli, Italy, August 31, 2023.

Gleason, Patrick P., Benjamin Y. Urick, Landon Z. Marshall, Nicholas Friedlander, Yang Qiu, and R. Scott Leslie. "Real-World Persistence and Adherence to Glucagon-Like Peptide-1 Receptor Agonists Among Obese Commercially Insured Adults Without Diabetes." *J Manag Care Spec Pharm* 30, no. 8 (August 2024): 860–67. DOI: 10.18553/jmcp.2024.23332.

Gorgojo-Martínez, J. J., P. Mezquita-Raya, J. Carretero-Gómez, et al. "Clinical Recommendations to Manage Gastrointestinal Adverse Events in Patients Treated with GLP-1 Receptor Agonists: A Multidisciplinary Expert Consensus." *J Clin Med* 12, no. 1 (2022): 145. https://www.ncbi.nlm.nih.gov/pmc/articles/PMC9821052/.

Hampl, S. E., S. G. Hassink, A. C. Skinner, et al. "Clinical Practice Guideline for the Evaluation and Treatment of Children and Adolescents with Obesity." *Pediatrics* 151, no. 2 (February 1, 2023): e2022060640. DOI: 10.1542/peds.2022-060640. Erratum in *Pediatrics* 153, no. 1 (January 1, 2024): e2023064612. https://doi.org/10.1542/peds.2022-060640. PMID: 36622115.

Jalleh, Ryan J., Chris K. Rayner, Trygve Hausken, et al. "Gastrointestinal Effects of GLP-1 Receptor Agonists: Mechanisms, Management, and Future Directions." *Lancet Gastroenterol and Hepatol* 9, no. 10 (2024): 957–64.

Jastreboff, Ania M., Louis J. Aronne, Nadia N. Ahmad, et al., for the SURMOUNT-1 Investigators. "Tirzepatide Once Weekly for the Treatment of Obesity." *New Eng J Med* 387, no. 3 (2022): 205–16. DOI: 10.1056/NEJMoa2206038.

Ji, Yu, Hangii Lee, Shawn Kaura, et al. "Effect of Bariatric Surgery on Metabolic Diseases and Underlying Mechanisms." *Biomolecules* 11, no. 11 (2021): 1582. DOI: 10.3390/biom11111582.

Jo, D., G. Yoon, and J. Song. "Role of Exendin-4 in Brain Insulin Resistance, Mitochondrial Function, and Neurite Outgrowth in Neurons Under Palmitic Acid–Induced Oxidative Stress." *Antioxidants* (Basel, Switzerland) 10, no. 1 (January 9, 2021): 78. DOI: 10.3390/antiox10010078. PMID: 33435277; PMCID: PMC7827489.

Kalm, L. M., and R. D. Semba. "They Starved So That Others Be Better Fed: Remembering Ancel Keys and the Minnesota Experiment." *J Nutr* 135, no. 6 (June 2005): 1347–52. DOI: 10.1093/jn/135.6.1347. PMID: 15930436.

Kang, D.-H., S.-H. Kwon, W.-Y. Sim, and B.-L. Lew. "Telogen Effluvium Associated with Weight Loss: A Single Center Retrospective Study." *Ann Dermatol* 36 (2024).

Kaplan, Lee M. "The Physiology of Bariatric and Metabolic Surgery." Lecture presented at the Boston Course in Obesity Medicine, Boston, MA, June 16, 2023.

Kauppila, Joonas H., Sheraz Markar, Giola Santoni, Dag Holmberg, and Jesper Lagergren. "Temporal Changes in Obesity-Related Medication After Bariatric Surgery vs. No Surgery for Obesity." *JAMA Surg* 158, no. 8 (2023): 817–23. DOI: 10.1001/jamasurg.2023.0252.

Klijs, Bart, et al. "Obesity, Smoking, Alcohol Consumption and Years Lived with Disability: A Sullivan Life Table Approach." *BMC Public Health* 11, no. 378. DOI: 10.1186/1471-2458-11-378.

Kolata, Gina. "How Fen-Phen, a Diet 'Miracle,' Rose and Fell." *New York Times*, September 23, 1997. https://www.nytimes.com/1997/09/23/science/how-fen-phen-a-diet-miracle-rose-and-fell.html.

Korner, Judith. "Side Effects of Pharmacologic Treatment and Their Management." Lecture presented at 2024 Columbia Cornell Obesity: Etiology, Prevention, and Treatment, May 1–4, 2024.

Kral, John G., Simon Biron, Serge Simard, et al. "Large Maternal Weight Loss from Obesity Surgery Prevents Transmission of Obesity to Children Who Were Followed for 2 to 18 Years." *Pediatr* 118, no. 6 (2006): e1644–49. DOI: 10.1542/peds.2006–1379.

Kraljevic, Marko, Julian Süsstrunk, Marc Slawik, et al., "Outcomes Beyond 10 Years of Laparoscopic Roux-en-Y Gastric Bypass vs. Laparoscopic Sleeve Gastrectomy for Obesity: Weight Loss, Comorbidities, and Reoperations of the SM-BOSS Trial." Lecture presented at IFSO Melbourne 2024, September 3–6, 2024.

Lassailly, Guillaume, Robert Calazzo, David Buob, et al. "Bariatric Surgery Reduces Features of Nonalcoholic Steatohepatitis in Morbidly Obese Patients." *J. Gastroenterol* 149, no. 2 (2015): 379–88. DOI: 10.1053/j.gastro.2015.04.014.

Lauti, Melanie, Malsha Kularatna, Andrew G. Hill, and Andrew D. MacCormick. "Weight Regain Following Sleeve Gastrectomy—A Systematic Review." *Obes Surg* 26 (2016): 1326–34.

Le Roux, Carel W., Simon J. B. Aylwin, Rachel L. Batterham, et al. "Gut Hormone Profiles Following Bariatric Surgery Favor an Anorectic State, Facilitate Weight Loss, and Improve Metabolic Parameters." *Ann Surg* 243, no. 1 (2006). DOI: 10.1097/01.sla.0000183349.16877.84.

Lin, Kevin, Ateev Mehrotra, and Thomas C. Tsai. "Metabolic Bariatric Surgery in the Era of GLP-1 Receptor Agonists for Obesity Management." *JAMA Netw Open* 7, no. 10 (2024): e2441380. DOI: 10.1001/jamanetworkopen.2024.41380.

Lincoff, A. M., K. Brown-Frandsen, H. M. Colhoun, et al., for the SELECT Trial Investigators. "Semaglutide and Cardiovascular Outcomes in Obesity Without Diabetes." *N Engl J Med* 389, no. 24 (December 14, 2023): 2221–32. DOI: 10.1056/NEJMoa2307563. Epub November 11, 2023. PMID: 37952131.

Liss, D. T., M. Cherupally, M. J. O'Brien, et al. "Treatment Modification After Initiating Second-Line Medication for Type 2 Diabetes." *Am J Manag Care* 29, no. 12 (December 2023): 661–68. DOI: 10.37765/ajmc.2023.89466. PMID: 38170483.

Long, He, Li Qiuyu, Yang Yongfeng, et al. "Pharmacovigilance Study of GLP-1 Receptor Agonists for Metabolic and Nutritional Adverse Events." *Front Pharmacol* 15 (2024): 1416985. DOI: 10.3389/fphar.2024.1416985.

Lu, J., H. Liu, Q. Zhou, M. W. Wang, and Z. Li. "A Potentially Serious Adverse Effect of GLP-1 Receptor Agonists." *Acta Pharm Sin B* 13, no. 5 (2023): 2291–93. https://www.ncbi.nlm.nih.gov/pmc/articles/PMC10213739/.

Marx, Nikolaus, Mansoor Husain, Michael Lehrke, Subodh Verma, and Naveed Sattar. "GLP-1 Receptor Agonists for the Reduction of Atherosclerotic Cardiovascular Risk in Patients with Type 2 Diabetes." *Circulation* 146, no. 24 (2022): 1882–94. DOI: 10.1161/CIRCULATIONAHA.122.059595.

Mayo Clinic. "Sleeve Gastrectomy." August 2, 2024. https://www.mayoclinic.org/tests-procedures/sleeve-gastrectomy/about/pac-20385183.

Montero, Alex, Grace Sparks, Marley Presiado, and Liza Hamel. "KFF Health Tracking Poll May 2024: The Public's Use and Views of GLP-1 Drugs." KFF, May 10, 2024.

https://www.kff.org/health-costs/poll-finding/kff-health-tracking-poll-may-2024-the-publics-use-and-views-of-glp-1-drugs/.

Naqvi, Jeanean B., Ashley Berthoumieux, and Jeanna Napoleone. "GLP-1 Discontinuation: Real-World Perspectives on a Complex Journey." Omada Health white paper, 2024.

Nevola, R., R. Epifani, S. Imbriani, et al. "GLP-1 Receptor Agonists in Non-alcoholic Fatty Liver Disease: Current Evidence and Future Perspectives." *Int J Mol Sci* 24, no. 2 (January 15, 2023): 1703. DOI: 10.3390/ijms24021703. PMID: 36675217; PMCID: PMC9865319.

Nicholson, Wanda. Interviewed in Elizabeth Cooney, "To Treat Obesity in Children, Task Force Favors Behavioral Therapy over Drugs Like Wegovy." *Stat News*, June 18, 2024. https://www.statnews.com/2024/06/18/children-obesity-behavioral-therapy-wegovy-recommendations/.

Nicholson, Wanda K., Michael Silverstein, John B. Wong, et al. "Interventions for High Body Mass Index in Children and Adolescents: US Preventive Services Task Force Recommendation Statement." *JAMA* 332, no. 3 (2024): 226–32.

O'Brien, P. E., A. Hindle, L. Brennan, S. Skinner, P. Burton, A. Smith, G. Crosthwaite, and W. Brown. "Long-Term Outcomes After Bariatric Surgery: A Systematic Review and Meta-analysis of Weight Loss at 10 or More Years for All Bariatric Procedures and a Single-Centre Review of 20-Year Outcomes After Adjustable Gastric Banding." *Obes Surg* 29, no. 1 (January 2019): 3–14. DOI: 10.1007/s11695-018-3525-0. PMID: 30293134; PMCID: PMC6320354.

Passman, Jesse E., Elizabeth Wall-Wieler, Yuki Liu, Feibi Zheng, and Jordana B. Cohen. "Antihypertensive Medication Use Trajectories After Bariatric Surgery: A Matched Cohort Study." *Hypertension* 81, no. 8 (2024): 1737–46. DOI: 10.1161/HYPERTENSIONAHA.124.23054.

Peterli, Ralph, Robert E. Steinert, Bettina Woelnerhanssen, et al. "Metabolic and Hormonal Changes After Laparoscopic Roux-en-Y Gastric Bypass and Sleeve Gastrectomy: A Randomized, Prospective Trial." *Obes Surg* 22, no. 5 (2012): 740–48. DOI: 10.1007/s11695-012-0622-3.

Phillips, Blaine T., and Scott A. Shikora. "The History of Metabolic and Bariatric Surgery: Development of Standards for Patient Safety and Efficacy." *J Metab* 79 (2018): 97–107. DOI: 10.1016/j.metabol.2017.12.010.

Powell, W., X. Song, Y. Mohamed, D. Walsh, E. J. Parks, T. M. McMahon, M. Khan, and L. R. Waitman. "Medications and Conditions Associated with Weight Loss in Patients Prescribed Semaglutide Based on Real-World Data." *Obesity* (Silver Spring, MD) 31, no. 10 (October 2023): 2482–92. DOI: 10.1002/oby.23859. Epub August 18, 2023. PMID: 37593896; PMCID: PMC10702395.

Raffat, Umer. "GLP-1: Demand Issue? What's Going On with the Rx Trends? Where Is 2025 Tracking?" Presentation for Evercor GLP-1 Demand Webinar, January 24, 2025. https://bdadvanced.ipreo.com/OpenFileLink.aspx?ID1=85be7bfa-d43c-46e5-805b-5497d4ce5343&ID2=955992021/.

Roberts, Sue. "How Do Energy Requirements Change During Aging, and Implications for Eating a Healthy Diet." Lecture presented as part of Tufts University's HNRCA Monday Seminar Series, Boston, MA, October 4, 2021.

Rodriguez, P. J., B. M. Goodwin Cartwright, S. Gratzl, et al. "Semaglutide vs. Tirzepatide for Weight Loss in Adults with Overweight or Obesity." *JAMA Intern Med* 184, no. 9 (2024): 1056–64. https://www.ncbi.nlm.nih.gov/pmc/articles/PMC11231910/.

Rubino, D., N. Abrahamsson, M. Davies, et al., and STEP 4 Investigators. "Effect of

Continued Weekly Subcutaneous Semaglutide vs. Placebo on Weight Loss Maintenance in Adults with Overweight or Obesity: The STEP 4 Randomized Clinical Trial." *JAMA* 325, no. 14 (April 13, 2021): 1414–25. DOI: 10.1001/jama.2021.3224. PMID: 33755728; PMCID: PMC7988425.

Shah, Shashank, Poonam Shah, Jayashree Todkar, Michel Gagner, S. Sonar, and S. Solav. "Prospective Controlled Study of Effect of Laparoscopic Sleeve Gastrectomy on Small Bowel Transit Time and Gastric Emptying Half-Time in Morbidly Obese Patients with Type 2 Diabetes Mellitus." *Surg Obes Relat Dis* 6, no. 2 (2010): 152–57. DOI: 10.1016/j.soard.2009.11.019.

Siddeeque, Nabeela, Mohammad H. Hussein, Ahmed Abdelmaksoud, et al. "Neuroprotective Effects of GLP-1 Receptor Agonists in Neurogenerative Disorders: A Large-Scale Propensity-Matched Cohort Study." *Int Immunopharmacol* 143, no. 3 (October 2024): 11357. DOI: 10.1016/j.intimp.2024.113537.

Singhal, Vibha. Interviewed in Vanessa Villafuerte, "Are GLP-1 Drugs Safe for Children? Doctors Say Despite High Use Among Youth, No Unique Health Risks Detected." UCLA Health, July 10, 2024. https://www.uclahealth.org/news/release/are-glp-1-drugs-safe-children-doctors-say-despite-high-use.

Sjöström, L., K. Narbro, C. D. Sjöström, et al. "Swedish Obese Subjects Study: Effects of Bariatric Surgery on Mortality in Swedish Obese Subjects." *N Engl J Med* 357, no. 8 (August 23, 2007): 741–52. DOI: 10.1056/NEJMoa066254. PMID: 17715408.

Sole-Smith, Virginia. Interviewed in Erica Schwiegershausen, "What If You Weren't Scared of Your Kid Being Fat?" *New York Magazine*, April 20, 2023. https://www.thecut.com/article/interview-virginia-sole-smith-parenting-fatphobia.html?origSession=D2412170n3hNnyk5TCNXHqVuOUYBczocaRDvroPZ6sCvoe5fPc%3D.

Sole-Smith, Virginia. "Why the New Obesity Guidelines for Kids Terrify Me." *New York Times*, January 26, 2023. https://www.nytimes.com/2023/01/26/opinion/aap-obesity-guidelines-bmi-wegovy-ozempic.html.

Sorice-Virk, Sarah. "Beyond the Weight Loss: Implementing GLP-1 Agonists Safely and Effectively." Lecture presented at Ninety-Third Plastic Surgery, San Diego, CA, September 26–29, 2024.

Syn, Nicholas L., David E. Commings, Louis Z. Wang, et al. "Association of Metabolic-Bariatric Surgery with Long-Term Survival in Adults With and Without Diabetes: A One-Stage Meta-analysis of Matched Cohort and Prospective Controlled Studies with 174,772 Participants." *Lancet* 397, no. 10287 (2021): 1830–41. DOI: 10.1016/S0140–6736(21)00591–2.

Tajeu, G. S., E. Johnson, M. Buccilla, et al. "Changes in Antihypertensive Medication Following Bariatric Surgery." *Obes Surg* 32, no. 4 (April 2022): 1312–24. DOI: 10.1007/s11695-022-05893-5. Epub January 26, 2022. PMID: 35083703; PMCID: PMC9070659.

Tajeu, Gabriel S., Emily Johnson, Mason Buccilla, et al. "Changes in Antihypertensive Medication Following Bariatric Surgery." *Obes Surg* 32, no. 4 (2022): 1312–24. DOI: 10.1007/s11695-022-05893-5.

Terhune, Chad. "Exclusive: Most Patients Stop Using Wegovy, Ozempic for Weight Loss Within Two Years." Reuters, July 10, 2024. https://www.reuters.com/business/healthcare-pharmaceuticals/most-patients-stop-using-wegovy-ozempic-weight-loss-within-two-years-analysis-2024–07–10/.

Turker, Y., D. Baltaci, Y. Turker, S. Ozturk, C. I. Sonmez, M. H. Deler, Y. C. Sariguzel, F. Sariguzel, and H. Ankarali. "Investigation of Relationship of Visceral Body Fat and Inflammatory Markers with Metabolic Syndrome and Its Components Among

Apparently Healthy Individuals." *Int J Clin Exp Med* 8, no. 8 (August 15, 2015): 13067–77. PMID: 26550229; PMCID: PMC4612914.

Tzoulis, Ploutarchos, and Stephanie E. Baldeweg. "Semaglutide for Weight Loss: Unanswered Questions." *Front Endocrinol* 15 (2024): 1382814.

UCSF Health. "Dietary Guidelines After Bariatric Surgery." n.d. https://www.ucsfhealth.org/education/dietary-guidelines-after-bariatric-surgery.

Umans, Benjamin D., and Stephen D. Liberles. "Neural Sensing of Organ Volume." *Trends Neurosci* 41, no. 12 (2018): 911–24. DOI: 10.1016/j.tins.2018.07.008.

Umashanker, Devika. "Very Low Calorie Diet: In a Patient Care Setting." Lecture presented at the Overcoming Obesity 2022 Conference by Obesity Medicine Association, Anaheim, CA, October 12–16, 2022.

US Food and Drug Administration. "Federal Food, Drug, and Cosmetic Act (FD&C Act)." March 29, 2018. https://www.fda.gov/regulatory-information/laws-enforced-fda/federal-food-drug-and-cosmetic-act-fdc-act.

US Government Accountability Office. "Drug Safety: FDA Should Take Additional Steps to Improve Its Foreign Inspection Program." February 7, 2022. https://www.gao.gov/products/gao-22-103611.

US Senate Health, Education, Labor and Pensions Committee. "Media Advisory: Sanders to Lead HELP Committee Hearing on Outrageous Ozempic and Wegovy Prices with Novo Nordisk CEO." September 20, 2024. https://www.help.senate.gov/chair/newsroom/press/media-advisory-sanders-to-lead-help-committee-hearing-on-outrageous-ozempic-and-wegovy-prices-with-novo-nordisk-ceo.

Villafuerte, Vanessa. "Are GLP-1 Drugs Safe for Children? Doctors Say Despite High Use Among Youth, No Unique Health Risks Detected." UCLA Health, July 10, 2024. https://www.uclahealth.org/news/release/are-glp-1-drugs-safe-children-doctors-say-despite-high-use.

Wang, Guocheng, Yan Huang, Haojun Yang, Huang Lin, Shengfang Zhou, and Jun Qian. "Impacts of Bariatric Surgery on Adverse Liver Outcomes: A Systematic Review and Meta-analysis." *Surg Obes Relat Dis* 19, no. 7 (20232): 717–26. DOI: 10.1016/j.soard.2022.12.025.

Warren, Karon. "How Much Does Wegovy Cost?" GoodRx. https://www.goodrx.com/wegovy/wegovy-for-weight-loss-cost-coverage.

Weiss, T., R. D. Carr, S. Pal, et al. "Real-World Adherence and Discontinuation of Glucagon-Like Peptide-1 Receptor Agonists Therapy in Type 2 Diabetes Mellitus Patients in the United States." *Patient Pref Adherence* 14 (November 27, 2020): 2337–45. DOI: 10.2147/PPA.S277676.

Wharton, S., M. Davies, D. Dicker, I. Lingvay, O. Mosenzon, D. M. Rubino, and S. D. Pedersen. "Managing the Gastrointestinal Side Effects of GLP-1 Receptor Agonists in Obesity: Recommendations for Clinical Practice. *Postgrad Med* 134, no. 1 (January 2022): 14–19. DOI: 10.1080/00325481.2021.2002616. Epub November 29, 2021. PMID: 34775881.

Wilding, John P. H., Rachel L. Batterham, Salvatore Calanna, et al., STEP 1 Study Group. "Once-Weekly Semaglutide in Adults with Overweight or Obesity." *New Eng J Med* 384, no. 11 (2021): 989–1002. DOI: 10.1056/NEJMoa2032183.

Wilding, J. P. H., R. L. Batterham, M. Davies, et al. "Weight Regain and Cardiometabolic Effects After Withdrawal of Semaglutide: The STEP 1 Trial Extension." *Diab Obes Metab* 24, no. 8 (2022): 1553–64. https://www.ncbi.nlm.nih.gov/pmc/articles/PMC9542252/.

Wilson, Robert B., Dhruvi Lathigara, and Devesh Kaushal. "Systematic Review and Meta-analysis of the Impact of Bariatric Surgery on Future Cancer Risk." *Int J Mol Sci* 24, no. 7 (2023): 6192. DOI: 10.3390/ijms24076192.

Wingrove, Patrick. "Fake Ozempic: How Batch Numbers Help Criminal Groups Spread Dangerous Weight Loss Drugs." Reuters, September 6, 2024. https://www.reuters .com/business/healthcare-pharmaceuticals/fake-ozempic-how-batch-numbers-help -criminal-groups-spread-dangerous-drugs-2024–09–05/.

World Health Organization. "WHO Issues Warning on Falsified Medicines Used for Diabetes Treatment and Weight Loss." June 20, 2024. https://www.who.int/news/item /20–06–2024-who-issues-warning-on-falsified-medicines-used-for-diabetes-treatment -and-weight-loss.

Woronow, D., C. Chamberlain, A. Niak, M. Avigan, M. Houstoun, and C. Kortepeter. "Acute Cholecystitis Associated with the Use of Glucagon-Like Peptide-1 Receptor Agonists Reported to the US Food and Drug Administration." *JAMA Intern Med* 182, no. 10 (October 1, 2022): 1104–6. DOI: 10.1001/jamainternmed.2022.3810. PMID: 36036939; PMCID: PMC9425280.

Wyszomirski, K., M. Waledziak, and A. Róża-ska-Walędziak. "Obesity, Bariatric Surgery and Obstructive Sleep Apnea—A Narrative Literature Review." *Medicina* (Kaunas, Lithuania) 59, no. 7 (2023): 1266. DOI: 10.3390/medicina59071266.

Interviews and Correspondence with the Author

Atwater, Jason [not his real name] (September 2024).

Batterham, Rachel (August 2023).

Dennis, Kim (September 2024).

Gaudiani, Jennifer (August 2024).

Kushner, Robert (April 2024).

Rosenbaum, Michael (September 2024).

Skibicka, Karolina (August 2024).

Notes

130 **is SMART: specific, measurable, achievable:** Doran, "There's a S.M.A.R.T. Way to Write Management's Goals and Objectives."

131 **advised to avoid GLP-1s:** US Food and Drug Administration, "WEGOVY (semaglutide) Injection, for Subcutaneous Use."

131 **a very real risk:** "Dehydration was the most frequent AE contributing to serious outcomes for liraglutide (n = 318, 23.93%), dulaglutide (n = 434, 20.90%), semaglutide (n = 370, 25.10%) and tirzepatide (n = 70, 32.86%)." From Long et al., "Pharmacovigilance Study of GLP-1 Receptor Agonists for Metabolic and Nutritional Adverse Events."

131 **FDA originally approved the use:** US Food and Drug Administration, "WEGOVY (semaglutide) Injection, for Subcutaneous Use."

132 **reduced cardiovascular risk:** Lincoff et al., "Semaglutide and Cardiovascular Outcomes in Obesity Without Diabetes."

132 **three additional years of disability:** Klijs et al., "Obesity, Smoking, Alcohol Consumption and Years Lived with Disability: A Sullivan Life Table Approach."

132 **Dr. Sue Roberts:** Roberts, "How Do Energy Requirements Change During Aging, and Implications for Eating a Healthy Diet."

133 **0.25 mg weekly for semaglutide:** Novo Nordisk, "Wegovy® Dosing Schedule."

133 **2.5 mg weekly for tirzepatide:** Eli Lilly, "How to Prescribe Mounjaro."

133 **says regarding dose:** In an assessment of the risk of thyroid cancer, Dr. Judy Korner, professor of medicine at Columbia University, states, "Official box warning for thyroid C-cell tumors in the US: GLP-1RAs are contraindicated in patients with a personal or family history of MTC, as well as in patients with multiple endocrine neoplasia (MEN) type 2. In rodents, the thyroid C cells (neuroendocrine parafollicular cells which secrete calcitonin) highly express the GLP-1 receptor. Stimulation leads to upregulation of the calcitonin gene expression, calcitonin synthesis, C-cell hyperplasia, and increased risk of medullary adenomas and carcinomas. GLP-1 receptor is only marginally expressed in thyroids of non-human primates and humans. Monkeys treated with >60 times the human dose of liraglutide do not develop C-cell abnormalities after 20 months. A study by Bezin et al., 'GLP-1 Receptor Agonists and the Risk of Thyroid Cancer,' analyzed use of GLP-1 RA in 2,562 cases of thyroid cancer and 45,184 controls without thyroid cancer. The conclusion was: Increased risk of all thyroid cancer and medullary thyroid cancer with use of GLP-1 RA, in particular after 1–3 years of treatment. Detection bias: Use of GLP-1RAs may be associated with increased monitoring and imaging. Given the evidence, it is unclear whether GLP-1RAs cause an increase in thyroid cancer. MTC is rare (estimated incidence of 0.2 cases per 100,000 patient-years), and as such, it is very difficult to definitively rule out an association between GLP-1RA and thyroid malignancies. Pharmacovigilance of cases is ongoing." From Korner, "Side Effects of Pharmacologic Treatment and Their Management."

133 **the clinical trials:** Real-world clinical data show the percentage weight loss for tirzepatide at three, six, and twelve months was 6, 10, and 15% respectively, and for semaglutide, 4, 6, and 8% respectively.

133 **patients on semaglutide:** Wilding, et al., "Once-Weekly Semaglutide in Adults with Overweight or Obesity."

133 **Patients on tirzepatide:** Jastreboff, et al., "Tirzepatide Once Weekly for the Treatment of Obesity."

133 **"super responders":** Tzoulis and Baldeweg, "Semaglutide for Weight Loss."

133 **"non-responders":** Clinicians have anecdotally stated that patients with thyroid conditions, anxiety, depression, and binge-eating disorders that have not been addressed may not respond as well. Physicians—again, anecdotally—recommend cardiovascular and resistance training in patients who have failed to respond. This is an area that needs further study.

134 **Weight plateaus:** Tzoulis and Baldeweg, "Semaglutide for Weight Loss."

134 **experience some gastrointestinal issues:** Wharton et al., "Managing the Gastrointestinal Side Effects of GLP-1 Receptor Agonists in Obesity."

135 **GLP-1s is reduced appetite:** Aldawsari et al., "The Efficacy of GLP-1 Analogues on Appetite Parameters, Gastric Emptying, Food Preference and Taste Among Adults with Obesity."

135 **slowed-down transfer of stomach contents:** Jalleh et al., "Gastrointestinal Effects of GLP-1 Receptor Agonists."

135 **serious effect is cholelithiasis (gallstones):** Woronow et al., "Acute Cholecystitis Associated with the Use of Glucagon-Like Peptide-1 Receptor Agonists . . ."

135 **very-low-calorie:** Umashanker, "Very Low Calorie Diet."

135 **may experience is malnutrition:** Powell et al., "Medications and Conditions Associated with Weight Loss in Patients Prescribed Semaglutide."

136 **toxic visceral body fat:** Turker et al., "Investigation of Relationship of Visceral Body Fat and Inflammatory Markers."

136 **FDA has changed the indications:** US Food and Drug Administration, "WEGOVY (semaglutide) Injection, for Subcutaneous Use."

136 **Dr. Jason Atwater:** not his real name.

136 **"I wasn't obese":** Author interview with Atwater, September 2024.

137 **30% of people who discontinue:** Raffat, "GLP-1: Demand Issue?"

138 **statistics from the CDC:** CDC, "Childhood Obesity Facts."

138 **"should offer adolescents":** Hampl et al., "Clinical Practice Guideline for the Evaluation and Treatment of Children and Adolescents with Obesity."

139 **"Severe obesity" is:** Kral et al., "Large Maternal Weight Loss from Obesity Surgery Prevents Transmission of Obesity to Children Who Were Followed for 2 to 18 Years."

139 **Virginia Sole-Smith:** Sole-Smith, "Why the New Obesity Guidelines for Kids Terrify Me."

139 **Some psychologists worried:** Gaffney, "Could New Childhood Obesity Guidelines Fuel Eating Disorders?"

139 **"we need more evidence":** Wanda Nicholson, in Cooney, "To Treat Obesity in Children."

139 **make a recommendation:** Nicholson, "To Treat Obesity in Children."

139 **mainly gastrointestinal distress:** Villafuerte, "Are GLP-1 Drugs Safe for Children?"

139 **"When young patients":** Singhal, "Are GLP-1 Drugs Safe for Children?"

139 **"apply a double standard":** Fox and Kelly, "Pharmacotherapy for Obesity in Youth."

140 **The fact that GLP-1s:** Author interview with Rosenbaum, September 2024.

140 **have a two-year:** Villafuerte, "Are GLP-1 Drugs Safe for Children?"

140 **It took around five:** Kolata, "How Fen-Phen, a Diet 'Miracle,' Rose and Fell."

141 **can't yet match:** Dicker et al., "Bariatric Metabolic Surgery vs Glucagon-Like Peptide-1 Receptor Agonists."

141 **takes an entire team:** Elder and Wolfe, "Bariatric Surgery."

141 **most recent guidelines:** Eisenberg et al., "2022 American Society for Metabolic and Bariatric Surgery."

141 **surgery is recommended:** Eisenberg et al., "2022 American Society of Metabolic and Bariatric Surgery."

141 **weight loss of up to 30%:** Alfadda et al., "Long-Term Weight Outcomes After Bariatric Surgery."

141 **about a 25% drop:** Tajeu et al., "Changes in Antihypertensive Medication Following Bariatric Surgery."

141 **about a 3–7% drop:** Kauppila et al., "Temporal Changes in Obesity-Related Medication After Bariatric Surgery vs. No Surgery for Obesity."

141 **obstructive sleep apnea:** Wyszomirski et al., "Obesity, Bariatric Surgery and Obstructive Sleep Apnea."

141 **cancer:** Adams et al., "Cancer Incidence and Mortality After Gastric Bypass Surgery."

141 **decrease in all-cause mortality:** Syn et al., "Association of Metabolic-Bariatric Surgery with Long-Term Survival in Adults With and Without Diabetes."

141   **all-cause mortality of about 50%:** Sjöström et al., "Effects of Bariatric Surgery on Mortality in Swedish Obese Subjects."

141   **reduce the size of the stomach:** Ji et al., "Effect of Bariatric Surgery on Metabolic Diseases and Underlying Mechanisms."

142   **causing malabsorption:** Ji et al., "Effect of Bariatric Surgery on Metabolic Diseases and Underlying Mechanisms."

142   **Approximately 60%:** Felsenreich et al., "Weight Loss, Weight Regain, and Conversions to Roux-en-Y Gastric Bypass"; Lauti et al., "Weight Regain Following Sleeve Gastrectomy."

142   **sleeve gastrectomy:** Kraljevic et al., "Outcomes Beyond 10 Years of Laparoscopic Roux-en-Y Gastric Bypass vs. Laparoscopic Sleeve Gastrectomy for Obesity."

142   **150,000 such operations:** American Society for Metabolic Bariatric Surgery, "Estimate of Bariatric Surgery Numbers, 2011–2022."

142   **sleeve gastrectomy group:** Kraljevic et al., "Outcomes Beyond 10 Years of Laparoscopic Roux-en-Y Gastric Bypass vs. Laparoscopic Sleeve Gastrectomy for Obesity."

143   **25% drop:** Lin et al., "Metabolic Bariatric Surgery in the Era of GLP-1 Receptor Agonists for Obesity Management."

143   **on average, for six to eight months:** Raffat, "GLP-1: Demand Issue?"

143   **two-thirds of the weight:** Wilding et al., "Weight Regain and Cardiometabolic Effects After Withdrawal of Semaglutide."

144   **A survey taken:** Sorice-Virk, "Beyond the Weight Loss."

144   **cost of these medications:** Warren, "How Much Does Wegovy Cost?"; Eli Lilly, "How Much Should I Expect to Pay for Mounjaro®?"

144   **discontinuation rates:** Liss et al., "Treatment Modification After Initiating Second-Line Medication for Type 2 Diabetes."

144   **23% of test subjects dropped out:** Lincoff et al., "Semaglutide and Cardiovascular Outcomes in Obesity Without Diabetes."

144   **less than one-third:** Gleason et al., "Real-World Persistence and Adherence to Glucagon-Like Peptide-1 Receptor Agonists Among Obese Commercially Insured Adults Without Diabetes."

144   **Blue Cross Blue Shield:** Blue Health Intelligence, *Real-World Trends in GLP-1 Treatment Persistence and Prescribing for Weight Management.*

15: Managing Major Weight Loss

Sources
Works Referenced

Ahtiainen, Juha P., Simon Walker, Heikki Peltonen, et al. "Heterogeneity in Resistance Training-Induced Muscle Strength and Mass Responses in Men and Women of Different Ages." *Age* (Dordrecht, Netherlands) 38, no. 10 (2016): 1–13. DOI: 10.1007/s11357-015-9870-1.

Albrechtsen, N. J. W., R. Albrechtsen, L. Bremholm, et al. "Glucagon-Like Peptide 1 Receptor Signaling in Acinar Cells Causes Growth-Dependent Release of Pancreatic Enzymes." *Cell Rep* 17, no. 11 (2016): 2845–56.

Alduraibi, R. K., Y. M. Alrebdi, and Y. F. Altowayan. "Euglycemic Diabetic Ketoacidosis

After the Initiation of Dulaglutide in Patient with Type 2 Diabetes." *Medicine* (Baltimore) 102, no. 23 (2023): e34027. https://www.ncbi.nlm.nih.gov/pmc/articles/PMC10256347/.

Almandoz, Jaime. "Practical Aspects of Using Anti-obesity Medications." Lecture presented at UT Southwestern Weight Wellness Day, Dallas, TX, September 14, 2024.

Aronne, L. J., N. Sattar, D. B. Horn, et al. "Continued Treatment with Tirzepatide for Maintenance of Weight Reduction in Adults with Obesity: The SURMOUNT-4 Randomized Clinical Trial." *JAMA* 331, no. 1 (2024): 38–48.

Baraki, Austin, Jordan Feigenbaum, and Jonathon Sullivan. "Practical Guidelines for Implementing a Strength Training Program for Adults." UpToDate, November 2024. https://www.uptodate.com/contents/practical-guidelines-for-implementing-a-strength -training-program-for-adults.

Barbagallo, M., and L. J. Dominguez. "Magnesium and Aging." *Current Pharm Des* 16, no. 7 (2010): 832–39. DOI: 10.2174/138161210790883679.

Bezin, Julien, Amandine Gouverneur, Marine Pénichon, et al. "GLP-1 Receptor Agonists and the Risk of Thyroid Cancer." *Diab Care* 46, no. 2 (2023): 384–90. DOI: 10.2337 /dc22–1148.

Bovend'Eerdt, Thamar J. H., Rachel E. Botell, and Derick T. Wade. "Writing SMART Rehabilitation Goals and Achieving Goal Attainment Scaling: A Practical Guide." *Clin Rehab* 23, no. 4 (2009): 352–61. DOI: 10.1177/0269215508101741.

Bray, George A., and Donna H. Ryan. "Evidence-Based Weight Loss Interventions: Individualized Treatment Options to Maximize Patient Outcomes." *Diab Obes Metab* 23, Suppl. 1 (2021): 50–62. DOI: 10.1111/dom.14200.

Chomko, Maureen. "Protocol in Practice—Standing Orders for RD/RN Management of GLP-1/GIP Receptor Agonist." American Diabetes Association 84th Scientific Session, Orlando, FL, June 22, 2024.

Christensen, S., K. Robinson, S. Thomas, and D. R. Williams. "Dietary Intake by Patients Taking GLP-1 and Dual GIP/GLP-1 Receptor Agonists: A Narrative Review and Discussion of Research Needs." *Obes Pillars* (2024): 100121.

ConsumerLab.com. "Ad-Free. Independent. Powered by Members Like You." 2024. https://www.consumerlab.com/.

Feigenbaum, Jordan, Austin Baraki, Derek Miles, Leah Lutz, and Tom Campitelli. *Barbell Medicine Seminar Attendee Handbook*, 2023.

Francavilla, Carolyn. "Nutrition Therapy: Fundamentals of Obesity Treatment." Lecture presented at Obesity Medicine Association, 2024.

Friedrichsen, M., A. Breitschaft, S. Tadayon, A. Wizert, and D. Skovgaard. "The Effect of Semaglutide 2.4 mg Once Weekly on Energy Intake, Appetite, Control of Eating, and Gastric Emptying in Adults with Obesity." *Diab Obes Metab* 23, no. 3 (2021): 754–62.

Garvey, Timothy W., Rachel L. Batterham, Meena Bhatta, et al. "Two-Year Effects of Semaglutide in Adults with Overweight or Obesity: The STEP 5 Trial." *Nature* 28 (2022): 2083–91.

Gorgojo-Martínez, J. J., P. Mezquita-Raya, J. Carretero-Gómez, et al. "Clinical Recommendations to Manage Gastrointestinal Adverse Events in Patients Treated with GLP-1 Receptor Agonists: A Multidisciplinary Expert Consensus." *J Clin Med* 12, no. 1 (2022): 145. https://www.ncbi.nlm.nih.gov/pmc/articles/PMC9821052/.

Gross, Katharina, and Christian Brinkmann. "Why You Should Not Skip Tailored

Exercise Interventions When Using Incretin Mimetics for Weight Loss." *Front Endocrinol* 15 (July 22, 2024). https://doi.org/10.3389/fendo.2024.1449653.

Gudzune, Kimberly A., Lee M. Kaplan, Scott Kahan, et al., and OBSERVE Study. "Weight-Reduction Preferences Among OBSERVE Study Participants with Obesity or Overweight: Opportunities for Shared Decision-Making." *Endocr Pract* 30, no. 10 (October 2024): 917–26. DOI: 10.1016/j.eprac.2024.06.009.

Hathaway, J. T., M. P. Shah, D. B. Hathaway, et al. "Risk of Nonarteritic Anterior Ischemic Optic Neuropathy in Patients Prescribed Semaglutide." *JAMA Ophthalmol* 142, no. 8 (2024): 732–39.

He, L., J. Wang, F. Ping, et al. "Association of Glucagon-Like Peptide-1 Receptor Agonist Use with Risk of Gallbladder and Biliary Diseases: A Systematic Review and Meta-analysis of Randomized Clinical Trials." *JAMA Int Med* 182, no. 5 (2022): 513–19.

Hussain, Amna. Letter to author from Novo Nordisk medical information specialist, June 27, 2023.

Kalm, Leah M., and Richard D. Semba. "They Starved So That Others Be Better Fed: Remembering Ancel Keys and the Minnesota Experiment." *J Nutr* 135, no. 6 (June 1, 2005): 1347–52. https://doi.org/https://doi.org/10.1093/jn/135.6.1347; https://www.sciencedirect.com/science/article/pii/S002231662210249X.

Kanu, E. O., D. K. Kim, R. Menon, C. Burke, and N. Vicknair. "Euglycemic Ketoacidosis After the Addition of Glucagon-Like Peptide-1 Receptor Agonist: A Case Report." *AIMCC* 3, no. 6 (2024): e230565.

Keogh, Justin W. L., and Paul W. Winwood. "The Epidemiology of Injuries Across the Weight-Training Sports." *Sports Med* (Auckland) 47, no. 3 (2017): 479–501. DOI: 10.1007/s40279-016-0575-0.

Keys, Ancel. *The Biology of Human Starvation*. University of Minnesota Press, 1950.

Korner, Judith. "Side Effects of Pharmacologic Treatment and Their Management." Lecture presented at 2024 Columbia Cornell Obesity: Etiology, Prevention, and Treatment, May 1–4, 2024.

Kushner, Robert. "Beyond Medication: The Role of Behavior Change." Lecture presented at Obesity Medicine 2024 by Obesity Medicine Association Academy, May 2024.

Lauti, Melanie, Malsha Kularatna, Andrew G. Hill, and Andrew D. MacCormick. "Weight Regain Following Sleeve Gastrectomy—A Systematic Review." *Obes Surg* 26 (2016): 1326–34.

Long, He, Li Qiuyu, Yongfeng Yang, et al. "Pharmacovigilance Study of GLP-1 Receptor Agonists for Metabolic and Nutritional Adverse Events." *Front Pharmacol* 15 (2024): 1416985. DOI: 10.3389/fphar.2024.1416985.

Lu J., H. Liu, Q. Zhou, M. W. Wang, and Z. Li. "A Potentially Serious Adverse Effect of GLP-1 Receptor Agonists." *Acta Pharm Sin B* 13, no. 5 (2023): 2291–93. https://www.ncbi.nlm.nih.gov/pmc/articles/PMC10213739/.

Martini, M., P. Longo, T. Tamarin, et al. "Exploring Caloric Restriction in Inpatients with Eating Disorders: Cross-Sectional and Longitudinal Associations with Body Dissatisfaction, Body Avoidance, Clinical Factors, and Psychopathology." *Nutrients* 15, no. 15 (July 31, 2023): 3409. DOI: 10.3390/nu15153409. PMID: 37571346; PMCID: PMC10420884.

Marzuca-Nassr, Gabriel N., Andrea Alegría-Molina, Yuri SanMartín-Calísto, et al. "Muscle Mass and Strength Gains Following Resistance Exercise Training in Older Adults 65–75 Years and Older Adults Above 85 Years." *Int J Sport Nutr Exerc Metab* 34, no. 1 (2023): 11–19. DOI: 10.1123/ijsnem.2023–0087.

Rodriguez, P. J., B. M. Goodwin Cartwright, S. Gratzl, et al. "Semaglutide vs. Tirzepatide for Weight Loss in Adults with Overweight or Obesity." *JAMA Intern Med* 184, no. 9 (2024): 1056–64. https://www.ncbi.nlm.nih.gov/pmc/articles/PMC11231910/.

Schoenfeld, Brad J. "The Mechanisms of Muscle Hypertrophy and Their Application to Resistance Training." *J Strength Cond Res* 24, no. 10 (2010): 2857–72. DOI: 10.1519/JSC.0b013e3181e840f3.

Silverii, Giovanni A., Matteo Monami, Marco Gallo, et al. "Glucagon-Like Peptide-1 Receptor Agonists and Risk of Thyroid Cancer: A Systematic Review and Meta-analysis of Randomized Controlled Trials." *Diabetes Obes Metab* 26, no. 3 (2024): 891–900. DOI: 10.1111/dom.15382.

Soligard, Torbjørn, Martin Schwellnus, Juan-Manuel Alonso, et al. "How Much Is Too Much? (Part 1): International Olympic Committee Consensus Statement on Load in Sport and Risk of Injury." *Br J Sports Med* 50, no. 17 (2016): 1030–41. DOI: 10.1136/bjsports-2016-096581.

Sorice-Virk, Sarah. "Beyond the Weight Loss: Implementing GLP-1 Agonists Safely and Effectively." Lecture presented at Ninety-Third Plastic Surgery, San Diego, CA, September 26–29, 2024.

Terhune, Chad. "Exclusive: Most Patients Stop Using Wegovy, Ozempic for Weight Loss Within Two Years." Reuters, July 10, 2024. https://www.reuters.com/business/healthcare-pharmaceuticals/most-patients-stop-using-wegovy-ozempic-weight-loss-within-two-years-analysis-2024–07–10/.

Thompson, Caroline A., and Til Stürmer. "Putting GLP-1 RAs and Thyroid Cancer in Context: Additional Evidence and Remaining Doubts." *Diabetes Care* 46, no. 2 (2023): 249–51. DOI: 10.2337/dci22–0052.

Tinsley, Grant. "Obesity Treatment and Body Composition." Lecture presented at the Thirty-Seventh Annual Blackborn Course in Obesity Medicine: Treating Obesity 2024, Boston, MA, June 10–13, 2024.

Tsai, Adam Gilden, and Thomas A. Wadden. "The Evolution of Very-Low-Calorie Diets: An Update and Meta-analysis." *Obesity* 14, no. 8 (2006): 1283–93.

Tucker, Todd. *The Great Starvation Experiment: Ancel Keys and the Men Who Starved for Science.* University of Minnesota Press, 2007.

Wang, Z., Z. Ying, A. Bosy-Westphal, et al. "Specific Metabolic Rates of Major Organs and Tissues Across Adulthood: Evaluation by Mechanistic Model of Resting Energy Expenditure." *Am J Clin Nutr* 92, no. 6 (December 2010): 1369–77. DOI: 10.3945/ajcn.2010.29885. Epub October 20, 2010. PMID: 20962155; PMCID: PMC2980962.

Wing, R. R., K. Strohacker, and J. McCaffery. "Long-Term Hormonal Adaptions to Weight Loss." *N Eng J Med* 366, no. 4 (2012): 381.

Interviews and Correspondence with the Author

Dennis, Kim (September 2024).

Gaudiani, Jennifer (August 2024).

Jacoby, Wendy (September 2024).

Kanu, Ernest (August 2024).

Plutzky, Jorge (November 2024).

Skibicka, Karolina (August 2024).

Notes

146 **"we would suspect":** Chomko, "Protocol in Practice—Standing Orders for RD/RN Management of GLP-1/GIP Receptor Agonist."

147 **reported a reduction:** Christensen, "Dietary Intake by Patients Taking GLP-1 and Dual GIP/GLP-1 Receptor Agonists."

147 **In another study:** Friedrichsen, "The Effect of Semaglutide 2.4 mg Once Weekly on Energy Intake, Appetite, Control of Eating, and Gastric Emptying in Adults with Obesity."

147 **being treated for anorexia:** Martini et al., "Exploring Caloric Restriction in Inpatients with Eating Disorders: Cross-Sectional and Longitudinal Associations with Body Dissatisfaction, Body Avoidance, Clinical Factors, and Psychopathology."

147 **nutritional needs, according to US:** US Department of Agriculture and US Department of Health and Human Services, *Dietary Guidelines for Americans, 2020–2025*.

147 **Minnesota Starvation Experiment:** Kalm and Semba, "They Starved So That Others Be Better Fed"; Tucker, *The Great Starvation Experiment*; Keys, *The Biology of Human Starvation*.

147 **At a conference:** Almandoz, "Practical Aspects of Using Anti-obesity Medications."

149 **an expert in eating disorders:** Author interview with Dennis, September 2024.

149 **euglycemic ketoacidosis:** Kanu et al., "Euglycemic Ketoacidosis After the Addition of Glucagon-Like Peptide-1 Receptor Agonist."

149 **forty-four-year-old diabetic:** Kanu et al., "Euglycemic Ketoacidosis After the Addition of Glucagon-Like Peptide-1 Receptor Agonist."

150 **In their published paper:** Kanu et al., "Euglycemic Ketoacidosis After the Addition of Glucagon-Like Peptide-1 Receptor Agonist."

150 **"I suspect that we":** Author interview with Kanu, August 2024.

150 **bump in pancreatic enzymes:** Albrechtsen, "Glucagon-Like Peptide 1 Receptor Signaling in Acinar Cells Causes Growth-Dependent Release of Pancreatic Enzymes."

150 **increased risk of gallstones:** He et al., "Association of Glucagon-Like Peptide-1 Receptor Agonist Use with Risk of Gallbladder and Biliary Diseases."

150 **nonarteritic anterior ischemic optic neuropathy:** Hathaway et al., "Risk of Nonarteritic Anterior Ischemic Optic Neuropathy in Patients Prescribed Semaglutide."

150 **telogen effluvium:** Author interview with Jacoby, September 2024.

151 **"At this time":** Amna Hussain, at Novo Nordisk, letter to author, June 27, 2023.

151 **drugs and chills:** Author interview with Skibicka, August 2024.

151 **could be an early:** Author interview with Gaudiani, August 2024.

152 **40% of the weight:** Tinsley, "Obesity Treatment and Body Composition."

152 **for maintenance:** Wang et al., "Specific Metabolic Rates of Major Organs and Tissues Across Adulthood."

153 **found an evidence-based:** Baraki et al., "Practical Guidelines for Implementing a Strength Training Program for Adults."

154 **Yet that seemingly small:** Schoenfeld, "The Mechanisms of Muscle Hypertrophy and Their Application to Resistance Training."

154 **strength training is less:** Keogh and Winwood, "The Epidemiology of Injuries Across the Weight-Training Sports."

154 **using weights that:** Soligard et al., "How Much Is Too Much?"

155 **Older people are:** Marzuca-Nassr et al., "Muscle Mass and Strength Gains Following Resistance Exercise Training in Older Adults 65–75 Years and Older Adults Above 85 Years."

16: The Path Toward Healthy Eating

Sources
Works Referenced

Aggarwal, Monica, Stephen Devries, Andrew M. Freeman, et al. "The Deficit of Nutrition Education of Physicians." *American Journal of Medicine* 131, no. 4 (April 2018): 339–45. doi 10.1016/j.amjmed.2017.11.036.

Aguilera, José Miguel. "The Food Matrix: Implications in Processing, Nutrition and Health." *Crit Rev Food Sci* 59, no. 22 (2019): 3612–29. DOI: 10.1080/10408398.2018.1502743.

Almandoz, Jaime P., Thomas A. Wadden, Colleen Tewksbury, et al. "Nutritional Considerations with Antiobesity Medications." *Obesity* (Silver Spring, MD) 32, no. 9 (2024): 1613–31. DOI: 10.1002/oby.24067.

Anderson, James W., Pat Baird, Richard H. Davis Jr., et al. "Health Benefits of Dietary Fiber." *Nutr Rev* 67, no. 4 (April 2009): 188–205. doi 10.1111/j.1753–4887.2009.00189.x.

Annie E. Casey Foundation. "Communities with Limited Food Access in the United States." August 4, 2024. https://www.aecf.org/blog/communities-with-limited-food-access-in-the-united-states.

Ard, Jamy, Angela Fitch, Sharon Fruh, and Lawrence Herman. "Weight Loss and Maintenance Related to the Mechanism of Action of Glucagon-Like Peptide 1 Receptor Agonists." *Adv Ther* 38, no. 6 (June 2021): 2821–39. DOI: 10.1007/s12325-021-01710-0.

Barbagallo, M., and L. J. Dominguez. "Magnesium and Aging." *Current Pharm Des* 16, no. 7 (2010): 832–39. DOI: 10.2174/138161210790883679.

Bays, Harold. "Role of Nutrition Intervention in the Age of Highly Effective Antiobesity Medications." Lecture presented at Obesity Week 2024 by the Obesity Society, Atlanta, GA, November 4–7, 2024.

Benton, David, and Hayley A. Young. "Reducing Calorie Intake May Not Help You Lose Body Weight." *Perspect Psychol Sci* 12, no. 5 (September 2017): 703–14. DOI: 10.1177/1745691617690878.

Burt, Kate. "The Whiteness of the Mediterranean Diet: A Historical, Sociopolitical, and Dietary Analysis Using Critical Race Theory." *J Critical Dietetics* 5, no. 2 (2021): 41–52.

Capuano, Edoardo, and Anja E. M. Janssen. "Food Matrix and Macronutrient Digestion." *Annu Rev Food Sci Technol* 12, no. 1 (2021): 193–212. https://doi.org/10.1146/annurev-food-032519-051646.

Cooperman, Tod. "Multivitamin and Multimineral Supplements Review." ConsumerLab.com. Updated October 24, 2024. https://www.consumerlab.com/reviews/multivitamin-review-comparisons/multivitamins/.

Cornell University. "Lactose Intolerance Linked to Ancestral Environment." *ScienceDaily*, June 2, 2005. www.sciencedaily.com/releases/2005/06/050602012109.htm.

Craig, Winston J., Ann Reed Mangels, Ujué Fresán, et al. "The Safe and Effective Use of Plant-Based Diets with Guidelines for Health Professionals." *Nutrients* 13, no. 11 (November 2021): 4144. DOI: 10.3390/nu13114144.

Damms-Machado, Antje, Gesine Weser, and Stephan C. Bischoff. "Micronutrient Deficiency in Obese Subjects Undergoing Low Calorie Diet." *Nutr J* 11, no. 34 (2012). DOI: 10.1186/1475–2891–11–34.

Da Poian, Andrea T., Tatiana El-Bacha, and Mauricio R. M. P. Luz. "Nutrient Utilization in Humans: Metabolism Pathways." *Nature Ed* 3, no. 9 (2010): 11. https://www.nature.com/scitable/topicpage/nutrient-utilization-in-humans-metabolism-pathways-14234029/.

de Jesus, Janet M. "2025 Dietary Guidelines Advisory Committee: Meeting 6, Day 2." Virtual lecture presented by the National Institutes of Health, September 26, 2024. https://videocast.nih.gov/watch=55079.

Department of Health and Aged Care. "How Are Vitamins Regulated in Australia?" Australian Government, February 13, 2019. https://www.tga.gov.au/news/blog/how-are-vitamins-regulated-australia.

Despain, David, and Brenda L. Hoffman. "Optimizing Nutrition, Diet, and Lifestyle Communication in GLP-1 Medication Therapy for Weight Management: A Qualitative Research Study with Registered Dietitians." *Obes Pillars* 12 (October 2024): 100–143. DOI: 10.1016/j.obpill.2024.100143.

Devahastin, Sakamon, ed. *Food Microstructure and Its Relationship with Quality and Stability.* Elsevier, 2018.

Drake, Victoria. "Micronutrient Inadequacies in the US Population: An Overview." Linus Pauling Institute at Oregon State University, November 2017. Reviewed by Balz Frei, March 2018. https://lpi.oregonstate.edu/mic/micronutrient-inadequacies/overview.

Fang, Zhe, Sinara L. Rossato, Dong Hang, et al. "Association of Ultra-processed Food Consumption with All Cause and Cause Specific Mortality: Population Based Cohort Study." *Br Med J (Clin Res Ed)* 385 (2024): e078476. DOI: 10.1136/bmj-2023–078476.

Forde, Ciarán G., and Kees de Graaf. "Influence of Sensory Properties in Moderating Eating Behaviors and Food Intake." *Front Nutr* 21, no. 9 (February 2022): 841–44. DOI: 10.3389/fnut.2022.841444.

Fuhrman, Joel, and Robert B. Phillips. *Fast Food Genocide: How Processed Food Is Killing Us and What We Can Do About It.* HarperOne, 2017.

Gardner, Christopher D., John F. Trepanowski, Del Gobbo, et al. "Effect of Low-Fat vs. Low-Carbohydrate Diet on 12-Month Weight Loss in Overweight Adults and the Association with Genotype Pattern or Insulin Secretion: The DIETFITS Randomized Clinical Trial." *JAMA* 319, no. 7 (2018): 667–79. DOI: 10.1001/jama.2018.0245.

Grassby, Terri, Giuseppina Mandalari Grundy, Cathrina H. Edwards, et al. "In Vitro and In Vivo Modeling of Lipid Bioaccessibility and Digestion from Almond Muffins: The Importance of the Cell-Wall Barrier Mechanism." *J Funct Foods* 37 (2017): 263–71. DOI: 10.1016/j.jff.2017.07.046.

Holick, Michael F., and Tai C. Chen. "Vitamin D Deficiency: A Worldwide Problem with Health Consequences." *Am J Clin Nutr* 87, no. 4 (2008): 1080S–1086S. DOI: 10.1093/ajcn/87.4.1080S.

Huppertz, Thom, Blerina Shkembi, Lea Brader, and Jan Geurts. "Dairy Matrix Effects: Physicochemical Properties Underlying a Multifaceted Paradigm." *Nutrients* 16, no. 7 (2024): 943. DOI: 10.3390/nu16070943.

Johnston, Bradley C., Steve Kanters, Kristofer Bandayrel, et al. "Comparison of Weight Loss Among Named Diet Programs in Overweight and Obese Adults: A Meta-analysis." *JAMA* 312, no. 9 (2014): 923–33. DOI: 10.1001/jama.2014.10397.

Ju, Se-Young. "Changes in Eating-Out Frequency According to Sociodemographic Characteristics and Nutrient Intakes Among Korean Adults." *Iran J Pub Health* 49, no. 1 (January 2020): 46–55.

Kalab, Miloslav. "Microstructure of Dairy Foods." *J Dairy Sci* 68, no. 12 (December 1985): 3234–48. DOI: 10.3168/jds.S0022–0302(85)81232–7.

Kessler, David. *Fast Carbs, Slow Carbs*. HarperCollins, 2020.

Kessler, David A. *Your Food Is Fooling You: How Your Brain Is Hijacked by Sugar, Fat, and Salt*. Roaring Brook, 2013.

Khodayari, Shadhayegh, Omid Sadeghi, Maryam Safabahksh, and Hassan Mozaffari Khosravi. "Meat Consumption and the Risk of General and Central Obesity: The Shahedieh Study." *BMC Res Notes* 15, no. 1 (November 2022): 339. DOI: 10.1186/s13104-022-06235–5.

Klurfeld, David M. "The Whole Food Beef Matrix Is More Than the Sum of Its Parts." *Crit Rev Food Sci* 64, no. 14 (2024): 4523–31.

LaFata, E. M., Kelly C. Allison, Janet Audrain-McGovern, and Evan M. Forman. "Ultra-processed Food Addiction: A Research Update." *Current Obesity Reports* 13 (2024): 214–23. https://doi.org/10.1007/s13679-024-00569-w.

Leroy, Frédéric, Nick W. Smith, Adegbola T. Adesogan, et al. "The Role of Meat in the Human Diet: Evolutionary Aspects and Nutritional Value." *Anim Front* 13, no. 2 (2023): 11–18. DOI: 10.1093/af/vfac093.

Levine, Allen S., and Job Ubbink. "Ultra-processed Foods: Processing versus Formulation." *Obes Sci Prac* 9, no. 4 (January 2023): 435–39. DOI: 10.1002/osp4.657.

Li, Yuhan, Yanping Li, Xiao Gu, et al. "A Prospective Study of Long-Term Red Meat Intake, Risk of Dementia, and Cognitive Function in US Adults." Alzheimer's Association International Conference, ALZ, 2024.

Mackie, Alan. "Food: More Than the Sum of Its Parts." *Curr Opin Food Sci* 16 (2017): 120–24. https://doi.org/10.1016/j.cofs.2017.07.004.

Martin, Corby. "Effects of Tirzepatide on Eating Behavior: A Phase 1 Study in People Living with Obesity." Lecture presented at Obesity Week 2023 by the Obesity Society, Dallas, TX, October 14–17, 2023.

Masoodi, Ameen. "Who Can Take GLP-1 Medications for Weight Loss? Exploring Eligibility and Safety." Noom, November 22, 2024. https://www.noom.com/blog/weight-management/who-can-take-glp-1-medications-for-weight-loss-exploring-eligibility-and-safety/.

Medlineplus. "Magnesium in Diet." National Library of Medicine, January 19, 2023. https://medlineplus.gov/ency/article/002423.htm.

Mendoza, Kenny, Stephanie A. Smith-Warner, Sinara Laurini Rossato, et al. "Ultra-processed Foods and Cardiovascular Disease: Analysis of Three Large US Prospective Cohorts and a Systematic Review and Meta-analysis of Prospective Cohort Studies." *Lancet Reg Health Am* 37 (September 2024): 100859. DOI: 10.1016/j.lana.2024.100859.

Mysonhimer, Annemarie R., and Hannah D. Holscher. "Gastrointestinal Effects and Tolerance of Nondigestible Carbohydrate Consumption." *Adv Nutr* 13, no. 6 (December 2022): 2237–76. DOI: 10.1093/advances/nmac094.

Onvani, Shokouh, Fahimeh Haghighatdoost, Pamela J. Surkan, and Leila Azadbakht. "Dairy Products, Satiety, and Food Intake: A Meta-analysis of Clinical Trials." *Clin Nutr* 36, no. 2 (April 2017): 389–98. DOI: 10.1016/j.clnu.2016.01.017.

Pollan, Michael. *Cooked: A Natural History of Transformation*. Penguin Books, 2014.

Pomeranz, Jennifer L., Jerold R. Mande, and Dariush Mozaffarian. "U.S. Policies Addressing Ultraprocessed Foods, 1980–2022." *Am J Prev Med* 65, no. 6 (December 2023): 1134–41. DOI: 10.1016/j.amepre.2023.07.006.

Popoviciu, Mihaela-Simona, Lorena Paduraru, Galal Yahya, Kamel Metwally, and Simona Cavalu. "Emerging Role of GLP-1 Agonists in Obesity: A Comprehensive Review of Randomised Controlled Trials." *Int J Mol Sci* 24, no. 13 (May 2023): 10449. https://doi.org/10.3390/ijms241310449.

Qaid, Mohammed M., and Khalid A. Abdoun. "Safety and Concerns of Hormonal Application in Farm Animal Production: A Review." *J Appl Animal Res* 50 no. 1 (June 2022): 426–39. https://doi.org/10.1080/09712119.2022.2089149.

Sen, Mousumi. *Food Chemistry: The Role of Additives, Preservatives, and Adulteration.* Wiley, 2021.

Shkembi, Blerina, and Thom Huppertz. "Calcium Absorption from Food Products: Food Matrix Effects." *Nutrients* 14, no. 1 (2021): 180. DOI: 10.3390/nu14010180.

Simsek, Miray, and Kristin Whitney. "Examination of Primary and Secondary Metabolites Associated with a Plant-Based Diet and Their Impact on Human Health." *Foods* 13, no. 7 (2024): 1020. https://doi.org/10.3390/foods13071020.

Skorbiansky, Sharon Raszap, Andrea Carlson, and Ashley Spalding. "Rising Consumer Demand Reshapes Landscape for U.S. Organic Farmers." US Department of Agriculture, Economic Research Service, November 14, 2023. https://www.ers.usda.gov/amber-waves/2023/november/rising-consumer-demand-reshapes-landscape-for-u-s-organic-farmers/.

Sparks, J. R., Erin E. Kishman, Mark A. Karzynski, et al. "Glycemic Variability: Importance, Relationship with Physical Activity, and the Influence of Exercise." *Sports Med Health Sci* 3, no. 4 (October 2021): 183–93. DOI: 10.1016/j.smhs.2021.09.004.

State of California, Health and Human Services Agency, Department of Health Care Services. "California Advancing and Innovating Medi-Cal (CalAIM) Proposal." January 2021. https://www.dhcs.ca.gov/provgovpart/Documents/CalAIM-Proposal-Updated-02172021.pdf.

Teo, Pey Sze, Rob M. van Dam, Clare Whitton, et al. "Consumption of Foods with Higher Energy Intake Rates Is Associated with Greater Energy Intake, Adiposity, and Cardiovascular Risk Factors in Adults." *J Nutr* 151, no. 2 (2021): 370–78. DOI: 10.1093/jn/nxaa344.

Umashanker, Dr. Devika. "Dr. Devika Umashanker: Why Diet, Exercise Isn't a Weight-Loss Formula for Everyone." Hartford Hospital Healthcare, January 22, 2018. https://hartfordhospital.org/about-hh/news-center/news-detail?articleId=12150.

US Department of Agriculture and US Department of Health and Human Services. *Dietary Guidelines for Americans, 2020–2025.* Ninth edition. USDA and US HHS, 2020. https://www.dietaryguidelines.gov/.

US Food and Drug Administration. "FDA Adverse Event Reporting System (FAERS) Public Dashboard." https://www.fda.gov/drugs/fdas-adverse-event-reporting-system-faers/fda-adverse-event-reporting-system-faers-public-dashboard.

US Food and Drug Administration. "Questions and Answers on Dietary Supplements." February 21, 2024. https://www.fda.gov/food/information-consumers-using-dietary-supplements/questions-and-answers-dietary-supplements.

Wadden, Thomas, Sheri Volger, David B. Sarwer, et al. "A Two-Year Randomized Trial of Obesity Treatment in Primary Care Practice." *N Eng J Med* 365, no. 21 (November 2011): 1969–79.

Wan, Zifan, Sucheta Khubber, Madhuresh Dwivedi, and N. N. Misra. "Strategies for Lowering the Added Sugar in Yogurts." *Food Chem* 15 (May 2021): 344. DOI: 10.1016/j.foodchem.2020.128573.

Weaver, C. M. "Calcium Requirements of Physically Active People." *Am J Clin Nutr* 72, no. 2 Suppl. (2000): 579S–584S. DOI: 10.1093/ajcn/72.2.579S.

Wharton, S., R. L. Batterham, M. Bhatta, et al. "Two-Year Effect of Semaglutide 2.4 mg on Control of Eating in Adults with Overweight/Obesity: STEP 5." *Obesity* (Silver Spring, MD) 31, no. 3 (March 2023): 703–15. DOI: 10.1002/oby.23673. Epub January 18, 2023. PMID: 36655300.

Zhang, Yin, and Edward L. Giovannucci. "Ultra-processed Foods and Health: A Comprehensive Review." *Crit Rev Food Sci Nutr* 63, no. 31 (2023): 10836–48. DOI: 10.1080/10408398.2022.2084359.

Zhou, Hualu, Yuying Hu, Yunbing Tan, Zhiyun Zhang, and David Julian McClements. "Digestibility and Gastrointestinal Fate of Meat Versus Plant-Based Meat Analogs: An In Vitro Comparison." *Food Chem* 364 (2021): 130439. DOI: 10.1016/j.foodchem.2021.130439.

Interviews and Correspondence with the Author

Baker, Christian (September 2024).

Bloomgarden, Eve (September 2024).

Cooperman, Tod (September 2024).

Hu, Frank (December 2023).

Kushner, Robert (April 2024).

Lazarus, Ethan (April 2024).

Papuckovski, Marko (September 2024).

Plutzky, Jorge (November 2024).

Wharton, Sean (May 2024).

Wyatt, Holly (January 2024).

Notes

157 **"We actually showed it clinically":** Author interview with Wharton, May 2024.

157 **The authors found:** Wharton, "Two-Year Effect of Semaglutide 2.4 mg on Control of Eating."

157 **examined the impact:** Martin, "Effects of Tirzepatide on Eating Behavior."

158 **that people taking:** Bays, "Role of Nutrition Intervention in the Age of Highly Effective Anti-obesity Medications."

160 **More than half:** Holick et al., "Vitamin D Deficiency."

160 **30 to 50%:** Weaver, "Calcium Requirements of Physically Active People."

160 **30% are deficient:** Weaver, "Calcium Requirements of Physically Active People."

160 **20 to 30% have:** Barbagallo and Dominguez, "Magnesium and Aging."

161 **4 to 7% weight loss:** Johnston et al., "Comparison of Weight Loss Among Named Diet Programs in Overweight and Obese Adults."

161 **GLP-1s are unlikely to be a permanent solution:** Ard et al., "Weight Loss and Maintenance Related to the Mechanism of Action of Glucagon-Like Peptide 1 Receptor Agonists."

161 **nutrition therapy can add:** Despain and Hoffman, "Optimizing Nutrition, Diet, and Lifestyle Communication in GLP-1 Medication Therapy."

162 **glycemic variability:** Sparks et al., "Glycemic Variability."

162 **their chemical trickery is hidden:** Fuhrman and Phillips, *Fast Food Genocide.*

164 **the food industry has gone well beyond:** Kessler, *Your Food Is Fooling You.*

164 **rich in phytic acid:** Leroy et al., "The Role of Meat in the Human Diet."

165 **entrapped plant proteins:** Zhou et al., "Digestibility and Gastrointestinal Fate of Meat Versus Plant-Based Meat Analogs."

165 **Slow digestion:** Grassby et al., "In Vitro and In Vivo Modeling of Lipid Bioaccessibility and Digestion from Almond Muffins."

165 **rich in starches:** Capuano and Janssen, "Food Matrix and Macronutrient Digestion."

165 **Soluble fibers:** Mackie, "Food."

165 **increasing our feelings of fullness:** Anderson et al., "Health Benefits of Dietary Fiber."

166 **Animal proteins:** Zhou et al., "Digestibility and Gastrointestinal Fate of Meat Versus Plant-Based Meat Analogs."

166 **Unlike plant proteins:** Klurfeld, "The Whole Food Beef Matrix Is More Than the Sum of Its Parts."

166 **In animal tissue:** Klurfeld, "The Whole Food Beef Matrix Is More Than the Sum of Its Parts."

166 **The iron in meat:** Leroy et al., "The Role of Meat in the Human Diet."

167 **increased overall risk:** Fang et al., "Association of Ultra-processed Food Consumption with All Cause and Cause Specific Mortality."

167 **processed meats:** Li et al., "A Prospective Study of Long-Term Red Meat Intake, Risk of Dementia, and Cognitive Function in US Adults."

167 **examined ten categories:** Mendoza et al., "Ultra-processed Foods and Cardiovascular Disease: Analysis."

167 **Whey proteins:** Capuano and Janssen, "Food Matrix and Macronutrient Digestion."

167 **proteins form a gel:** Mackie, "Food."

167 **dairy products like yogurt lead to:** Onvani et al., "Dairy Products, Satiety and Food Intake."

167 **Solid and semi-solid:** Aguilera, "The Food Matrix."

168 **The dispersed fat droplets:** Mackie, "Food."

168 **condition is often linked to ancestry:** Cornell University, "Lactose Intolerance Linked to Ancestral Environment."

168 **Lactose can enhance:** Shkembi and Huppertz, "Calcium Absorption from Food Products."

168 **calcium and phosphorus:** Huppertz et al., "Dairy Matrix Effects."

170 **foundations of a healthy diet:** Author interview with Hu, December 2023.

17: The Role of Insulin Resistance

Sources
Works Referenced

Astrup, Arne. "Precision Dietary Management of Obesity and Type 2 Diabetes." Great Debates in Nutrition, Jean Mayer USDA Human Nutrition Research Center on Aging, February 13, 2023.

Bojsen-Møller, Kirstine N., Annemarie Lundsgaard, Sten Madsbad, et al. "Hepatic Insulin Clearance in Regulation of Systemic Insulin Concentrations—Role of Carbohydrate and Energy Availability." *J Diabetes* 67, no. 11 (2018): 2129–36. https://doi.org/10.2337/db18–0539.

Chow, Lisa. "Possibilities of Fasting in Patients with Diabetes." Presented at the American Diabetes Association Eighty-Fourth Scientific Sessions, June 22, 2024.

DiMaggio, D. M., I. Abersone, and A. F. Porto. "Infant Consumption of 100% Lactose-Based and Reduced Lactose Infant Formula in the United States: Review of NHANES Data from 1999 to 2020." *J Pediatr Gastroenterol Nutr* 29, no. 5 (November 2024): 10171023. DOI: 10.1002/jpn3.12292. Epub June 27, 2024. PMID: 38934419.

Gardner, Christopher D., John F. Trepanowski, Liana C. Del Gobbo, et al. "Effect of Low-Fat vs. Low-Carbohydrate Diet on 12-Month Weight Loss in Overweight Adults and the Association with Genotype Pattern or Insulin Secretion: The DIETFITS Randomized Clinical Trial." *JAMA* 319, no. 7 (2018): 667–79. DOI: 10.1001/jama.2018.0245.

Garr Barry, Valene, Mariah Stewart, Taraneh Soleymani, Renee A. Desmond, Amy M. Goss, and Barbara A. Gower. "Greater Loss of Central Adiposity from Low-Carbohydrate versus Low-Fat Diet in Middle-Aged Adults with Overweight and Obesity." *Nutrients* 13, no. 2 (2021): 475.

Gołąbek, Katarzyna Daria, and Bożena Regulska-Ilow. "Dietary Support in Insulin Resistance: An Overview of Current Scientific Reports." *Adv Clin Exp Med* 28, no. 11 (2019): 1577–85.

Gower, Barbara. "Beneficial Effects of Carbohydrate Restriction in Patients with Type 2 Diabetes Can Be Traced to Changes in Hepatic Metabolism." Lecture presented at Nutrition 2024 by the American Society for Nutrition, Chicago, IL, June 29–July 2, 2024.

Gower, Barbara. "Hepatic Ketone Production as the Governing Factor in Determining Fatty Liver and Type 2 Diabetes." Lecture presented at Nutrition 2024 by the American Society for Nutrition, Chicago, IL, June 29–July 2, 2024.

Gower, Barbara A., and Amy M. Goss. "A Lower-Carbohydrate, Higher-Fat Diet Reduces Abdominal and Intermuscular Fat and Increases Insulin Sensitivity in Adults at Risk of Type 2 Diabetes." *J Nutr* 145, no. 1 (2015): 177S–183S.

HCPLive. "Roy Taylor, MD: Using Personal Fat Thresholds to Reach Type 2 Diabetes Remission." June 5, 2022. https://www.hcplive.com/view/roy-taylor-personal-fat-thresholds-type-2-diabetes-remission.

Jamshed, Humaira, Felicia L. Steger, David R. Bryan, et al. "Effectiveness of Early Time-Restricted Eating for Weight Loss, Fat Loss, and Cardiometabolic Health in Adults with Obesity: A Randomized Clinical Trial." *JAMA Intern Med* 182, no. 9 (2022): 953–62.

Janssen, Joseph A. M. J. L. "Overnutrition, Hyperinsulinemia and Ectopic Fat: It Is Time for a Paradigm Shift in the Management of Type 2 Diabetes." *Int J Mol Sci* 25, no. 10 (2024): 5488.

Kahleova, Hana, Kitt Falk Petersen, Gerald I. Shulman, et al. "Effect of a Low-Fat Vegan

Diet on Body Weight, Insulin Sensitivity, Postprandial Metabolism, and Intramyocellular and Hepatocellular Lipid Levels in Overweight Adults: A Randomized Clinical Trial." *JAMA Netw Open* 3, no. 11 (2020): e2025454.

Kweh, Frederick A., Carlos R. Sulsona, Jennifer L. Miller, and Daniel J. Driscoll. "Hyperinsulinemia Is a Probable Trigger for Weight Gain and Hyperphagia in Individuals with Prader-Willi Syndrome." *Obes Sci Pract* 9, no. 4 (2023): 383–94. DOI: 10.1002/osp4.663.

Lundsgaard, Annemarie, Kirstine Nyvold Bojsen-Møller, and Bente Kiens. "Dietary Regulation of Hepatic Triacylglycerol Content: The Role of Eucaloric Carbohydrate Restriction with Fat or Protein Replacement." *Adv Nutr* 14, no. 6 (2023): 1359–73. DOI: 10.1016/j.advnut.2023.08.005.

Magkos, Faidon, Mads F. Hjorth, and Arne Astrup. "Diet and Exercise in the Prevention and Treatment of Type 2 Diabetes Mellitus." *Nat Rev Endocrinol* 16, no. 10 (2020): 545–55.

Miller, Jennifer L., Christy H. Lynn, Danielle C. Driscoll, et al. "Nutritional Phases in Prader-Willi Syndrome." *Am J Med Genet Part A* 155A, no. 5 (2011): 1040–49. DOI: 10.1002/ajmg.a.33951.

Mishra, Amrendra, and Valter D. Longo. "Fasting and Fasting Mimicking Diets in Obesity and Cardiometabolic Disease Prevention and Treatment." *Phys Med Rehabil Clin N Am* 33, no. 3 (2022): 699–717.

Mosley, Michael, and Mimi Spencer. *The Fast Diet.* Short Books, 2014.

Parcha, Vibhu, Brittain Heindl, Rajat Kalra, Peng Li, Barbara Gower, Garima Arora, and Pankaj Arora. "Insulin Resistance and Cardiometabolic Risk Profile Among Nondiabetic American Young Adults: Insights from NHANES." *J Clin Endocrinol Metab* 107, no. 1 (January 1, 2022): e25–e37. https://doi.org/10.1210/clinem/dgab645.

Peterson, Courtney. "Can Time-Restricted Eating Inhibit the Progression of Prediabetes?" Lecture presented at the American Diabetes Association Eighty-Fourth Scientific Sessions, Orlando, FL, June 22, 2024.

Ravussin, Eric. "Intermittent Fasting and Time Restrictive Feeding: Is It Superior to Caloric Restriction?" International Congress on Obesity, São Paulo, Brazil, June 27, 2024.

Spartano, Nicole. "I Would NOT Recommend Intermittent Fasting to Your Patients." American Diabetes Association Eighty-Third Scientific Sessions, Philadelphia, PA, June 22, 2023.

Taylor, Roy, Ambady Ramachandran, William S. Yancy, and Nita G. Forouhi. "Nutritional Basis of Type 2 Diabetes Remission." *BMI* 374 (2021).

US Centers for Disease Control and Prevention. "Fast Facts: Health and Economic Costs of Chronic Conditions." US Department of Health and Human Services, July 12, 2024. https://www.cdc.gov/chronic-disease/data-research/facts-stats/index.html.

Wang, L., E. Martínez Steele, M. Du, et al. "Trends in Consumption of Ultraprocessed Foods Among US Youths Aged 2–19 Years, 1999–2018." *JAMA* 326, no. 6 (2021): 519–30. DOI:10.1001/jama.2021.10238.

Young, B. E., M. Tang, K. Griese, et al. "Consumption of a Corn-Sugar Based Infant Formula Is Associated with Higher C-peptide Secretion Compared to Lactose Based Formula Among Exclusively Formula Fed Infants." *FASEB J* 30 (2016): 673.7–673.7. https://doi.org/10.1096/fasebj.30.1_supplement.673.7.

Yu, Z., F. Nan, L. Y. Wang, H. Jiang, W. Chen, and J. Jiang. "Effects of High-Protein Diet on Glycemic Control, Insulin Resistance, and Blood Pressure in Type 2 Diabetes: A Systematic Review and Meta-analysis of Randomized Controlled Trials." *Clin Nutr* 39, no. 6 (2020): 1724–34.

Interviews and Correspondence with the Author

Cantley, Lewis (January 2025).

Driscoll, Daniel (January 2024; June 2024).

Notes

173   **the body shifts:** Gower and Goss, "A Lower-Carbohydrate, Higher-Fat Diet Reduces Abdominal and Intermuscular Fat and Increases Insulin Sensitivity in Adults at Risk of Type 2 Diabetes."

173   **consistent reduction:** HCPLive, "Roy Taylor, MD."

174   **high carbohydrate consumption:** Bojsen-Møller et al., "Hepatic Insulin Clearance in Regulation of Systemic Insulin Concentrations."

174   **demonstrate that diets:** Lundsgaard et al., "Dietary Regulation of Hepatic Triacylglycerol Content."

174   **reduce insulin resistance:** Yu et al., "Effects of High-Protein Diet on Glycemic Control, Insulin Resistance, and Blood Pressure in Type 2 Diabetes."

175   **several distinct nutritional phases:** Miller et al., "Nutritional Phases in Prader-Willi Syndrome."

175   **"a remarkable syndrome":** Author interviews with Driscoll, January 2024 and June 2024.

176   **less than 10%:** O'Hearn et al., "Trends and Disparities in Cardiometabolic Health Among US Adults."

176   **consume 67% of their calories:** Wang et al., "Trends in Consumption of Ultraprocessed Foods Among US Youths Aged 2–19 Years."

176   **Dr. Dana DiMaggio:** DiMaggio et al., "Infant Consumption of 100% Lactose-Based and Reduced Lactose Infant Formula in the United States."

176   **Dr. Nancy Krebs:** Young et al., "Consumption of a Corn-Sugar Based Infant Formula Is Associated with Higher C-peptide Secretion."

176   **"I'm pretty convinced":** Author interview with Cantley, January 2025.

178   **reducing even a small:** Gołąbek and Regulska-Ilow, "Dietary Support in Insulin Resistance."

178   **low-fat vegan diet:** Kahleova et al., "Effect of a Low-Fat Vegan Diet on Body Weight, Insulin Sensitivity, Postprandial Metabolism, and Intramyocellular and Hepatocellular Lipid Levels in Overweight Adults."

178   **individual to maintain:** Gardner et al., "Effect of Low-Fat vs. Low-Carbohydrate Diet on 12-Month Weight Loss in Overweight Adults and the Association with Genotype Pattern or Insulin Secretion."

179   **fasting window:** Jamshed et al., "Effectiveness of Early Time-Restricted Eating for Weight Loss, Fat Loss, and Cardiometabolic Health in Adults with Obesity."

179   **"people are eating all the time":** Chow, "Possibilities of Fasting in Patients with Diabetes."

180   **body can mobilize:** Peterson, "Can Time-Restricted Eating Inhibit the Progression of Prediabetes?"

180   **Typically, it's followed:** Mishra and Longo, "Fasting and Fasting Mimicking Diets in Obesity and Cardiometabolic Disease Prevention and Treatment."

180 **"three cycles spread"**: Peterson, "Can Time-Restricted Eating Inhibit the Progression of Prediabetes?"

181 **"has a tendency toward"**: Spartano, "I Would NOT Recommend Intermittent Fasting to Your Patients."

18: Eating to Support Health

Sources
Works Referenced

Alexander, Lydia. "Lecture at Obesity Medicine 2024." May 2024, Denver, CO.

Athinarayanan, Shaminie J., Rebecca N. Adams, Britannie M. Volk, and Caroline G. P. Roberts. "Weight After Discontinuing Semaglutide and Tirzepatide in People with T2D on Carb-Restricted Therapy." SJA Obesity Week 2024, San Antonio, TX. https://onlinelibrary.wiley.com/doi/10.1002/oby.24195.

Boston Medical Center. "Haitian Epis." https://www.bmc.org/recipes/epis-haitian-seasoning-base.

Burt, Kate. "The Whiteness of the Mediterranean Diet: A Historical, Sociopolitical, and Dietary Analysis Using Critical Race Theory." *Critical Dietetics* 5, no. 2 (2021): 41–52.

CAP Profiles. "Christopher Gardner, Rehnborg Farguhar Professor." Stanford Medicine. https://med.stanford.edu/profiles/christopher-gardner.

Cena, Hellas, and Philip C. Calder. "Defining a Healthy Diet: Evidence for the Role of Contemporary Dietary Patterns in Health and Disease." *Nutrients* 12, no. 2 (January 2020): 334. DOI: 10.3390/nu12020334.

Chiavaroli, Laura, Danielle Lee, Amna Ahmed, et al. "Effect of Low Glycaemic Index or Load Dietary Patterns on Glycaemic Control and Cardiometabolic Risk Factors in Diabetes: Systematic Review and Meta-analysis of Randomised Controlled Trials." *BMJ* 374 (2021).

de Jesus, Janet M. "2025 Dietary Guidelines Advisory Committee: Meeting 6, Day 2." Virtual lecture presented by the National Institutes of Health, September 26, 2024. https://videocast.nih.gov/watch=55079.

DiNicolantonio, James J., and James O'Keefe. "The Importance of Maintaining a Low Omega-6/Omega-3 Ratio for Reducing the Risk of Autoimmune Diseases, Asthma, and Allergies." *Mo Med* 118, no. 5 (2021): 453.

Fratta Pasini, Anna Maria, and Luciano Cominacini. "Potential Benefits of Antioxidant Phytochemicals on Endogenous Antioxidants Defences in Chronic Diseases." *Antioxidants* 12, no. 4 (2023): 890.

Gardner, C. D., M. J. Landry, D. Perelman, et al. "Effect of a Ketogenic Diet Versus Mediterranean Diet on Glycated Hemoglobin in Individuals with Prediabetes and Type 2 Diabetes Mellitus: The Interventional Keto-Med Randomized Crossover Trial." *Am J Clin Nutr* 116, no. 3 (September 2, 2022): 640–52. https://doi.org/10.1093/ajcn/nqac154.

Hudson J. L., Y. Wang, R. E. Bergia III, and W. W. Campbell. "Protein Intake Greater Than the RDA Differentially Influences Whole-Body Lean Mass Responses to Purposeful Catabolic and Anabolic Stressors: A Systematic Review and Meta-analysis." *Adv Nutr* 11, no. 3 (2020): 548–58.

Khan, Safi U., Ahmad N. Lone, Muhammad Shahzeb Khan, et al. "Effect of Omega-3

Fatty Acids on Cardiovascular Outcomes: A Systematic Review and Meta-analysis." *EClinicalMedicine* 38 (2021).

Landry, Matthew J., Catherine P. Ward, Kristen M. Cunanan, et al. "Switching Diets After 6 Months Does Not Result in Renewed Weight Loss: A Secondary Analysis of a 12-Month Crossover Randomized Trial." *Sci Rep* 14, no. 1 (2024): 9865. DOI: 10.1038 /s41598-024-60547-z.

Ng, Jennifer. "Planting the Rainbow for Weight Loss." Lecture presented at the Obesity Medicine 2024 Spring Conference, Denver, CO, April 25–28, 2024.

Noakes, Tim, Tamzyn Murphy, Neville Wellington, Hassina Kajee, Jayne Bullen, Sarah Rice, and Candice Egnos. *Ketogenic: The Science of Therapeutic Carbohydrate Restriction in Human Health.* Elsevier, 2023.

O'Hearn, Meghan, Brianna N. Lauren, John B. Wong, David D. Kim, and Dariush Mozaffarian. "Trends and Disparities in Cardiometabolic Health Among US Adults, 1999– 2018." *J Am Coll Cardiol* 80, no. 2 (2022): 138–51.

Phillips, S. M., S. Chevalier, and H. J. Leidy. "Protein 'Requirements' Beyond the RDA: Implications for Optimizing Health." *Appl Physiol Nutr Metab* 41, no. 5 (2016): 565–72. [Addendum: *Appl Physiol Nutr Metab* 47, no. 5 (May 2022): 615. DOI: 10.1139/apnm -2022–0131.]

Phinney, Stephen D., and Jeff S. Volek. *The Art and Science of Low Carbohydrate Living: An Expert Guide to Making the Life-Saving Benefits of Carbohydrate Restriction Sustainable and Enjoyable.* Beyond Obesity, 2011.

Shai, Iris, Dan Schwarzfuchs, Yaakov Henkin, et al. "Weight Loss with a Low-Carbohydrate, Mediterranean, or Low-Fat Diet." *N Eng J Med* 359, no. 3 (2008): 229–41. DOI: 10.1056/NEJMoa0708681.

US Centers for Disease Control and Prevention. "Fast Facts: Health and Economic Costs of Chronic Conditions." https://www.cdc.gov/chronic-disease/data-research/facts-stats /index.html.

Interviews and Correspondence with the Author

Athinarayanan, Shaminie (November 2024).

Brand-Miller, Jennie (October 2024).

Ference, Brian (November 2024).

Ferreira, Lisa (April 2024).

Gardner, Christopher (August 2024).

Golden, Angela (April 2024).

Kushner, Robert (April 2024).

Landry, Matthew (July 2024).

Lazarus, Ethan (April 2024).

Libby, Peter (November 2024).

Ng, Jennifer (April 2024).

Nikitidis, Ioannas (August 2024).

Plutzky, Jorge (November 2024).

Westman, Eric (April 2024).

Willett, Walter (September 2024).

Notes

183 **"With the right support":** Author interview with Athinarayanan, November 2024.

184 ***quality* of carbohydrates":** Author interview with Willett, September 2024.

185 ***compared to what*":** Author interview with Gardner, August 2024.

185 **focused on the potential health:** Gardner et al., "Effect of Low-Fat vs. Low-Carbohydrate Diet on 12-Month Weight Loss in Overweight Adults and the Association with Genotype Pattern or Insulin Secretion."

185 **whether improvements in diet quality:** Gardner et al., "Effect of a Ketogenic Diet versus Mediterranean Diet on Glycated Hemoglobin in Individuals with Prediabetes and Type 2 Diabetes Mellitus."

185 **researching the optimal:** Author interview with Landry, July 2024.

186 **"There are two camps":** Author interview with Golden, April 2024.

186 **arguing that the formula:** Author interview with Westman, April 2024.

187 **Dr. Brian Ference:** Author interview with Ference, November 2024.

188 **"For most people":** Author interview with Plutzky, November 2024.

188 **"health benefits are":** Author interview with Libby, November 2024.

189 **good job of debunking:** Burt, "The Whiteness of the Mediterranean Diet."

190 **"The feeling of satiety":** Author interview with Nikitidis, August 2024.

191 **decouple energy intake from nutrition:** Alexander, "Lecture at Obesity Medicine 2024."

192 **the current RDA:** Phillips et al., "Protein 'Requirements' Beyond the RDA."

193 **Diets high in antioxidants:** Fratta Pasini and Cominacini, "Potential Benefits of Antioxidant Phytochemicals on Endogenous Antioxidants Defences in Chronic Diseases."

194 **"Plant-based is still":** Author interview with Ng, April 2024.

195 **omega-6 to omega-3:** DiNicolantonio and O'Keefe, "The Importance of Maintaining a Low Omega-6/Omega-3 Ratio for Reducing the Risk of Autoimmune Diseases, Asthma, and Allergies."

195 **A useful compensation:** Khan et al., "Effect of Omega-3 Fatty Acids on Cardiovascular Outcomes."

197 **"refined grains should not":** de Jesus, "2025 Dietary Guidelines Advisory Committee."

197 **Glycemic load:** Chiavaroli et al., "Effect of Low Glycaemic Index or Load Dietary Patterns on Glycaemic Control and Cardiometabolic Risk Factors in Diabetes."

198 **"Potatoes consistently have":** Author interview with Brand-Miller, October 2024.

19: A New Way of Viewing Behavioral Therapy

Sources
Works Referenced

Ainslie, George. "Intertemporal Bargaining in Addiction." *Front Psych* 4, no. 63 (2013): 1–5. DOI: 10.3389/fpsyt.2013.00063.

Borland, Ron. *Understanding Hard to Maintain Behaviour Change: A Dual Process Approach.* Wiley, 2014.

Brewer, Judson. "Mindfulness Training for Addictions: Has Neuroscience Revealed a Brain Hack by Which Awareness Subverts the Addictive Process?" *Curr Opin Psychol* 28 (2019): 198–203.

Burger, Kyle S. "Food Reinforcement Architecture: A Framework for Impulsive and Compulsive Overeating and Food Abuse." *Obesity* 31, no. 7 (July 2023): 1734–44. DOI: https://doi.org/10.1002/oby.23792.

Center for Weight and Eating Disorders. "Our History." Penn Psychiatry, n.d. https://www.med.upenn.edu/weight/history.html.

Cherry, Kendra. "What Is Behaviorism?" Very Well Mind, November 7, 2022. https://www.verywellmind.com/behavioral-psychology-4157183.

The Chicago School. "Any Positive Change." February 21, 2019. https://www.thechicagoschool.edu/insight/news/any-positive-change.

Christensen, E. L., I. H. Harding, K. Voigt, T. T. Chong, and A. Verdejo-Garcia. "Neural Underpinnings of Food Choice and Consumption in Obesity." *Int J Obes* (London) 46, no. 1 (January 2022): 194–201. doi: 10.1038/s41366-021-00974-4. Epub October 5, 2021. PMID: 34611286.

Dobbs, David. "Zen Gamma." *Sci Am*, April 1, 2005. https://shorturl.at/CtmNQ.

Fairburn, Christopher G. *Cognitive Behavior Therapy and Eating Disorders.* Guilford Press, 2008.

Kessler, David A. *Capture: Unraveling the Mystery of Mental Suffering.* HarperCollins, 2016.

Krause, Florian, Nikos Kogias, Martin Krentz, et al. "Self-Regulation of Stress-Related Large-Scale Brain Network Balance Using Real-Time fMRI Neurofeedback." *Neuroimage* 243 (2021): 118527. DOI: 10.1016/j.neuroimage.2021.118527.

Lembke, Anna. *Dopamine Nation: Finding Balance in the Age of Indulgence.* Penguin, 2021.

Levitz, Leonard S., and Albert J. Stunkard. "A Therapeutic Coalition for Obesity: Behavior Modification and Patient Self-help." *Am J Psych* 131, no. 4 (1974): 423–27.

Manejwala, Omar. *Craving: Why We Can't Seem to Get Enough.* Hazelden, 2013.

Michaelsen, Maren M., and Tobias Esch. "Functional Mechanisms of Health Behavior Change Techniques: A Conceptual Review." *Front Psychol* 13 (2022): 725644. https://doi.org/10.3389/fpsyg.2022.725644.

Michaelsen, Maren M., and Tobias Esch. "Motivation and Reward Mechanisms in Health Behavior Change Processes." *Brain Res* 1757 (April 15, 2021): 147309. DOI: 10.1016/j.brainres.2021.147309.

Michaelsen, Maren M., and Tobias Esch. "Understanding Health Behavior Change by Motivation and Reward Mechanisms: A Review of the Literature." *Front Behav Neurosci* 17 (2023): 1151918. DOI: 10.3389/fnbeh.2023.1151918.

Pates, Richard, and Diane Riley. *Harm Reduction in Substance Use and High-Risk Behaviour.* Wiley-Blackwell, 2012.

Pico Economics. "About George Ainslie." n.d. https://www.picoeconomics.org/personal.html.

Rodríguez-Martín, Boris C., and Belén Gallego-Arjiz. "Overeaters Anonymous: A Mutual-Help Fellowship for Food Addiction Recovery." *Front Psychol* 9, no. 1491 (2018): 1–5. DOI: 10.3389/fpsyg.2018.01491.

Schelling, Thomas C. "Self-Command in Practice, in Policy, and in a Theory of Rational Choice." *Am Econ Rev* 74, no. 2 (1984): 1–11.

Stunkard, A. J. "Presidential Address—1974: From Explanation to Action in Psychosomatic Medicine: The Case of Obesity." *Psychosom Med* 37, no. 3 (1975): 195–236.

Stunkard, Albert J. "The Success of TOPS, a Self-Help Group." *Postgrad Med* 51, no. 5 (1972): 143–47.

Stunkard, Albert, Harold Levine, and Sonja Fox. "The Management of Obesity: Patient Self-help and Medical Treatment." *Arch Int Med* 125, no. 6 (1970): 1067–72.

Stunkard, Albert J., and Sydnor B. Penick. "Behavior Modification in the Treatment of Obesity: The Problem of Maintaining Weight Loss." *Arch Gen Psych* 36, no. 7 (1979): 801–6.

Tarman, Vera. "About Addictions Unplugged." Addictions Unplugged: The Power Is Ours. https://addictionsunplugged.com/sweet-enough-september-challenge/about/.

Tatarsky, Andrew. "Demystifying Harm Reduction Addiction Treatment." Lecture presented at Cambridge Health Alliance, Treating the Addictions, Boston, MA, March 1–2, 2024.

TOPS. "History of TOPS." n.d. https://www.tops.org/tops/tops/History2.aspx.

Vakharia, Sheila P. *The Harm Reduction Gap: Helping Individuals Left Behind by Conventional Drug Prevention and Abstinence-Only Addiction Treatment.* Routledge, 2024.

Vitello, Paul. "Dr. Albert J. Stunkard, Destigmatizer of Fat, Dies at 92." *New York Times,* July 20, 2014. https://www.nytimes.com/2014/07/21/us/21stunkard.html.

Wadden, Thomas A., Timothy S. Bailey, Liana K. Billings, et al. "Effect of Subcutaneous Semaglutide vs. Placebo as an Adjunct to Intensive Behavioral Therapy on Body Weight in Adults with Overweight or Obesity: The STEP 3 Randomized Clinical Trial." *JAMA* 325, no. 14 (2021): 1403–13.

Wharton Medical Clinic. "About Dr. Wharton." n.d. https://whartonmedicalclinic.com/about/.

Wonderlich, Stephen A. "Eating Disorders, Emotions, and Recovery." Virtual lecture presented at Sanford Promise Community Lecture Series, November 16, 2021.

Wonderlich, Stephen A., Carol B. Peterson, and Tracey Leone Smith. *Integrative Cognitive-Affective Therapy for Bulimia Nervosa: A Treatment Manual.* Guilford, 2015.

Young, Lisa R. "Behavioral Treatment of Obesity: Portion Control, Mindful Eating, and Other Lifestyle Strategies." Lecture presented at 2023 Columbia Cornell Obesity: Etiology, Prevention, and Treatment, New York, May 3–6, 2023.

Interviews and Correspondence with the Author

Libby, Peter (November 2024).

Manejwala, Omar (July 2024).

Nikitidis, Ioannis (August 2024).

Stunkard, Albert (2005).

Notes

200   **puts it more bluntly:** Brewer, "Mindfulness Training for Addictions."

201   **the most emotionally impactful stimulus:** Burger, "Food Reinforcement Architecture"; Christensen et al., "Neural Underpinnings of Food Choice and Consumption in Obesity"; Devoto et al., "How Images of Food Become Cravingly Salient in Obesity."

201   **Salient stimuli:** Kessler, *Capture.*

202 **change how we feel:** I want to acknowledge Dr. Stephen A. Wonderlich for creating a diagram from which this diagram was developed. Wonderlich, "Eating Disorders, Emotions, and Recovery"; Wonderlich et al., *Integrative Cognitive-Affective Therapy for Bulimia Nervosa.*

202 **automatic behaviors take over:** Krause et al., "Self-Regulation of Stress-Related Large-Scale Brain Network Balance Using Real-Time fMRI Neurofeedback."

202 **searched scientific literature:** Michaelsen and Esch, "Understanding Health Behavior Change by Motivation and Reward Mechanisms."

203 **first physicians:** Center for Weight and Eating Disorders, "Our History."

204 **school of thought:** Cherry, "What Is Behaviorism?"

204 **first to connect:** Vitello, "Dr. Albert J. Stunkard."

205 **"self-binding":** Schelling, "Self-Command in Practice, in Policy, and in a Theory of Rational Choice."

205 **three categories:** Lembke, *Dopamine Nation.*

205 **only nurtures:** Tatarsky, "Demystifying Harm Reduction Addiction Treatment."

206 **"any positive change":** Chicago School, "Any Positive Change."

206 **meeting at Columbia University:** Young, "Behavioral Treatment of Obesity."

207 **helps educate the public:** Tarman, "About Addictions Unplugged."

207 **Overeaters Anonymous:** Rodríguez-Martín and Gallego-Arjiz, "Overeaters Anonymous."

207 **Sometimes it seems:** Manejwala, *Craving,* 14.

207 **designed to "lie":** Manejwala, *Craving,* 27.

208 **"change the brain":** Author interview with Manejwala, July 2024.

208 **"an autopsy":** Author interview with Manejwala, July 2024.

208 **"The challenge becomes":** Author interview with Manejwala, July 2024.

208 **"Build logs, build patterns":** Author interview with Manejwala, July 2024.

208 **"Very little of dealing":** Author interview with Manejwala, July 2024.

209 **suggests engaging in:** Manejwala, *Craving.*

209 **"This is the reason":** Author interview with Manejwala, July 2024.

20: Tricks of the Mind

Sources
Works Referenced

Aggarwal, Monica, Stephen Devries, Andrew M. Freeman, et al. "The Deficit of Nutrition Education of Physicians." *Am J Med* 131, no. 4 (2018): 339–45. https://www.amjmed.com/article/S0002-9343(17)31229-9/fulltext.

Ainslie, G. "Intertemporal Bargaining in Addiction." *Front Psych* 4 (August 13, 2013). https://www.frontiersin.org/journals/psychiatry/articles/10.3389/fpsyt.2013.00063/full.

Ainslie, George. "Picoeconomics in a Nutshell." Picoeconomics, n.d. https://www.picoeconomics.org/Nut2/Nutshell2.html.

Allen Carr's Easyway. "About Allen Carr's Easyway." n.d. https://www.allencarr.com/en-us/about-allen-carrs-easyway/.

Brewer, Judson. *The Craving Mind: From Cigarettes to Smartphones to Love: Why We Get Hooked and How We Can Break Bad Habits.* Yale University Press, 2017.

Brewer, Judson. "Transcript: Ezra Klein Interviews Judson Brewer." *New York Times,* April 20, 2021. https://www.nytimes.com/2021/04/20/podcasts/ezra-klein-podcast -judson-brewer-transcript.html.

Brewer, Judson. *The Hunger Habit: Why We Eat When We're Not Hungry and How to Stop.* Penguin, 2024.

Brownell, Kelly D., and Mark S. Gold, eds. *Food and Addiction: A Comprehensive Handbook.* Oxford University Press, 2012.

Carr, Allen. *Allen Carr's Easy Way to Stop Smoking.* Clarity Marketing USA, 2011.

CDC Obesity. "Adult Obesity Prevalence Maps." September 12, 2024. https://www.cdc .gov/obesity/data-and-statistics/adult-obesity-prevalence-maps.html.

Centers for Disease Control and Prevention. "FastStats: Sleep in Adults." May 15, 2024. https://www.cdc.gov/sleep/data-research/facts-stats/adults-sleep-facts-and-stats.html.

Centers for Disease Control and Prevention. "Sleep." n.d. https://www.cdc.gov/cdi /indicator-definitions/sleep.html.

Covassin, Naima, Prachi Singh, Shelly K. McCrady-Spitzer, et al. "Effects of Experimen- tal Sleep Restriction on Energy Intake, Energy Expenditure, and Visceral Obesity." *J Am Coll Cardiol* 79, no. 13 (2022): 1254–65.

Dasgupta, Kaberi, Samantha Hajna, Lawrence Joseph, Deborah Da Costa, et al. "Effects of Meal Preparation Training on Body Weight, Glycemia, and Blood Pressure: Results of a Phase 2 Trial in Type 2 Diabetes." *Int J Behav Nutr Phys Act* 9, no. 125 (2012). DOI: 10.1186/1479–5868–9–125.

The Economist. "Obituary: Allen Carr." December 7, 2006. https://www.economist.com /obituary/2006/12/07/allen-carr.

Epstein, Lawrence. "Evaluating Sleep in Obesity and Diabetes." Lecture presented at Harvard Diabetes and Obesity: Patient-Centered Management, Boston, MA, 2023.

Fingarette, Herbert. *The Self in Transformation: Psychoanalysis, Philosophy, and the Life of the Spirit.* HarperCollins, 1963.

Galef, J. "Negotiating with Your Future Selves." George Ainslie, guest. *Rationally Speaking* (podcast), January 3, 2021. https://www.listennotes.com/podcasts/sped-up-rationally /rationally-speaking-158-dr-XQjKZpFTD3A/?srsltid=AfmBOooSaeEuN9NctNEzPx h0Cqc6Lgx9VZaO-J1_WkzlRAXgSO8CChH2.

Goldman, Rena. "Is Phosphoric Acid Bad for Me?" Healthline, August 3, 2022. https:// www.healthline.com/health/food-nutrition/is-phosphoric-acid-bad-for-me.

Grace, Annie. *This Naked Mind: Control Alcohol, Find Freedom, Discover Happiness and Change Your Life.* Avery, 2018.

He, Fan, Edward O. Bixler, Arthur Berg, et al. "Habitual Sleep Variability, Not Sleep Dura- tion, Is Associated with Caloric Intake in Adolescents." *Sleep Med* 16, no. 7 (2015): 856–61.

June. "New Cooking Survey Shows Dinner Table, Dinner Time Are Becoming Obsolete." PR Newswire, May 16, 2019. https://www.prnewswire.com/news-releases/new-cooking -survey-shows-dinner-table-dinner-time-are-becoming-obsolete-300851396.html.

Killgore, William D. S., Zachary J. Schwab, Mareen Weber, et al. "Daytime Sleepiness Affects Prefrontal Regulation of Food Intake." *NeuroImage* 71 (January 24, 2013): 216–23. https://doi.org/10.1016/j.neuroimage.2013.01.018.

Krans, Brian. "Two Things You'd Rather Not Know About Chicken Nuggets." Healthline, September 19, 2013. https://www.healthline.com/health-news/strange-the-anatomy-of-a-chicken-nugget-091913.

Leith, William. "Obituary: Allen Carr." *Guardian*, December 1, 2006. https://www.theguardian.com/news/2006/dec/01/guardianobituaries.smoking.

Liu, Yong, Susan A. Carlson, Anne G. Wheaton, Kurt J. Greenlund, and Janet B. Croft. "Sleep Disorder Symptoms Among Adults in 8 States and the District of Columbia, 2017." *Prev Chronic Dis* 18 (December 30, 2021). https://doi.org/10.5888/pcd18.210305.

MedStar Health. "Paul Schwartz's Story—Healthy Eating Saves a Life." MedStar Health, February 11, 2020. https://www.youtube.com/watch?v=xF8KeWJcXlM&ab_channel=MedStarHealth.

Nibbles and Sprouts. "Transforming Childhood Anemia Detection: The Future Is Non-invasive." September 4, 2024. https://nibblesandsprouts.com/The-Inside-Scoop/Blog/Transforming-Childhood-Anemia-Detection.

Nolan, Laurence J., and Allan Geliebter. "Sleep Dysfunction, Night Eating, and Food Addiction." In *Food and Addiction: A Comprehensive Handbook*. Second ed. Ed. Ashley N. Gearhardt et al. Oxford Academic, 2024. Online edition September 19, 2024. https://doi.org/10.1093/oso/9780190671051.003.0009.

Orford, Jim. *Excessive Appetites: A Psychological View of Addictions*. Second ed. Wiley, 2001.

Peto, R., S. Darby, H. Deo, et al. "Smoking, Smoking Cessation, and Lung Cancer in the UK Since 1950: Combination of National Statistics with Two Case-Control Studies." *Br Med J (Clin Res Ed)* 321, no. 7257 (2000): 323–29. DOI: 10.1136/bmj.321.7257.323.

Picoeconomics. "About George Ainslie." n.d. https://www.picoeconomics.org/personal.html.

Ratcliffe, Dr. Denise. "About Me." n.d. https://www.drdeniseratcliffe.co.uk/about-me.

Ratcliffe, Denise. *Understanding and Managing Emotional Eating: A Psychological Skills Workbook*. Taylor and Francis, 2024.

Ricanati, Elizabeth H. W., Mladen Golubic, Dongshend Yang, et al. "Mitigating Preventable Chronic Disease: Progress Report of the Cleveland Clinic's Lifestyle 180 Program." *Nutr Metab* (London, UK) 8, no. 83 (2011). DOI: 10.1186/1743-7075-8-83.

Rihm, Julia S., Mareike M. Menz, Heidrun Schultz, et al. "Sleep Deprivation Selectively Upregulates an Amygdala-Hypothalamic Circuit Involved in Food Reward." *J Neurosci* 39, no. 5 (2019): 888–99. https://doi.org/10.1523/jneurosci.0250-18.2018. https://www.jneurosci.org/content/jneuro/39/5/888.full.pdf.

Ross, Don, Carla Sharp, Rudy E. Vuchinich, and David Spurrett. *Midbrain Mutiny: The Picoeconomics and Neuroeconomics of Disordered Gambling—Economic Theory and Cognitive Science*. Bradford Books, 2012.

Schweizer, Errol. "Why Now Is the Time to Reinvent Processed Foods." *Forbes*, August 20, 2024. https://www.forbes.com/sites/errolschweizer/2024/03/04/why-now-is-the-time-to-reinvent-processed-foods/.

Seldowitz, Dovi. "Yalta: The Story Arc of a Rabbinic Woman." Sefaria, n.d. https://www.sefaria.org/sheets/454889?lang=bi.

Somers, Virend K. "Sleep Disorders and Cardiometabolic Health." Presented at the 2024 Cardiometabolic Health Congress, Boston, MA, October 17–19, 2024.

Spaeth, Andrea M., David F. Dinges, and Namni Goel. "Resting Metabolic Rate Varies by Race and by Sleep Duration." *J Obes* 23, no. 12 (November 5, 2015): 2349–56. https://doi.org/10.1002/oby.21198.

Speaking.com. "Dr. John La Pluma." n.d. https://speaking.com/speakers/dr-john-la-puma/.

Steele, Tony D. "The History of Cigarette Advertising in the UK." Dr Fox, October 14, 2021. https://www.doctorfox.co.uk/news/the-history-of-cigarette-advertising-in-the-uk/.

St-Onge, M.-P. "Do Sleepy Brains Make Poor Food and Other Lifestyle Choices? Impact of Sleep on Weight Management." Presented at OMA 2023 Spring Summit, New York, April 21–23, 2023.

St-Onge, Marie-Pierre. "The Role of Sleep Duration in the Regulation of Energy Balance: Effects on Energy Intakes and Expenditure." *J Clin Sleep Med* 9, no. 1 (2013): 73–80.

St-Onge, Marie-Pierre, Andrew McReynolds, Zalak B. Trivedi, Amy L. Roberts, Melissa Sy, and Joy Hirsch. "Sleep Restriction Leads to Increased Activation of Brain Regions Sensitive to Food Stimuli." *Am J Clin Nutr* 95, no. 4 (February 23, 2012): 818–24. https://doi.org/10.3945/ajcn.111.027383.

Sun, Wendy, and Hedy Kober. "Regulating Food Craving: From Mechanisms to Interventions." *Physiol Behav* 222 (2020): 112878. DOI:10.1016/j.physbeh.2020.112878.

Taylor, Maija. "A Review of Food Craving Measures." *Eat Behav* 32 (2019): 101–10. DOI:10.1016/j.eatbeh.2019.01.005.

Vujović, Nina, Matthew J. Piron, Jingyi Qian, et al. "Late Isocaloric Eating Increases Hunger, Decreases Energy Expenditure, and Modifies Metabolic Pathways in Adults with Overweight and Obesity." *Cell Metab* 34, no. 10 (2022): 1486–98.

WCCO News. "Survey Shows How Often Americans Dine Out." CBS News, May 16, 2019. https://www.cbsnews.com/minnesota/news/survey-shows-how-often-americans-dine-out/.

Weinstein, Olivia. "Nutritional Plans for Patients." Lecture presented at the Obesity Medicine 2024 Spring Conference, Denver, CO, April 25–28, 2024.

Yoo, Seung-Schik, Ninad Gujar, Peter Hu, Ferenc A. Jolesz, and Matthew P. Walker. "The Human Emotional Brain Without Sleep—A Prefrontal Amygdala Disconnect." *Curr Biol* 17, no. 20 (2007): R877–R878. https://doi.org/10.1016/j.cub.2007.08.007.

Interviews and Correspondence with the Author

Badaracco, Christina (April 2024).

Davis, Heidi (April 2024).

Hart, Adante (April 2024).

McWhorter, John (April 2024).

Ratcliffe, Denise (August 2024).

Stone, Theresa (April 2024).

Weinstein, Olivia (April 2024).

Notes

211 **creating alternative routes:** Ratcliffe, *Understanding and Managing Emotional Eating.*

212 **"To feel uncomfortable":** Author interview with Ratcliffe, August 2024.

213 **"With the meds":** Author interview with Ratcliffe, August 2024.

213 **Behavioral economist George Ainslie:** Picoeconomics, "About George Ainslie."

213 **medical student working:** Picoeconomics, "About George Ainslie."

213 **overvalue a potential reward:** Ainslie, "Intertemporal Bargaining in Addiction."

213 **work with veterans:** Ainslie, "Intertemporal Bargaining in Addiction."

214 **compromises people make:** Ainslie, "Picoeconomics in a Nutshell."

214 **repeated failures to control:** Galef, "Negotiating with Your Future Selves."

214 **Three-quarters of Americans:** Liu et al., "Sleep Disorder Symptoms Among Adults in 8 States and the District of Columbia, 2017."

215 **"The less sleep you get":** Epstein, "Evaluating Sleep in Obesity and Diabetes."

215 **200 and 450 calories:** St-Onge, "Do Sleepy Brains Make Poor Food and Other Lifestyle Choices?"

215 **sleep-deprived body:** Spaeth et al., "Resting Metabolic Rate Varies by Race and by Sleep Duration."

215 **a small study in 2013:** Killgore et al., "Daytime Sleepiness Affects Prefrontal Regulation of Food Intake."

215 **reported more daytime sleepiness:** Killgore et al., "Daytime Sleepiness Affects Prefrontal Regulation of Food Intake."

215 **"Sleep problems may":** Nolan and Geliebter, "Sleep Dysfunction, Night Eating, and Food Addiction."

215 **fMRI research:** St-Onge et al., "Sleep Restriction Leads to Increased Activation of Brain Regions Sensitive to Food Stimuli."

216 **amygdala:** Yoo et al., "The Human Emotional Brain Without Sleep."

216 **hypothalamus:** Rihm et al., "Sleep Deprivation Selectively Upregulates an Amygdala-Hypothalamic Circuit Involved in Food Reward."

216 **Just one night:** St-Onge, "The Role of Sleep Duration in the Regulation of Energy Balance."

216 **high sleep variability:** He et al., "Habitual Sleep Variability, Not Sleep Duration, Is Associated with Caloric Intake in Adolescents."

216 **In a small 2022 study:** Covassin et al., "Effects of Experimental Sleep Restriction on Energy Intake, Energy Expenditure, and Visceral Obesity."

217 **designed an experiment:** Vujović et al., "Late Isocaloric Eating Increases Hunger, Decreases Energy Expenditure, and Modifies Metabolic Pathways in Adults with Overweight and Obesity."

218 **Born in 1932:** Leith, "Obituary: Allen Carr."

218 **By some estimates:** Peto et al., "Smoking, Smoking Cessation, and Lung Cancer in the UK Since 1950."

218 **People smoked in restaurants:** Steele, "The History of Cigarette Advertising in the UK."

218 **With little external:** *The Economist*, "Obituary: Allen Carr."

218 **Reflecting on the:** Allen Carr's Easyway, "About Allen Carr's Easyway."

220 **Although she spent:** Grace, *This Naked Mind.*

221 **But the body:** Grace, *This Naked Mind.*

221 **Carr calls cigarettes:** Allen Carr's Easyway, "About Allen Carr's Easyway."

221 **compares alcohol to:** Grace, *This Naked Mind.*

221 **Some addiction researchers:** Orford, *Excessive Appetites.*

222 **chicken nuggets made:** Krans, "Two Things You'd Rather Not Know About Chicken Nuggets."

222 **sodas containing phosphoric:** Goldman, "Is Phosphoric Acid Bad for Me?"

222 **"pleasure plateau":** Brewer, "Transcript: Ezra Klein Interviews Judson Brewer."

21: Continuing the Journey

Sources
Works Referenced

Athinarayanan, Shaminie J., Rebecca N. Adams, Britannie M. Volk, and Caroline G. P. Roberts. "Weight After Discontinuing Semaglutide and Tirzepatide in People with T2D on Carb-Restricted Therapy." SJA Obesity Week 2024, San Antonio, TX. https://onlinelibrary.wiley.com/doi/10.1002/oby.24195.

Shai, I., D. Schwarzfuchs, Y. Henkin, D. R. Shahar, S. Witkow, I. Greenberg, et al. "Weight Loss with a Low-Carbohydrate, Mediterranean, or Low-Fat Diet." *N Eng J Med* 359, no. 3 (July 17, 2008): 229–41. https://doi.org/10.1056/NEJMoa0708681.

Notes

224 **their original weight:** Figure 2 from Shai et al., "Weight Loss with a Low-Carbohydrate, Mediterranean, or Low-Fat Diet." Copyright © 2008 Massachusetts Medical Society. Reprinted with permission from Massachusetts Medical Society.

225 **adjust their eating patterns:** Graph with permission of the author.

22: A New Landscape

Sources
Works Referenced

Aaseth, Jan, Stian Ellefsen, Urban Alehagen, et al. "Diets and Drugs for Weight Loss and Health in Obesity: An Update." *Biomed Pharmacother* 140 (2021): 111789. DOI: 10.1016/j.biopha.2021.111789.

Anderson, G. Harvey, and Dianne Woodend. "Effect of Glycemic Carbohydrates on Short-Term Satiety and Food Intake." *Nutrient Review* 61, no. 5, part 2 (May 2023): S17–S26. DOI: 10.1301/nr.2003.may.S17-S26.

Baik, Ja-Hyun. "Dopamine Signaling in Reward-Related Behaviors." *Frontiers in Neural Circuits* 7 (2013): 152. DOI: 10.3389/fncir.2013.00152.

Beals, Joseph W., Brandon D. Kayser, Gordon Smith, et al. "Dietary Weight Loss–Induced Improvements in Metabolic Function Are Enhanced by Exercise in People with Obesity and Prediabetes." *Nat Metab* 5, no. 7 (2023): 1221–35. DOI: 10.1038/s42255-023-00829-4.

Brindisi, Marie-Claude, Laurent Brondel, Sophie Meillon, et al. "Proof of Concept: Effect of GLP-1 Agonist on Food Hedonic Responses and Taste Sensitivity in Poor Controlled Type 2 Diabetic Patients." *Diab Metab Synd* 13, no. 4 (2019): 2489–94. DOI: 10.1016/j.dsx.2019.06.021.

Bryant, Erin. "Most Covid-19 Hospitalizations Due to Four Conditions." NIH Research Matters, March 19, 2021. https://www.nih.gov/news-events/nih-research-matters/most-covid-19-hospitalizations-due-four-conditions#:~:text=A%20study%20estimated%20that%20nearly,to%20hospitalizations%20during%20the%20pandemic.

Center for Science in the Public Interest. "Why Good Nutrition Is Important." n.d. https://www.cspinet.org/eating-healthy/why-good-nutrition-important.

Columbia University Mailman School of Public Health. "Food Systems and Public Health." n.d. https://www.publichealth.columbia.edu/research/featured-research/food-systems-public-health.

Courtney, Hamish, Rahul Nayer, Chinnadorai Rajeswaran, et al. "Long-Term Management of Type 2 Diabetes with Glucagon-Like Peptide-1 Receptor Agonists." *Diab Metab Synd Obes* 10 (2017): 79–87. DOI: 10.2147/DMSO.S126763.

Farberman, Rhea. "State of Obesity 2024: Better Policies for a Healthier America." Trust for America's Health, September 12, 2024. https://www.tfah.org/report-details/state-of-obesity-2024/.

Filippatos, Theodosios D., Thalia V. Panagiotopoulou, Moses S. Elisaf, et al. "Adverse Effects of GLP-1 Receptor Agonists." *Rev Diab Stud* 11, no. 3–4 (2014): 202–30. DOI: 10.1900/RDS.2014.11.202.

Hall, Kevin D., Alexis Ayuketah, Robert Brychta, et al. "Ultra-processed Diets Cause Excess Calorie Intake and Weight Gain: An Inpatient Randomized Controlled Trial of Ad Libitum Food Intake." *Cell Metab* 30, no. 1 (July 2, 2019): 67–77.e3. DOI: 10.1016/j.cmet.2019.05.008.

Hayes, Tara O'Neill, and Rakeb Asres. "The Economic Costs of Poor Nutrition." American Action Forum, March 9, 2022. https://www.americanactionforum.org/research/the-economic-costs-of-poor-nutrition/.

Inaba, Hiroto, Mel Greaves, and Charles C. Mullighan. "Acute Lymphoblastic Leukaemia." *Lancet* 381, no. 9881 (2013): 1943–55. DOI: 10.1016/S0140-6736(12)62187-4.

Jenkins, Audrey Laganas. "Study Estimates Two-Thirds of COVID-19 Hospitalizations Due to Four Conditions." Tufts Now. February 25, 2021. https://now.tufts.edu/2021/02/25/study-estimates-two-thirds-covid-19-hospitalizations-due-four-conditions.

Kilian, Crawford. "'Health Populism' a Hazard to Public Health—and Yours." The Tyee, May 4, 2018. https://thetyee.ca/Opinion/2018/05/04/Health-Populism-Hazard-To-Public-Health/.

Kissin, Roger. "New Survey Finds Covid-19 Pandemic Changed Public's View of Obesity." American Society for Metabolic and Bariatric Surgery, March 22, 2023. https://asmbs.org/news_releases/new-survey-finds-covid-19-pandemic-changed-publics-view-of-obesity/.

Lakicevic, Nemanja, Roberto Roklicer, Antonino Bianco, et al. "Effects of Rapid Weight Loss on Judo Athletes: A Systematic Review." *Nutrients* 12, no. 5 (2020): 1220. DOI: 10.3390/nu12051220.

Lizzo, Jenna M., Jennifer Goldin, and Sara Cortes. *Pediatric Asthma*. StatPearls, 2024.

Lowe, Derek. "Compounded (and Counterfeit) Semaglutide." *Science*. January 2, 2024. https://www.science.org/content/blog-post/compounded-and-counterfeit-semaglutide.

Mallapaty, Smriti. "Cheaper Versions of Blockbuster Obesity Drugs Are Being Created in India and China." *Nature* 630 (June 19, 2024): 797–98. https://doi.org/10.1038/d41586-024-02044-x.

Mande, Jerold. "Processed Foods Are Making Us Sick: It's Time for the FDA and USDA to Step In." *Food Safety News*, March 6, 2023. https://www.foodsafetynews.com/2023/03/processed-foods-are-making-us-sick-its-time-for-the-fda-and-usda-to-step-in/.

Marrone, A. K. "Food and Drug Administration's Perspective on Medical Devices Intended for Weight Loss: A Guide for the Interventional Radiologist." *Tech Vasc Interv Radiol* 1 (2020): 100661. DOI: 10.1016/j.tvir.2020.100661.

Melson, Eka, Usma Ashraf, Dimitris Papamargaritis, and Melanie J. Davies. "What Is the Pipeline for Future Medications for Obesity?" *Int J Obes* (2024). DOI: 10.1038 /s41366-024-01473-y.

Menéndez-Arias, Luis, and Rafael Delgado. "Update and Latest Advances in Antiretroviral Therapy." *Trends Pharmacol Sci* 43, no. 1 (2022): 16–29. DOI: 10.1016/j.tips.2021.10.004.

National Institute of Diabetes and Digestive and Kidney Diseases. "Definition and Facts of NAFLD and NASH in Children." December 2021. https://www.niddk.nih .gov/health-information/liver-disease/nafld-nash-children/definition-facts#:~:text =NASH%20is%20the%20form%20of,is%20scarred%20and%20permanently%20dam aged.

National Institutes of Health. "Childhood Acute Lymphoblastic Leukemia (PDQ)—Patient Version." November 7, 2024. https://www.cancer.gov/types/leukemia/patient /child-all-treatment-pdq.

O'Neill Hayes, Tara, and Rakeb Asres. "The Economic Costs of Poor Nutrition." American Action Forum, March 9, 2022. https://www.americanactionforum.org/.

Roser, Max. "Why Is Life Expectancy in the US Lower Than in Other Rich Countries?" Our World in Data, October 29, 2020. https://ourworldindata.org/.

Sandsdal, Rasmus M., Christian R. Juhl, Simon B. K. Jensen, et al. "Combination of Exercise and GLP-1 Receptor Agonist Treatment Reduces Severity of Metabolic Syndrome, Abdominal Obesity, and Inflammation: A Randomized Controlled Trial." *Cardiovasc Diabetol* 22, no. 1 (2023): 41. DOI: 10.1186/s12933-023-01765-z.

Temneanu, O. R., L. M. Trandafir, and M. R. Purcarea. "Type 2 Diabetes Mellitus in Children and Adolescents: A Relatively New Clinical Problem Within Pediatric Practice." *J Med Life* 9, no. 3 (2016): 235–39.

van Zuylen, Mark L., Sarah E. Siegelaar, Mark P. Plummer, Adam M. Deane, Jeroen Hermanides, and Abraham H. Hulst. "Perioperative Management of Long-Acting Glucagon-Like Peptide-1 (GLP-1) Receptor Agonists: Concerns for Delayed Gastric Emptying and Pulmonary Aspiration." *Br J Anaesth* 132, no. 4 (2024): 644–48. DOI: 10.1016/j.bja.2024.01.001.

Zafiri, Daphne, and Sevil Duvarci. "Dopaminergic Circuits Underlying Associative Aversive Learning." *Front Behav Neurosci* 16 (2022): 1041929. DOI: 10.3389/fnbeh.2022.1041929.

Notes

231 **most common cancer in children:** National Institutes of Health, "Childhood Acute Lymphoblastic Leukemia (PDQ)—Patient Version."

231 **multiple mechanisms:** Inaba et al., "Acute Lymphoblastic Leukaemia"; Menéndez-Arias and Delgado, "Update and Latest Advances in Antiretroviral Therapy."

231 **aversive circuits:** Zafiri and Duvarci, "Dopaminergic Circuits Underlying Associative Aversive Learning."

231 **raise glucose and affect insulin levels:** Anderson and Woodend, "Effect of Glycemic Carbohydrates on Short-Term Satiety and Food Intake."

231 **ultraformulated foods that trigger continued eating:** Hall et al., "Ultraprocessed Diets Cause Excess Calorie Intake and Weight Gain."

232 **improved metabolic health:** Beals et al., "Dietary Weight Loss–Induced Improvements in Metabolic Function Are Enhanced by Exercise in People with Obesity and Prediabetes."

232 **potentially dangerous:** Filippatos et al., "Adverse Effects of GLP-1 Receptor Agonists."

232 **joy of eating:** Brindisi et al., "Proof of Concept."

232 **adequate strength training:** Sandsdal et al., "Combination of Exercise and GLP-1 Receptor Agonist Treatment Reduces Severity of Metabolic Syndrome"; Aaseth et al., "Diets and Drugs for Weight Loss and Health in Obesity."

232 **lose up to 25%:** Melson et al., "What Is the Pipeline for Future Medications for Obesity?"

233 **including gastroparesis:** van Zuylen et al., "Perioperative Management of Long-Acting Glucagon-Like Peptide-1 (GLP-1) Receptor Agonists."

233 **dangers of rapid weight loss:** Lakicevic et al., "Effects of Rapid Weight Loss on Judo Athletes."

233 **about five years of data:** Courtney et al., "Long-Term Management of Type 2 Diabetes with Glucagon-Like Peptide-1 Receptor Agonists."

233 **safety of compounded pharmaceutical drugs:** Lowe, "Compounded (and Counterfeit) Semaglutide."

233 **imported from China and elsewhere:** Mallapaty, "Cheaper Versions of Blockbuster Obesity Drugs Are Being Created in India and China."

233 **medical devices that are promoted:** Marrone, "Food and Drug Administration's Perspective on Medical Devices Intended for Weight Loss."

234 **addictive circuits:** Baik, "Dopamine Signaling in Reward-Related Behaviors."

234 **Our health:** Mande, "Processed Foods Are Making Us Sick."

234 **lowest average lifespan:** Roser, "Why Is Life Expectancy in the US Lower Than in Other Rich Countries?"

234 **two-thirds of hospitalizations:** Jenkins, "Study Estimates Two-Thirds of COVID-19 Hospitalizations Due to Four Conditions."

234 **678,000 deaths annually:** Center for Science in the Public Interest, "Why Good Nutrition Is Important."

234 **$16 trillion:** Hayes and Asres, "The Economic Costs of Poor Nutrition."

234 **One in five children:** Farberman, "State of Obesity 2024."

234 **5 to 10% of children:** NIH—National Institute of Diabetes and Digestive and Kidney Diseases, "Definition & Facts of NAFLD & NASH in Children."

234 **common as asthma:** Lizzo, *Pediatric Asthma.*

234 **health populism movement:** Kilian, "'Health Populism' a Hazard to Public Health—and Yours."

23: You Couldn't Have Designed a Better Weapon

Sources
Works Referenced

Aggarwal, Monica, Stephen Devries, Andrew M. Freeman, et al. "The Deficit of Nutrition Education of Physicians." *Am J Med* 131, no. 4 (2018): 339–45. https://www.amjmed.com/article/S0002-9343(17)31229-9/fulltext.

Arnold, Amanda R., and Benoit Chassaing. "Maltodextrin, Modern Stressor of the

Intestinal Environment." *Cell Mol Gastroenterol Hepatol* 7, no. 2 (2019): 475–76. doi:10.1016/j.jcmgh.2018.09.014.

Badaracco, Christina. "Introduction to Culinary Medicine." Lecture presented at the Obesity Medicine 2024 Spring Conference, Denver, CO, April 25–28, 2024.

Barnes, Mollie. "7 Fruits That Can Help You Lose (or Maintain Your) Weight." Keck Medicine of USC, August 7, 2024. https://www.keckmedicine.org/blog/7-fruits-that-can-help-you-lose-or-maintain-your-weight/.

Batchelor, Melissa. "Health Meets Food: Culinary Medicine with Dr. Timothy S. Harlan." *This Is Getting Old: Moving Towards an Age-Friendly World* (podcast), May 11, 2021. https://www.youtube.com/watch?v=z9Mh31EN2lM&t=255s&ab_channel=MelissaBPhD.

Bolhuis, Dieuwerke P., and Ciarán G. Forde. "Application of Food Texture to Moderate Oral Processing Behaviors and Energy Intake." *Trends Food Sci Technol* 106 (2020): 445–56. https://doi.org/10.1016/j.tifs.2020.10.021.

Carpentier, Francesca R. Dillman, Lindsey Smith Taillie, and Teresa Correa. "Chile's Comprehensive Food Policy Offers Global Lesson in Tackling Unhealthy Foods." Health Policy Watch, August 8, 2023. https://healthpolicy-watch.news/chiles-comprehensive-food-policy/#:~:text=Sweeping%20food%20policy%20reforms&text=First%2C%20it%20mandates%20black%2C%20octagonal,a%20high%20proportion%20of%20children.

Chandon, Pierre, and Brian Wansink. "Does Food Marketing Need to Make Us Fat? A Review and Solutions." *Nutr Rev* 70, no. 10 (2012): 571–93. DOI: 10.1111/j.1753-4887.2012.00518.x.

Cleveland Clinic. "The Health Benefits of Blueberries." May 27, 2022. https://health.clevelandclinic.org/benefits-of-blueberries.

Colleen. "To Die For Blueberry Muffins." Allrecipes, September 27, 2024. https://www.allrecipes.com/recipe/6865/to-die-for-blueberry-muffins/.

Dasgupta, Kaberi, Samantha Hajna, Lawrence Joseph, et al. "Effects of Meal Preparation Training on Body Weight, Glycemia, and Blood Pressure: Results of a Phase 2 Trial in Type 2 Diabetes." *Int J Behav Nutr Phys Act* 9, no. 125 (2012). DOI: 10.1186/1479-5868-9-125.

Devezeaux de Lavergne, Marine, Fred van de Velde, and Markus Stieger. "Bolus Matters: The Influence of Food Oral Breakdown on Dynamic Texture Perception." *Food Funct* 8, no. 2 (2017): 464–80. DOI: 10.1039/c6fo01005a.

Eat This Much. "Cheese Crackers: Regular." n.d. https://www.eatthismuch.com/calories/cheese-crackers-4134.

Eat This Much. "Chocolate Chip Cookies: Refrigerated Dough." n.d. https://www.eatthismuch.com/calories/chocolate-chip-cookies-4087.

Eisenberg, David. "Teaching Kitchens and Culinary Medicine: Envisioning Obesity Management Strategies Which Combine Drug and Lifestyle Interventions." Lecture presented at the 2024 Blackburn Course in Obesity Medicine: Treating Obesity, Harvard Medical School, Cambridge, MA, June 13–16, 2024.

Fardet, A. "Minimally Processed Foods Are More Satiating and Less Hyperglycemic Than Ultra-processed Foods: A Preliminary Study with 98 Ready-to-Eat Foods." *Food Funct* 7, no. 5 (2016): 2338–46. DOI: 10.1039/c6fo00107f.

Fatsecret. "Spaghetti/Marinara Pasta Sauce." n.d. https://www.fatsecret.com/calories-nutrition/usda/spaghetti-marinara-pasta-sauce.

Fazzino, Tera L., K. Rohde, and D. K. Sullivan. "Hyper-palatable Foods: Development of a Quantitative Definition and Application to the US Food System Database." *Obesity* (Silver Spring, MD) 27, no. 11 (2019): 1761–68. DOI: 10.1002/oby.22639.

Forde, Ciarán G., and Dieuwerke Bolhuis. "Interrelations Between Food Form, Texture, and Matrix Influence Energy Intake and Metabolic Responses." *Curr Nutr Rep* 11, no. 2 (2022): 124–32. DOI: 10.1007/s13668-022-00413-4.

Gitalis, Josh. "The Dark Side of White Flour." *From the Desk of Josh Gitalis* (blog). https://joshgitalis.com/dark-side-white-sugar-flour/#:~:text=Refined%20white%20 flour%20has%20a,sugar%20into%20cells%20for%20energy.

Global Health Advocacy Incubator. "A Victory for Public Health Information Campaigns in Colombia: The Role of Legal Strategies for Health Promotion." July 2020. https://dfweawn6ylvgz.cloudfront.net/uploads/2020/08/GHAI-Case-Study_FPP _Colombia.pdf.

Gupta, S., T. Hawk, A. Aggarwal, and A. Drewnowski. "Characterizing Ultra-processed Foods by Energy Density, Nutrient Density, and Cost." *Front Nutr* 6 (May 28, 2019): 70. DOI: 10.3389/fnut.2019.00070.

Guo, Qing, Aiqian Ye, Nick Bellissimo, Harjinder Singh, and Dérrick Rousseau. "Modulating Fat Digestion Through Food Structure Design." *Prog Lipid Res* 68 (2017): 109–18. DOI: 10.1016/j.plipres.2017.10.001.

Hall, Kevin D., A. Ayuketah, R. Brychta, et al. "Ultra-processed Diets Cause Excess Calorie Intake and Weight Gain: An Inpatient Randomized Controlled Trial of Ad Libitum Food Intake." *Cell Metab* 30, no. 1 (2019): 67–77.e3. DOI: 10.1016/j.cmet.2019.05.008.

Horbatch, Faith. "You'll Never Believe How Much Sugar Is Lurking in Your Favorite Marinara Sauces." Spoon University at University of Michigan, December 21, 2016. https://spoonuniversity.com/school/u-mich/marinara-sauceyou-won-t-believe-how -much-sugar-is-in-your-favorite/.

Julson, Erica. "Cranberries 101: Nutrition Facts and Health Benefits." Healthline, April 18, 2023. https://www.healthline.com/nutrition/foods/cranberries.

June. "New Cooking Survey Shows Dinner Table, Dinner Time Are Becoming Obsolete." PR Newswire, May 16, 2019. https://www.prnewswire.com/news-releases/new -cooking-survey-shows-dinner-table-dinner-time-are-becoming-obsolete-300851396 .html.

Knorr, Dietrich, and Mary Ann Augustin. "Preserving the Food Preservation Legacy." *Crit Rev Food Sci Nutr* 63, no. 28 (2023): 9519–38. DOI: 10.1080/10408398.2022.2065459.

La Puma, John. "What Is Culinary Medicine and What Does It Do?" *Pop Health Manag* 19, no. 1 (2016): 1–3. DOI: 10.1089/pop.2015.0003.

Laudisi, Federica, Davide Di Fusco, Vincenzo Dinallo, et al. "The Food Additive Maltodextrin Promotes Endoplasmic Reticulum Stress-Driven Mucus Depletion and Exacerbates Intestinal Inflammation." *Cell Mol Gastroenterol Hepatol* 7, no. 2 (2019): 457–73. DOI:10.1016/j.jcmgh.2018.09.002.

Levine, Allen S., and Job Ubbink. "Ultra-processed Foods: Processing Versus Formulation." *Obes Sci Pract* 9, no. 4 (2023): 435–39. DOI:10.1002/osp4.657.

Magargal, Kate. "The Cost of Cooking for Foragers." *J Hum Evol* 162 (2022): 103091. DOI: 10.1016/j.jhevol.2021.103091.

Mark, Jorie. "Nutritionist Explains Why Cheetos Are So Addictive." Mashed, February 28, 2023. https://www.mashed.com/220445/nutritionist-explains-why-cheetos-are-so -addictive/#:~:text=%22It%20activates%20the%20glutamate%20receptors,would%20 taste%20like%20without%20it.%22.

MedStar Health. "Paul Schwartz's Story—Healthy Eating Saves a Life." February 11, 2020. https://www.youtube.com/watch?v=xF8KeWJcXlM&ab_channel=MedStarHealth.

Monteiro, C. A., J.-C. Moubarac, G. Cannon, et al. "Ultra-processed Products Are Becoming Dominant in the Global Food System." *Obes Rev* 14, Suppl. 2 (2013): 21–28. DOI: 10.1111/obr.12107.

Morin, Jean-Pascal, Luis F. Rodríguez-Durán, Kioko Guzmán-Ramos, et al. "Palatable Hyper-caloric Foods' Impact on Neuronal Plasticity." *Front Behav Neurosci* 11 (2017): 19. DOI: 10.3389/fnbeh.2017.00019.

National Institute of Diabetes and Digestive and Kidney Diseases. "Continuous Glucose Monitoring." NIH, June 2023. https://www.niddk.nih.gov/health-information/diabetes /overview/managing-diabetes/continuous-glucose-monitoring.

Newman, Courtney, Justin Yan, Sarah E. Messiah, and Jaclyn Albin. "Culinary Medicine as Innovative Nutrition Education for Medical Students: A Scoping Review." *J Acad Med* 98, no. 2 (February 2023): 274–86. DOI: 10.1097/ACM.0000000000004895.

Nibbles and Sprouts. "Transforming Childhood Anemia Detection: The Future Is Noninvasive." September 4, 2024. https://nibblesandsprouts.com/The-Inside-Scoop/Blog /Transforming-Childhood-Anemia-Detection.

Perko, Jim. "Culinary Medicine Demonstration with Chef Jim Perko." Cleveland Clinic, April 14, 2022. https://www.youtube.com/watch?v=bwdG3Z5YHvo&t=514s&ab _channel=ClevelandClinic.

Ricanati, Elizabeth H. W., Mladen Golubic, Dongshend Yang, et al. "Mitigating Preventable Chronic Disease: Progress Report of the Cleveland Clinic's Lifestyle 180 Program." *Nutr Metab* (London, UK) 8, no. 83 (2011). DOI: 10.1186/1743–7075–8–83.

Sagili, Venkata Sai, Priyadarshini Chakrabarti, Sastri Jayanty, Hemant Kardile, and Vidyasagar Sathuvalli. "The Glycemic Index and Human Health with an Emphasis on Potatoes." *Foods* 11, no. 15 (2022): 2302. DOI: 10.3390/foods11152302.

Spalvieri, Stefano. "Ultra-processed Foods: How Does Policy Respond?" Health Policy Partnership, October 17, 2024. https://www.healthpolicypartnership.com/ultra-processed -foods-how-does-policy-respond/.

Speaking.com. "Dr. John La Pluma." n.d. https://speaking.com/speakers/dr-john-la -puma/.

Sutton, Cassandra A., Matthew Stratton, Alex M. L'Insalata, and Tera L. Fazzino. "Ultraprocessed, Hyper-palatable, and High Energy Density Foods: Prevalence and Distinction Across 30 Years in the United States." *Obesity* 32, no. 1 (2024): 166–75. DOI: 10.1002/oby.23897.

Teo, Pey Sze, Rob M. Van Dam, Clare Whitton, et al. "Consumption of Foods with Higher Energy Intake Rates Is Associated with Greater Energy Intake, Adiposity, and Cardiovascular Risk Factors in Adults." *J Nutr* 151, no. 2 (2021): 370–78. DOI: 10.1093 /jn/nxaa344.

Thymann, Thomas, Hanne K. Møller, Barbara Stoll, et al. "Carbohydrate Maldigestion Induces Necrotizing Enterocolitis in Preterm Pigs." *Am J Physiol Gastrointest Liver Physiol* 297, no. 6 (2009): G1115–25. DOI:10.1152/ajpgi.00261.2009.

US Department of Agriculture. "Grapes." n.d. https://fdc.nal.usda.gov/food-details /174682/nutrients.

van Eck, Arianne, Erin Franks, Christopher J. Vinyard, et al. "Sauce It Up: Influence of Condiment Properties on Oral Processing Behavior, Bolus Formation and Sensory Perception of Solid Foods." *Food Funct* 11, no. 7 (2020): 6186–201. DOI: 10.1039/d0fo00821d.

WCCO News. "Survey Shows How Often Americans Dine Out." CBS News, May 16, 2019. https://www.cbsnews.com/minnesota/news/survey-shows-how-often-americans -dine-out/.

Whelan, Kevin, Aaron S. Bancil, James O. Lindsay, and Benoit Chassaing. "Ultra-processed Foods and Food Additives in Gut Health and Disease." *Nat Rev Gastroenterol Hepatol* 21, no. 6 (2024): 406–27. DOI:10.1038/s41575-024-00893-5.

Wu, Yong, Zhiwen Zhao, Xu Jiang, et al. "Effect of Extrusion on the Modification of Wheat Flour Proteins Related to Celiac Disease." *J Food Sci Technol* 59, no. 7 (2022): 2655–65. DOI: 10.1007/s13197-021-05285-0.

Zangara, Megan T., András K. Ponti, Noah D. Miller, Morgan J. Engelhart, et al. "Maltodextrin Consumption Impairs the Intestinal Mucus Barrier and Accelerates Colitis Through Direct Actions on the Epithelium." *Front Immunol* 13, no. 841188 (2022). DOI:10.3389/fimmu.2022.841188.

Interviews by the Author

Aleppo, Grazia (November 2024).

Badaracco, Christina (April 2024).

Davis, Heidi (April 2024).

Hart, Adante (April 2024).

McWhorter, John (April 2024).

Stone, Theresa (April 2024).

Weinstein, Olivia (April 2024).

A Note on Culinary Medicine

A big challenge that people face in changing their food preferences is that they require good guidance from a doctor or other medical practitioner, yet many doctors still have only limited understanding of diet, nutrition, and the complexities of obesity medicine. Starting in the late 1990s, a varied group—mostly doctors with a personal interest or professional background in restaurants and cooking—became concerned about how poorly medicine addressed the issue of nutrition, and they decided to do something about it. They began advocating for a new field of "culinary medicine," built around the idea that teaching nutrition and cooking skills should be an integral part of modern healthcare.

In April 2024, I joined a conversation with several leaders in the culinary medicine movement, chatting in a restaurant in Denver after a meeting of the Obesity Medicine Association. Around the table was a group of people with diverse skill sets—internists, dietitians, masters of public health, social workers—who, earlier in the day, had led a series of presentations on culinary medicine to a roomful of rapt physicians.

Culinary medicine, as dietitian Christina Badaracco defined it in her introductory presentation, is an "evidence-based field of medicine that blends the art of food and cooking with the science of medicine." The presentations that day had encompassed the breadth of topics culinary medicine touches upon: the appropriate application of specific diets, the role of food insecurity in the rise of obesity, how to make a tasty mocktail that isn't rife with sugar, and (of course) the role of GLP-1s in obesity medicine.

Dr. David Eisenberg, a passionate amateur chef who is now the director of culinary nutrition at the Harvard T. H. Chan School of Public Health, was dismayed to learn that so few of his colleagues shared his interest in food. "As a medical student and resident in the 1970s and '80s, I observed that few doctors knew anything about nutrition, and fewer knew anything about food or cooking," he said. "But don't all patients eat, and don't foods affect health?" It seems not much has changed on that front. In a 2018 study published in the *American Journal of Medicine*, roughly 73% of physicians reported receiving minimal or no instruction in nutrition.

At Tulane University, in New Orleans, Dr. Timothy Harlan, who had owned a restaurant prior to becoming an internist, started to contemplate the value of "making food part of the discussion and part of our therapy." Dr. John LaPuma studied at a Le Cordon Bleu–affiliated culinary school while working as a physician in Chicago with the idea that he would eventually start incorporating nutrition education into his medical practice. He later authored several bestselling books about nutrition and started his own regenerative farm.

These people and others started developing ideas about how to disseminate valuable information about nutrition to doctors and the general public alike. One idea was "teaching kitchens," venues to provide instruction on nutrition and cooking. In 2003, Harvard University partnered with the Culinary Institute of America at Greystone, in California, to launch the Healthy Kitchens, Healthy Lives program, in which doctors learned how to dice and sauté alongside nutritional information, such as the benefits of eating healthy grains. Tulane built its teaching kitchen in 2013 as part of the first ever culinary medicine center at a US medical school. Teaching kitchens soon followed at Yale, New York University, multiple University of California campuses, and the University of Texas.

While most teaching kitchens were originally used by medical students and doctors, over time their target audience and their goals have expanded. They now can be found in community centers, Veterans Affairs facilities, libraries, high schools, and YMCAs, with programming tailored for children, pregnant women, people with physical or mental disabilities, and others. One program in Philadelphia, paid for by the city, combines cooking classes with English lessons for recent immigrants. Some companies have started to build teaching kitchens in their offices; Google has teaching kitchens in seventeen of its campuses worldwide. The movement has also gone digital. You can watch culinary medicine demonstrations on YouTube, for example, or download apps like Pursuit, which allows users to create custom grocery lists and recipes.

No two culinary medicine courses look alike, though most are group classes that meet regularly for a set number of weeks. Some are more targeted to people with specific nutritional needs. A class for those diagnosed with anemia would focus on foods that are iron-rich, for example, while a person with Crohn's disease might need help determining which foods trigger their symptoms, such as high-fiber foods, and how to find good substitutes. A videotaped sample demonstration for diabetic patients led by Chef Jim Perko, executive chef at the Cleveland Clinic, and nutritionist and diabetes education specialist Kim Pierce shows viewers not only how to make broccoli and bean salad, but also provides helpful commentary as to the nutritional benefits of each ingredient and how the person cooking could maximize flavor.

"We're going to use less oil because we're going to add beans to [the broccoli]," Chef Perko said, adding that beans are "loaded with protein and dietary fiber." Later, Perko advised people not to squash their garlic too hard, lest they inadvertently lose its natural oil, which has been shown to have health benefits. This is what distinguishes a culinary medicine program from a standard cooking class or a boilerplate lecture about healthy eating from a primary care physician. By teaching people how to make delicious, wholesome meals and by elucidating the connection between those foods and various health outcomes, culinary medicine professionals have armed their patients with the tools they need to take control of their well-being.

A key component to culinary medicine is the somatic experience of eating. As social worker Heidi Davis, who manages a teaching kitchen in Oregon, told me that evening, after the Obesity Medicine Association conference, "One of the things that we focus on is making sure that food tastes good first, so that we can hook people with the flavor (recognizing what we are up against) and maybe trigger the same dopamine response a person might get from eating ultraprocessed food." If you can expose someone to the sensory pleasures of biting into a piece of crunchy, well-seasoned cauliflower and nudge them toward noticing how good their body feels afterward, they might lose their desire for a textural equivalent, like a Cheeto. "We're giving people options. You're bringing them the joy of cooking, the joy of taste, the vibrant colors, and then they lose the taste for the hyperpalatable food," added Dr. Theresa Stone, an internal medicine practitioner who uses teaching kitchens in her practice. "And we do it all without shame."

Practitioners will rarely advise a patient to follow one specific diet, as they see that as a potentially denigrating approach to weight loss. (There are exceptions in cases of medical conditions that have been shown to improve with specific nutritional regimens.) For example, "The way obesity was treated for decades was putting people on a 1,000-calorie diet," dietitian Olivia Weinstein, who runs a teaching kitchen at the Boston Medical Center, says.

Culinary medicine practitioners also try to be sensitive to cultural needs. "What we see a lot is when people migrate to the US, they can't find foods that are familiar," Weinstein said. "When they talk to healthcare providers, they're given a handout that says the Mediterranean diet is ideal. Now they have the perception that they have to change their food plan further and further from what they know, and what they're finding is more processed, more convenient, and more delicious than the things the doctor might suggest." A culinary medicine provider can point a person in the direction of nutritional foods from their own culture. (Weinstein gave the example of épis, a Haitian seasoning made from vegetables, as a superior choice to commercial barbecue sauce.)

Given what we know about premade, packaged, and restaurant food being laden with salt, sugar, and fat—and over 50% of Americans eat out three or more times a week, while just 20% cook daily, and usually not from scratch—it seems eminently reasonable that teaching a person how to make their own food at home would likely end up with that person seeing health benefits, regardless of whether they had any preexisting conditions. "Food is a simple human need that's become dominated by industry, and it's coming back to something we've known," Weinstein said.

The relatively few studies conducted on culinary medicine have shown positive results. In one 2012 study conducted by McGill University, in Montreal, fulfillment of a twenty-four-week culinary medicine course helped patients with type 2 diabetes improve their eating, lose weight, and reduce their blood pressure; in another study, from the prior year, participants with a variety of chronic weight-related conditions who enrolled in the Cleveland Clinic's Lifestyle 180 program, which combines nutrition, exercise, and stress management classes, saw a reduction in weight, waist circumference, and glucose levels, among other markers of poor metabolic health.

Though there are less data on this, many of the doctors, dietitians, chefs, and others who work in the field of culinary medicine believe that giving their patients this kind of instruction might also motivate them to commit to making healthier choices in other areas of their lives, like adopting an exercise routine or examining their sleep habits or incorporating more outdoor activities into their routines. "Having a little bit of agency in one area could lead to change in other areas," registered dietitian Adante Hart advised.

But culinary medicine faces a lot of obstacles, with our environment so heavily fortified with ultraformulated foods and a populace that's become dependent on their products. There is also the issue of scale. Doctors meet with patients individually, usually after a problem has already become apparent. Dietitians and doctors can't enable people to find sources of fresh food in food deserts. They also cannot correct insurance companies' lack of coverage for preventive healthcare, although at least there has been some progress on that front, such as in California, where Medicare will subsidize "nutritional education."

"I have hope for an individual-level change, of trying and tasting different things and improving flavors on an individual scale, with cooking and healthier food options," said Dr. John "Wesley" McWhorter, the director of lifestyle medicine at a primary care practice for Medicare patients and a chef, cookbook author, and strength and conditioning specialist. "I still think it takes higher-level shifts in the way we prepare foods, in restaurants or as packaged products, to make the changes necessary to combat obesity nationally."

The good news is that on their own, people appear to be eager to develop just the kinds of skills culinary medicine teaches. "Americans are more and more interested in understanding different aspects of their food," Heidi Davis said, citing increased concerns over issues like the use of hormones and antibiotics in meat and the presence of plastics and chemicals in other products. In the past few decades, the market for organic products has grown exponentially, and diners have expressed increased desire for "local" fare. Young people, particularly, are seen as increasingly health-conscious and suspicious of corporate involvement in all areas of life, including food and nutrition. "A lot of times, people feel their hands are being forced," Adante Hart said. "I think culinary medicine's giving people hope that they can change at least one part of their environment that they may not have otherwise felt they could change."

As we parted ways that evening, I wondered if perhaps the small changes made by individuals were finally adding up to something big, a genuinely new way of looking at nutrition. In contrast to the 1980s, when processed foods began to dominate and consumers had little means of investigating, today anyone can go online and listen to a culinary medicine practitioner give a talk about the downsides of ultraformulated food, or watch a demonstration on how to make kimchee, or curate a grocery list to build meals made of quality ingredients for their family for the week ahead. People can be reached in these grassroots ways even before they develop problems or, if that fails, find help more efficiently once they have.

The food industry has seemingly bottomless resources and can sway governments as a result, but consumer desire, too, can shape their agendas. As fears over climate change have mounted, for example, there has been increased focus on sustainable manufacturing and "eco-friendly" products, requiring many companies to change direction. Maybe it's too ideal a scenario, but it's not impossible to imagine a future in which a critical mass of consumers, educated on the benefits of wholesome foods and unwilling to pay for a pale impression of that food, demands something better than what they currently have.

Notes

236 **blueberry is a rich source:** Cleveland Clinic, "The Health Benefits of Blueberries."

236 **combined with sugar:** Colleen, "To Die For Blueberry Muffins."

236 **eat roots, stems, leaves:** Magargal, "The Cost of Cooking for Foragers."

236 **Simple forms of preservation:** Knorr and Augustin, "Preserving the Food Preservation Legacy."

237 **Extreme processing techniques:** Sutton et al., "Ultraprocessed, Hyper-palatable, and High Energy Density Foods."

237 **saturated and processed fats:** Guo et al., "Modulating Fat Digestion Through Food Structure Design."

238 **Professor Adam Drewnowski:** Gupta et al., "Characterizing Ultra-processed Foods by Energy Density, Nutrient Density, and Cost."

238 **higher energy density:** Monteiro et al., "Ultra-processed Products Are Becoming Dominant in the Global Food System."

238 **considerable amount of added sugar:** Horbatch, "You'll Never Believe How Much Sugar Is Lurking in Your Favorite Marinara Sauces."

239 **study by researchers:** Bolhuis and Forde, "Application of Food Texture to Moderate Oral Processing Behaviors and Energy Intake."

239 **Research indicates:** Forde and Bolhuis, "Interrelations Between Food Form, Texture, and Matrix Influence Energy Intake and Metabolic Responses."

239 **liquid foods:** Teo et al., "Consumption of Foods with Higher Energy Intake Rates Is Associated with Greater Energy Intake."

239 **weaker satiety response:** Bolhuis and Forde, "Application of Food Texture to Moderate Oral Processing Behaviors and Energy Intake."

239 **seamless transition from crunch to melt:** Mark, "Nutritionist Explains Why Cheetos Are So Addictive."

240 **refined into white flour:** Gitalis, "The Dark Side of White Flour."

240 **processed through extrusion:** Wu et al., "Effect of Extrusion on the Modification of Wheat Flour Proteins Related to Celiac Disease."

240 **around 4% natural sugar:** Julson, "Cranberries 101."

241 **significantly more calories:** Hall et al., "Ultra-processed Diets Cause Excess Calorie Intake and Weight Gain."

241 **67 calories per 100 grams:** US Department of Agriculture, "Grapes."

241 **cheese crackers:** Eat This Much, "Cheese Crackers: Regular."

241 **chocolate chip cookies:** Eat This Much, "Chocolate Chip Cookies: Refrigerated Dough."

241 **public health campaigns:** Global Health Advocacy Incubator, "A Victory for Public Health Information Campaigns in Colombia."

241 **Chile's attempts:** Carpentier et al., "Chile's Comprehensive Food Policy Offers Global Lesson in Tackling Unhealthy Foods."

241 **invest heavily in marketing and lobbying:** Spalvieri, "Ultra-processed Foods: How Does Policy Respond?"

242 **continuous glucose monitor:** National Institute of Diabetes and Digestive and Kidney Diseases, "Continuous Glucose Monitoring."

242 **"If you start eating cereal":** Author interview with Aleppo, November 2024.

24: The Food Industry Has Us in Its Sights

Sources
Works Referenced

Blum, Deborah. *The Poison Squad: One Chemist's Single-Minded Crusade for Food Safety at the Turn of the Twentieth Century.* Penguin, 2019.

Bottemiller, Helena. "The FDA's Food Failure." Organic Consumers Association, April 8, 2022. https://organicconsumers.org/the-fdas-food-failure/.

Boudreau, Catherine, and Helena Bottemiller Evich. "How Washington Keeps America

Sick and Fat." *Politico*, November 4, 2019. https://www.politico.com/news/agenda/2019 /11/04/why-we-dont-know-what-to-eat-060299.

Carolina Alumni Review. "Advancing Nutrition Research and Innovation." May/June 2023.

Carpentier, Francesca R. Dillman, Lindsey Smith Taillie, and Teresa Correa. "Chile's Comprehensive Food Policy Offers Global Lesson in Tackling Unhealthy Foods." Health Policy Watch, August 8, 2023. https://healthpolicy-watch.news/chiles-comprehensive-food-policy/#:~:text=Sweeping%20food%20policy%20reforms&text=First%2C%20 it%20mandates%20black%2C%20octagonal,a%20high%20proportion%20of%20 children.

Center for Science in the Public Interest. "Why Good Nutrition Is Important." n.d. https:// www.cspinet.org/eating-healthy/why-good-nutrition-important.

Centers for Disease Control and Prevention. "Nutritional Factors and the Development of Metabolic Diseases." *Emerg Infect Dis* 17, no. 1 (January 2011): 7–15. https://wwwnc .cdc.gov/eid/article/17/1/p1–1101_article.

Centers for Disease Control and Prevention. "Youth Tobacco Use Remains a Public Health Concern." October 17, 2024. https://www.cdc.gov/media/releases/2024/p1017 -youth-tobacco-use.html.

CSPI. "Why Good Nutrition Is Important: Unhealthy Eating and Physical Inactivity Are Leading Causes of Death in the U.S." https://www.cspinet.org/eating-healthy /why-good-nutrition-important.

Diamond, Dan. "America Has a Life Expectancy Crisis. But It's Not a Political Priority." *Washington Post*, December 28, 2023. https://www.washingtonpost.com /health/2023/12/28/life-expectancy-no-political-response/.

Donohue, Dane. "What Is Insulin Resistance and Why Do 80% of Americans Have It?" 8 Weeks to Wellness, March 15, 2023. https://www.8ww.com/post/what-is-insulin -resistance-and-why-do-80-of-americans-have-it.

Food Safety Authority of Ireland. "Labelling—Quantitative Ingredient Declaration (QUID)." n.d. https://www.fsai.ie/business-advice/labelling/labelling-general-labelling /quid.

Gaples Institute. "5 Misleading Nutrition Labels." n.d. https://www.gaplesinstitute .org/5-misleading-food-labels/.

Global Food Research Program. "Front-of-Package (FOP) Food Labelling: Empowering Consumers and Promoting Healthy Diets." October 2021. https://www .globalfoodresearchprogram.org/wp-content/uploads/2021/10/FOP_Factsheet _UNCGFRP.pdf.

Kessler, David A. "Toward More Comprehensive Food Labeling." *N Eng J Med* 371, no. 3 (2014): 193–95. DOI: 10.1056/NEJMp1402971.

Majmudar, Aman. "Poor Diets Are Killing Us. Better Spending on Nutrition Research Can Help." Harvard Public Health, October 16, 2024. https://harvardpublichealth.org /policy-practice/nutrition-research-is-underfunded-why-arent-we-spending-more/.

McFadden, Brandon. "'Gluten-Free Water' and Other Absurd Labelling Trends." BBC, January 26, 2018. https://www.bbc.com/worklife/article/20180126-gluten-free-water -and-absurd-labelling-of-whats-absent.

Mr. Breakfast. "2002 Frosted Flakes Olympics Ad." April 23, 2011. https://www .mrbreakfast.com/cereal_ucp_slideshow.asp?id=144&picid=2752.

National Institutes of Health. "Budget." October 3, 2024. https://www.nih.gov/about -nih/what-we-do/budget.

National Institutes of Health. *NIH Nutrition Research Report 2024*. November 2024. https://dpcpsi.nih.gov/sites/default/files/2024–11/NIH-Nutrition-Report-508-FV-508.pdf.

Nourish: Food Marketing. "Nourish Food Marketing's 2025 Trend Report Featured in the Globe and Mail." November 21, 2024. https://www.nourish.marketing/news/nourish-food-marketing-2025-trend-report-the-globe-and-mail.

Pampel, Fred C., and Jade Aguilar. "Changes in Youth Smoking, 1976–2002: A Time-Series Analysis." *Youth Soc* 39, no. 4 (2008): 453–79. DOI: 10.1177/0044118X07308070.

Perrin, James M., Elizabeth Anderson, and Jeanne Van Cleave. "The Rise in Chronic Conditions Among Infants, Children, and Youth Can Be Met with Continued Health System Innovations." *Health Aff* 33, no. 12 (2014): 2099–105. DOI: 10.1377/hlthaff.2014.0832.

Poinski, Megan. "Sugar Association Asks FDA to Overhaul Sweetener Labeling Rules." Food Dive, June 4, 2020. https://www.fooddive.com/news/sugar-association-asks-fda-to-overhaul-sweetener-labeling-rules/579151/#:~:text=The%20Sugar%20Association%20is%20asking,the%20front%20of%20food%20packages.

Politico. "The FDA Fails to Regulate Food Health and Safety Hazards." 2022. https://www.politico.com/interactives/2022/fda-fails-regulate-food-health-safety-hazards/.

Riddle, Holly. "The Untold Truth of Frosted Flakes." Mashed, January 25, 2023. https://www.mashed.com/199577/the-untold-truth-of-frosted-flakes/.

Rumrill, Joe. "Everything We Know About Tony the Tiger (Including His Height)." Sporked, July 31, 2023. https://sporked.com/article/tony-the-tiger-height-age-catchphrase/.

Scallan, E., Robert M. Hoekstra, Frederick J. Angulo, et al. "Foodborne Illness Acquired in the United States—Major Pathogens." *Emerg Infect Dis* 17, no. 1 (2011): 7–15. DOI: 10.3201/eid1701.P11101.

Schweizer, Errol. "Why Now Is the Time to Reinvent Processed Foods." *Forbes*, August 20, 2024. https://www.forbes.com/sites/errolschweizer/2024/03/04/why-now-is-the-time-to-reinvent-processed-foods/.

Spencer, George. "Just the Facts." *Carolina Alumni Review*, May/June 2023. https://alumni.unc.edu/news-publications/. https://www.carolinaalumnireview.com/carolinaalumnireview/20230506/MobilePagedArticle.action?articleId=1881716&app=false&cmsId=4099616#articleId1881716.

State of Childhood Obesity. "Food Marketing to Children." n.d. https://stateofchildhoodobesity.org/policy-topic/food-marketing-to-children/#:~:text=Children%20see%20ads%20every%20day,%2C%20candy%2C%20and%20unhealthy%20snacks.

Stokes, Kris. "Fitness Truth Behind 'Fat-Free' Labeled Foods by Custom Fitness: Amarillo Personal Trainers." Custom Fitness, July 6, 2017. https://customfitness.biz/fitness-truth-behind-fat-free-labeled-foods-custom-fitness-amarillo-personal-trainers/.

Taillie, Lindsey Smith, Marcela Reyes, M. Arantxa Colchero, et al. "An Evaluation of Chile's Law of Food Labeling and Advertising on Sugar-Sweetened Beverage Purchases from 2015 to 2017: A Before-and-After Study." *PLoS Med* 17, no. 2 (2020): e1003015.

US Department of Health and Human Services, Food and Drug Administration. *Proposed Rule: 21 CFR 101*. Docket No. FDA-2024-N-2910. RIN 0910-AI80. Document No. 2025-00778. 90 FR 5426, January 16, 2025, pp. 5426–63.

US Food and Drug Administration. *Quantitative Research on Front of Package Labeling on Packaged Foods*. May 2024. https://www.fda.gov/media/185007/download.

Washington Post. "Life Expectancy and the Lack of a Political Response." December

28, 2023. https://www.washingtonpost.com/health/2023/12/28/life-expectancy-no
-political-response/.

Washington Post Live. "Former FDA Commissioner David Kessler: Obesity Problem Is
Worse Than We Think." *Washington Post*, June 20, 2018. https://www.washingtonpost
.com/video/postlive/wplive/former-fda-commissioner-david-kessler-obesity-problem-is
-worse-than-we-think/2018/06/20/a98edecc-74c7–11e8-bda1–18e53a448a14_video.html.

Xu Jiaquan, Kenneth D. Kochanek, Sherry L. Murphy, et al. "Mortality in the United
States, 2012." Centers for Disease Control and Prevention: NCHS Brief, October 2024.
https://www.cdc.gov/nchs/data/databriefs/db168.pdf Kee.

Interviews by the Author

Pollay, Richard (August 2024).

Notes

245 **sat on opposite ends:** Author interview with Pollay, August 2024.

245 **Tony the Tiger:** Rumrill, "Everything We Know About Tony the Tiger (Including
His Height)."

246 **the word "sugar" was dropped:** Riddle, "The Untold Truth of Frosted Flakes."

246 **blurry streak of his orange tail:** Mr. Breakfast, "2002 Frosted Flakes Olympics Ad."

247 **spends $14 billion a year:** State of Childhood Obesity, "Food Marketing to
Children."

247 **hire market research firms:** Nourish: Food Marketing, "Nourish Food Marketing's 2025 Trend Report Featured in the Globe and Mail."

247 **"fat free" labels:** Stokes, "Fitness Truth Behind 'Fat-Free' Labeled Foods by Custom
Fitness."

247 **"gluten free" labels:** McFadden, "'Gluten-Free Water' and Other Absurd Labelling Trends."

248 **Government has also failed to act:** Diamond, "America Has a Life Expectancy
Crisis. But It's Not a Political Priority."

248 **consumers don't know:** McFadden, "'Gluten-Free Water' and Other Absurd Labelling Trends."

248 **often it is outright misleading:** Gaples Institute, "5 Misleading Nutrition
Labels."

249 **safety of our food:** Blum, *The Poison Squad.*

249 **no longer ensures the safety:** Bottemiller, "The FDA's Food Failure."

249 **80% of Americans:** Donohue, "What Is Insulin Resistance and Why Do 80% of
Americans Have It?"

249 **top three ingredients in packaged food:** Kessler, "Toward More Comprehensive
Food Labeling."

249 **warning labels on harmful foods:** Global Food Research Program, "Front-of-Package (FOP) Food Labelling: Empowering Consumers and Promoting Healthy Diets."

249 **a technique that has been shown:** Taillie et al., "An Evaluation of Chile's Law
of Food Labeling and Advertising on Sugar-Sweetened Beverage Purchases from
2015 to 2017: A Before-and-After Study."

249 **The agency has been testing:** US Food and Drug Administration, *Quantitative Research on Front of Package Labeling on Packaged Foods.*

249 **recently proposed:** US Department of Health and Human Services, Food and Drug Administration, *Proposed Rule: 21 CFR 101.*

249 **shown in studies to be ineffective:** Global Food Research Program, "Front-of-Package (FOP) Food Labelling."

251 **names that most consumers don't recognize:** Poinski, "Sugar Association Asks FDA to Overhaul Sweetener Labeling Rules."

251 **quantitative ingredient declarations:** Food Safety Authority of Ireland, "Labelling—Quantitative Ingredient Declaration (QUID)."

252 **chronically underinvest in nutrition research:** Boudreau and Bottemiller Evich, "How Washington Keeps America Sick and Fat."

252 **long argued:** *Washington Post Live*, "Former FDA Commissioner David Kessler: Obesity Problem Is Worse Than We Think."

252 **around $50 billion a year:** National Institutes of Health, "Budget."

252 **Less than 5%:** Majmudar, "Poor Diets Are Killing Us."

252 **FDA needs more nutrition resources:** Bottemiller, "The FDA's Food Failure."

252 **acute food illness deaths:** Scallan et al., "Foodborne Illness Acquired in the United States."

252 **more than that many people every day:** CSPI, "Why Good Nutrition Is Important: Unhealthy Eating and Physical Inactivity Are Leading Causes of Death in the U.S."

252 **rising incidence of chronic disease:** Perrin et al., "The Rise in Chronic Conditions Among Infants, Children, and Youth Can Be Met with Continued Health System Innovations."

252 **25% of young people smoked:** Pampel and Aguilar, "Changes in Youth Smoking."

252 **Today, our national youth smoking rate:** Centers for Disease Control and Prevention, "Youth Tobacco Use Remains a Public Health Concern."

25: The Gold Rush of Weight-Loss Drugs

Sources
Works Referenced

Ashraf, Amir Reza, Tim K. Mackey, János Schmidt, et al. "Safety and Risk Assessment of No-Prescription Online Semaglutide Purchases." *JAMA Netw Open* 7, no. 8 (2024): e2428280. DOI: 10.1001/jamanetworkopen.2024.28280.

Bigg, Matthew Mpoke. "Woman Who Sold Misbranded Ozempic on TikTok Faces Smuggling Charge." *New York Times*, May 2, 2024. https://www.nytimes.com/2024/05/02/nyregion/new-york-woman-charged-ozempic-tiktok.html.

Billingsley, Alyssa. "Is Semaglutide in Shortage? The Latest on Ozempic and Wegovy Availability." GoodRx, November 26, 2024. https://www.goodrx.com/classes/glp-1-agonists/semaglutide-shortage.

BizNews. "Novo Nordisk and Eli Lilly Dominate the $150bn Weight-Loss Drug Market." July 18, 2024. https://www.biznews.com/global-investing/2024/07/18/150bn-weight-loss-drug-market.

Buntz, Brian. "Lilly, Novo Nordisk Battle Surge in Copycat Weight-Loss Drugs amid Safety Concerns." Drug Discovery and Development, October 22, 2024. https://www .drugdiscoverytrends.com/lilly-novo-nordisk-battle-surge-in-copycat-weight-loss -drugs-amid-safety-concerns/.

Castro, M. Regina. "Diabetes Drugs and Weight Loss." Mayo Clinic, November 14, 2024. https://www.mayoclinic.org/diseases-conditions/type-2-diabetes/expert-answers /byetta/faq-20057955.

Chiappini, Stefania, Rachel Vickers-Smith, Daniel Harris, et al. "Is There a Risk for Semaglutide Misuse? Focus on the Food and Drug Administration's FDA Adverse Events Reporting System (FAERS) Pharmacovigilance Dataset." J Pharm 16, no. 7 (2023): 994. DOI: 10.3390/ph16070994.

Dickerson, Brian E., Anthony J. Calamunci, Nicole Hughes Waid, Amy L. Butler, and Katy Wane. "Pharmacist at Center of 2012 Fungal Meningitis Outbreak Sentenced to 9 Years in Prison." Lexology, June 30, 2017. https://www.lexology.com/library/detail.aspx ?g=7e7f4b81-ff5a-4691-94d9-92f9991c5d77.

Goodman, Brenda. "Poison Centers See Nearly 1,500% Increase in Calls Related to In-jected Weight-Loss Drugs as People Accidentally Overdose." CNN, December 18, 2023. https://www.cnn.com/2023/12/13/health/semaglutide-overdoses-wellness/index.html.

Gudeman, Jennifer, Michael Jozwiakowski, John Chollet, et al. "Potential Risks of Pharmacy Compounding." Drugs in R&D 13, no. 1 (2013): 1–8. DOI: 10.1007/s40268-013-0005-9.

Heinrich, Janet. "Prescription Drugs: State and Federal Oversight of Drug Compounding by Pharmacies." US Government Accountability Office, October 23, 2003. https://www .gao.gov/assets/gao-04-195t.pdf.

KnippeRx. "Offer Nationwide Pharmacy Services Under Your Brand." n.d. https:// www.knipperx.com/commercial-solutions/white-labeled-pharmacy/.

LaRosa, John. "U.S. Weight Loss Industry Grows to $90 Billion, Fueled by Obesity Drugs Demand." MarketResearch.com, March 6, 2024. https://blog.marketresearch .com/u.s.-weight-loss-industry-grows-to-90-billion-fueled-by-obesity-drugs-de mand.

LexisNexis. "Regulatory Challenges of Compounded Weight-Loss Drugs." State Net Insights, July 23, 2024. https://www.lexisnexis.com/community/insights/legal/capitol -journal/b/state-net/posts/regulatory-challenges-of-compounded-weight-loss-drugs-vt -s-lawsuit-against-major-pbms.

MarketResearch.com. "The Telehealth Weight Loss Market." April 2024. https:// www.marketresearch.com/Marketdata-Enterprises-Inc-v416/Telehealth-Weight-Loss -36701891/.

National Association of Boards of Pharmacy. "Prescription Drug Importation Is Not a Viable Solution to High Prescription Drug Costs." February 1, 2019. https:// nabp.pharmacy/news/news-releases/statement-on-prescription-drug-importation -proposals/.

National Association of Boards of Pharmacy. "Rogue RX Activity Report: Disrupting Illegal Online Pharmacies." NABP, 2022. https://nabp.pharmacy/wp-content/uploads/2022/10/ Rogue-Rx-Activity-Report-Disrupting-Illegal-Online-Pharmacies-2022.pdf.

National Cancer Institute. "Antineoplastons (PDQ®)—Patient Version." August 15, 2019. https://siteman.wustl.edu/ncipdq/antineoplastons-pdq-patient-version/.

OppGen Marketing. "The Ultimate Weight Loss Marketing Playbook." May 4, 2023. https://oppgen.com/blog/weight-loss/ultimate-weight-loss-marketing-playbook/.

Poisoncenters. "America's Poison Centers—GLP-1." n.d. https://poisoncenters.org/track/GLP-1.

Reuters Correspondents. "How Criminal Gangs Are Spreading Dangerous Fake Ozempic Across the World." *Independent*, September 5, 2024. https://www.independent.co.uk/health-and-wellbeing/fake-ozempic-fat-loss-injections-b2607568.html.

Ridge, Martin. "Disorder, Crime, and Punishment." *Montana: The Magazine of Western History* 49, no. 3, Special Gold Rush Issue (Autumn 1999): 12–27. http://www.jstor.org/stable/4520161.

Roche, Walter F., Jr. "Number Deaths Caused by the 2012 Fungal Meningitis Outbreak Underreported." *Tennessean*, December 31, 2018. https://www.tennessean.com/story/news/health/2018/12/31/number-deaths-caused-2012-fungal-meningitis-outbreak-underreported/2447091002/.

Satija, Bhanvi, and Patrick Wingrove. "Eli Lilly's Rare Sales Miss for Weight-Loss Drug Sends Shares Tumbling." Reuters, October 30, 2024. https://www.reuters.com/business/healthcare-pharmaceuticals/eli-lilly-misses-third-quarter-profit-amid-soaring-demand-weight-loss-drug-2024–10–30/.

Siwicki, Bill. "Will Telemedicine Stagnate Without Regulatory Reform?" Healthcare IT News, September 9, 2024. https://www.healthcareitnews.com/news/will-telemedicine-stagnate-without-regulatory-reform.

US Attorney. "Long Island Woman Arrested for Selling Misbranded and Adulterated Weight Loss Drugs, Including Ozempic, on TikTok." Justice.gov, May 1, 2024. https://www.justice.gov/usao-sdny/pr/long-island-woman-arrested-selling-misbranded-and-adulterated-weight-loss-drugs.

US Congress, House of Representatives. "FDA Foreign Drug Inspection Program: A System at Risk." Hearings Before the Subcommittee on Oversight and Investigations of the Committee on Energy and Commerce, 110th Congress, 1st sess., 2007, 110–74.

US Congress, House of Representatives. "Securing the US Drug Supply Chain: Oversight of FDA's Foreign Inspection Program." Hearings Before the Subcommittee on Oversight and Investigations of the Committee on Energy and Commerce, 116th Congress, 1st sess., 2019, 116–83.

US Department of Justice. "Former Owner of Defunct New England Compounding Center Resentenced to 14 Years in Prison in Connection with 2012 Fungal Meningitis Outbreak." FDA.gov, July 7, 2021. https://www.fda.gov/inspections-compliance-enforcement-and-criminal-investigations/press-releases/former-owner-defunct-new-england-compounding-center-resentenced-14-years-prison-connection-2012.

US Food and Drug Administration. "Compounding When Drugs Are on FDA's Drug Shortages List." FDA.gov, October 11, 2024. https://www.fda.gov/drugs/human-drug-compounding/compounding-when-drugs-are-fdas-drug-shortages-list.

US Food and Drug Administration. "Current and Resolved Drug Shortages and Discontinuations Reported to FDA." Data.gov, July 16, 2023. https://catalog.data.gov/dataset/current-and-resolved-drug-shortages-and-discontinuations-reported-to-fda.

US Food and Drug Administration. "FDA Alerts Health Care Providers, Compounders and Patients of Dosing Errors Associated with Compounded Injectable Semaglutide Products." FDA.gov, July 2024. https://www.fda.gov/drugs/human-drug-compounding/fda-alerts-health-care-providers-compounders-and-patients-dosing-errors-associated-compounded.

US Food and Drug Administration. "FDA's Concerns with Unapproved GLP-1 Drugs

Used for Weight Loss." FDA.gov, October 2, 2024. www.fda.gov/drugs/postmarket
-drug-safety-information-patients-and-providers/fdas-concerns-unapproved-glp-1
-drugs-used-weight-loss.

US Government Accountability Office. "Drug Safety: FDA Should Take Additional Steps to Improve Its Foreign Inspection Program." January 7, 2022. https://www.gao.gov/products/gao-22–103611.

Wingrove, Patrick. "Fake Ozempic: How Batch Numbers Help Criminal Groups Spread Dangerous Weight Loss Drugs." Reuters, September 6, 2024. https://www.reuters.com/business/healthcare-pharmaceuticals/fake-ozempic-how-batch-numbers-help-criminal-groups-spread-dangerous-drugs-2024–09–05/.

Wingrove, Patrick. "Lilly Sues Online Vendors, Medical Spa over Copycat Weight-Loss Drugs." Reuters, October 2, 2024. https://www.reuters.com/business/healthcare-pharmaceuticals/lilly-sues-online-vendors-medical-spa-over-copycat-weight-loss-drugs-2024–10–21/.

World Health Organization. "Full List of WHO Medical Product Alerts." n.d. https://www.who.int/teams/regulation-prequalification/incidents-and-SF/full-list-of-who-medical-product-alerts.

World Health Organization. "WHO Issues Warning on Falsified Medicines Used for Diabetes Treatment and Weight Loss." June 20, 2024. https://www.who.int/news/item/20–06–2024-who-issues-warning-on-falsified-medicines-used-for-diabetes-treatment-and-weight-loss.

Yetman, Daniel. "Compounded Semaglutide: Risks, Side Effects, and Insurance Coverage." Healthline, September 6, 2024. https://www.healthline.com/.

Interviews and Correspondence with the Author

FuturHealth. Email to Marc Smolonsky, September 19, 2024.

Notes

253 **The market for weight management:** LaRosa, "U.S. Weight Loss Industry Grows to $90 Billion, Fueled by Obesity Drugs Demand."

253 **The combined revenues:** BizNews, "Novo Nordisk and Eli Lilly Dominate the $150bn Weight-Loss Drug Market."

253 **between $80 and $150 billion:** Satija and Wingrove, "Eli Lilly's Rare Sales Miss for Weight-Loss Drug Sends Shares Tumbling."

253 **chaos and confusion:** Ridge, "Disorder, Crime, and Punishment."

254 **leading to misuse:** Chiappini et al., "Is There a Risk for Semaglutide Misuse?"

254 **copycat versions:** Buntz, "Lilly, Novo Nordisk Battle Surge in Copycat Weight-Loss Drugs amid Safety Concerns."

254 **unsure of the exact mechanisms:** Castro, "Diabetes Drugs and Weight Loss."

254 **officially declare shortages:** Billingsley, "Is Semaglutide in Shortage?"

254 **Four months later:** US Food and Drug Administration, "Current and Resolved Drug Shortages and Discontinuations Reported to FDA."

254 **Patients are caught:** US Food and Drug Administration, "FDA's Concerns with Unapproved GLP-1 Drugs Used for Weight Loss."

254 **many of them potentially dangerous:** Wingrove, "Lilly Sues Online Vendors, Medical Spa over Copycat Weight-Loss Drugs."

254   *The Ultimate Weight Loss Marketing Playbook*: OppGen Marketing, "The Ultimate Weight Loss Marketing Playbook."

254   **compensating revenue:** OppGen Marketing, "The Ultimate Weight Loss Marketing Playbook."

255   **15% weight loss:** FuturHealth, email to Marc Smolonsky, September 19, 2024.

255   **partner with compounding pharmacies:** KnippeRx, "Offer Nationwide Pharmacy Services Under Your Brand."

255   **less stringent safety requirements:** Gudeman et al., "Potential Risks of Pharmacy Compounding."

255   **The owner of the firm:** US Department of Justice, "Former Owner of Defunct New England Compounding Center Resentenced to 14 Years in Prison in Connection with 2012 Fungal Meningitis Outbreak."

255   **sentenced to prison:** Dickerson et al., "Pharmacist at Center of 2012 Fungal Meningitis Outbreak Sentenced to 9 Years in Prison."

255   **compounded versions now flooding:** LexisNexis, "Regulatory Challenges of Compounded Weight-Loss Drugs."

255   **many compounded versions:** Ashraf et al., "Safety and Risk Assessment of No-Prescription Online Semaglutide Purchases."

255   **traditionally has been underfunded:** US Congress, House of Representatives, "FDA Foreign Drug Inspection Program."

256   **"high-risk" federal programs:** US Congress, House of Representatives, "Securing the US Drug Supply Chain."

256   **public health safety:** US Government Accountability Office, "Drug Safety."

256   **1,500%:** Poisoncenters.org, "America's Poison Centers—GLP-1."

256   **half of the online pharmacies:** Ashraf et al., "Safety and Risk Assessment of No-Prescription Online Semaglutide Purchases."

256   **at least 35,000 online compound pharmacies:** National Association of Boards of Pharmacy, "Prescription Drug Importation Is Not a Viable Solution to High Prescription Drug Costs."

256   **acting illegally:** National Association of Boards of Pharmacy, "Rogue RX Activity Report: Disrupting Illegal Online Pharmacies."

256   **"adverse event reports":** US Food and Drug Administration, "FDA's Concerns with Unapproved GLP-1 Drugs Used for Weight Loss."

256   **The agency further warned:** US Food and Drug Administration, "FDA Alerts Health Care Providers, Compounders and Patients of Dosing Errors Associated with Compounded Injectable Semaglutide Products."

256   **largely unregulated:** Siwicki, "Will Telemedicine Stagnate Without Regulatory Reform?"

257   **"increased demand":** World Health Organization, "Full List of WHO Medical Product Alerts."

26: Economics and Equity

Sources
Works Referenced

American Medical Association, Council on Science and Public Health. "Recognition of Obesity as a Disease H-440.842." 2023. https://policysearch.ama-assn.org/policyfinder /detail/obesity?uri=%2FAMADoc%2FHOD.xml-0-3858.xml.

Aronne, Louis J., Naveed Sattar, Deborah Horn, et al. "Continued Treatment with Tirzepatide for Maintenance of Weight Reduction in Adults with Obesity: The SURMOUNT-4 Randomized Clinical Trial." *JAMA* 331, no. 1 (2024): 38–48. DOI: 10.1001/jama.2023.24945.

Arterburn, David. "Paradigm Shifts and Price Wars: The Bright and Bumpy Future of Obesity Treatment." Lecture presented at Obesity Medicine 2024: A New Path Forward, Denver, CO, April 25–28, 2024.

Garvey, Timothy W., Rachel L. Batterham, Meena Bhatta, et al. "Two-Year Effects of Semaglutide in Adults with Overweight or Obesity: The STEP 5 Trial." *Nature* 28 (2022): 2083–91.

Leach, Joseph, Marci Chodroff, Yang Qiu, et al. "Real-World Analysis of Glucagon-Like Peptide-1 Agonist (GLP-1a) Obesity Treatment One-Year Cost-Effectiveness and Therapy Adherence." Prime Therapeutics and MagellanRx, July 11, 2023. https://www .primetherapeutics.com/documents/d/primetherapeutics/glp-1a-obesity-treatment-1st -year-cost-effectiveness-study-abstract-final-7–11.

Lewis, Kristina H., Caroline E. Sloan, Daniel H. Bessesen, and David Arterburn. "Effectiveness and Safety of Drugs for Obesity." *BMJ* 384 (2024): e072686. DOI: https://doi .org/10.1136/bmj-2022–072686.

McMullin, Cara. "Employer Coverage of GLP-1 Drugs on the Rise." International Foundation of Employee Benefit Plans. *Word on Benefits* (blog), June 13, 2024. https:// blog.ifebp.org/employer-coverage-of-glp-1-drugs-on-the-rise/.

Pi-Sunyer, Xavier, Arne Astrup, Ken Fujioka, et al. "A Randomized, Controlled Trial of 3.0 mg of Liraglutide in Weight Management." *N Engl J Med* 373 (2015): 11–22. DOI: 10.1056/NEJMoa1411892.

Rodriguez, Patricia J., Brianna M. Goodwin Cartwright, Samuel Gratzl, et al. "Semaglutide vs. Tirzepatide for Weight Loss in Adults with Overweight or Obesity." *JAMA Intern Med* 184, no. 9 (2024): 1056–64. DOI: 10.1001/jamainternmed.2024.2525.

Syracuse University School of Law. "Professor Katherine Macfarlane Discusses State and Federal Efforts to Recognize Obesity as a Disability." October 1, 2024. https://law .syracuse.edu/news/professor-katherine-macfarlane-discusses-state-and-federal-efforts -to-recognize-obesity-as-a-disability/.

Interviews and Correspondence with the Author

Arterburn, David (August 2024).

Notes

262 **interest in obesity:** Author interview with Arterburn, August 2024.

262 **focus has shifted:** Arterburn, "Paradigm Shifts and Price Wars."

262 **upfront costs:** Lewis et al., "Effectiveness and Safety of Drugs for Obesity."

263 **price of these medications:** Author interview with Arterburn, August 2024.

263 **carefully controlled studies:** Garvey et al., "Two-Year Effects of Semaglutide in Adults with Overweight or Obesity"; Pi-Sunyer et al., "A Randomized, Controlled Trial of 3.0 mg of Liraglutide in Weight Management"; Aronne et al., "Continued Treatment with Tirzepatide for Maintenance of Weight Reduction in Adults with Obesity."

263 **when patients are:** Leach et al., "Real-World Analysis of Glucagon-Like Peptide-1 Agonist (GLP-1a) Obesity Treatment One-Year Cost-Effectiveness and Therapy Adherence"; Rodriguez et al., "Semaglutide vs. Tirzepatide for Weight Loss in Adults with Overweight or Obesity."

263 **"More than 90%":** Author interview with Arterburn, August 2024.

263 **"The slope of weight":** Author interview with Arterburn, August 2024.

264 **Given the high cost:** Arterburn, "Paradigm Shifts and Price Wars."

264 **prioritizing less expensive:** Arterburn, "Paradigm Shifts and Price Wars."

265 **Cigna Health and Life Insurance:** Syracuse University School of Law, "Professor Katherine Macfarlane."

265 **AMA recognized obesity:** American Medical Association, "Recognition of Obesity as a Disease H-440.842."

265 **International Foundation of Employee Benefit Plans:** McMullin, "Employer Coverage of GLP-1 Drugs on the Rise."

Epilogue

Sources
Works Referenced

Goedde, Lutz, Joshua Katz, Alexandre Ménard, and Julien Revellat. "Agriculture's Connected Future: How Technology Can Yield New Growth." McKinsey Global Institute, October 9, 2020. https://www.mckinsey.com/.

Juul, Filippa, Niyati Parekh, Euridice Martinez-Steele, Carlos Augusto Monteiro, and Virginia W. Chang. "Ultra-processed Food Consumption Among US Adults from 2001 to 2018." *Am J Clin Nutr* 115, no. 1 (2022): 211–21. DOI: 10.1093/ajcn/nqab305.

NCD Risk Factor Collaboration. "Worldwide Trends in Underweight and Obesity from 1990 to 2022: A Pooled Analysis of 3663 Population-Representative Studies with 222 Million Children, Adolescents, and Adults." *Lancet* 403, no. 10431 (2024): 1027–50. DOI: 10.1016/S0140–6736(23)02750–2.

Raut, Rabin, Pramir Maharjan, and Aliyar Cyrus Fouladkhah. "Practical Preventive Considerations for Reducing the Public Health Burden of Poultry-Related Salmonellosis." *Int J Environ Res Public Health* 20, no. 17 (2023): 6654. DOI: 10.3390/ijerph20176654.

Rossati, Antonella. "Global Warming and Its Health Impact." *Int J Occup Environ Med* 8, no. 1 (2017): 7–20. DOI: 10.15171/ijoem.2017.963.

Tilman, David, Christian Balzer, Jason Hill, and Belinda Belfort. "Global Food Demand and the Sustainable Intensification of Agriculture." *Proceedings of the National Academy of Sciences of the United States of America* 108, no. 50 (2011): 20260–64. DOI: 10.1073/pnas.1116437108.

Notes

266 **replaced with abundance:** Tilman, "Global Food Demand and the Sustainable Intensification of Agriculture."

266 **drastically increased agricultural productivity:** Goedde et al., "Agriculture's Connected Future."

266 **cornucopia of convenient snacks:** Juul et al., "Ultra-processed Food Consumption Among US Adults from 2001 to 2018."

266 **highest levels of obesity:** NCD Risk Factor Collaboration, "Worldwide Trends in Underweight and Obesity from 1990 to 2022."

267 **including floods and droughts:** Rossati, "Global Warming and Its Health Impact."

Index

About the Author

DAVID. A. KESSLER, MD, served as chief science officer of the White House COVID-19 Response Team and co-led Operation Warp Speed under President Joe Biden and previously served as commissioner of the US Food and Drug Administration under Presidents George H. W. Bush and Bill Clinton. He is the author of the *New York Times* bestsellers *The End of Overeating* and *Capture* as well as *Fast Carbs, Slow Carbs* and *A Question of Intent*. Dr. Kessler is a pediatrician and has been the dean of the medical schools at Yale and the University of California, San Francisco. He is a graduate of Amherst College, the University of Chicago Law School, and Harvard Medical School.